HEMATOLOGY - LATEST RESEARCH AND CLINICAL ADVANCES

Edited by **Margarita Guenova**
and **Gueorgui Balatzenko**

Hematology - Latest Research and Clinical Advances
http://dx.doi.org/10.5772/intechopen.70388
Edited by Margarita Guenova and Gueorgui Balatzenko

Contributors

Sridurga Mithraprabhu, Andrew Spencer, Vivek Kumar, Abhinav Chandra, Trishala Meghal, Makardhwaj Shrivastava, Vijaya Pilli, Marcelo Navarrete, Julieta Sepulveda, Pablo Oppezzo, Noe Seija, Bhaskar Kahali, Baba P.D. Inusa, Mariachiara Lodi, Kenneth Ataga, Giovanni Palazzi, Cecilia Lantos, Steven Mitchell Kornblau, Amina Ann Qutub, Margarita Guenova, Emmanuel Andres

First published in London, United Kingdom, 2018 by IntechOpen
IntechOpen is the global imprint of INTECHOPEN LIMITED, registered in England and Wales, registration number: 11086078, The Shard, 25th floor, 32 London Bridge Street
London, SE19SG – United Kingdom
Printed in Croatia

British Library Cataloguing-in-Publication Data
A catalogue record for this book is available from the British Library

Additional hard copies can be obtained from orders@intechopen.com

Hematology - Latest Research and Clinical Advances, Edited by Margarita Guenova and Gueorgui Balatzenko
p. cm.
Print ISBN 978-1-78923-350-6
Online ISBN 978-1-78923-351-3

For EU product safety concerns:
IN TECH d.o.o., Prolaz Marije Krucifikse Kozulić 3, 51000 Rijeka, Croatia,
info@intechopen.com or visit our website at intechopen.com.

Meet the editors

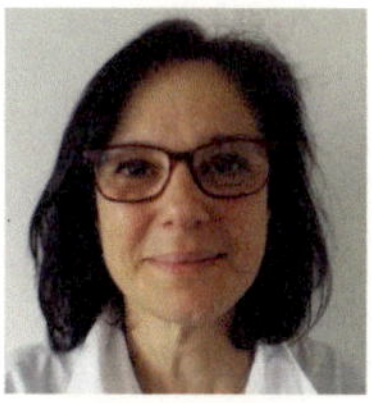

Professor Dr. Margarita Guenova received her medical training at the Medical University of Sofia and her PhD degree at the National Center of Haematology in 2000. She is employed as the head of the Laboratory of Haematopathology and Immunology and a professor of Haematology and Blood Transfusion at the National Specialised Hospital for Active Treatment of Haematological Diseases, Sofia, Bulgaria, teaching both undergraduate and graduate studies at the Medical University of Sofia. She specializes in the field of leukemia and lymphoma diagnostics. In regard to her scientific interests, she worked on the elucidation of critical mechanisms of leukemia pathogenesis and progression, investigation of clinically relevant biomarkers and potential targets for therapy in leukemias and lymphomas, characterization of leukemic stem cell populations, minimal residual disease, and implementation of a multifaceted approach in oncohematology. Dr. Guenova has authored and coauthored many abstracts, articles in peer-reviewed journals, and book chapters. She serves on editorial boards and is the president of the Bulgarian Society of Hematology, as well as a member of several professional societies such as the Bulgarian Society of Pathology, the Bulgarian Association of Clinical Immunology, the European Hematology Association, the European Association of Hematopathology, and the International Society of Hematology.

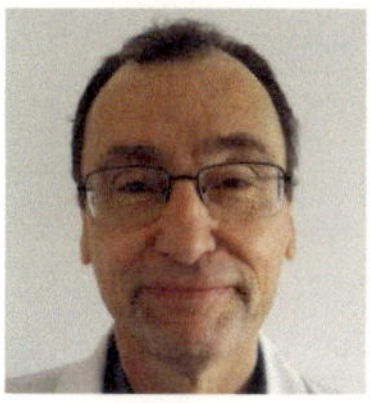

Professor Dr. Gueorgui Balatzenko received his medical training at the Medical University of Sofia and his PhD degree at the National Center of Haematology in 2002. He obtained additional qualifications at the Red Cross Blood Bank, Groningen-Drenth, the Netherlands; Institute Paoli-Calmettes Marseille, France; and Hôpital Necker-Enfants Malades, Paris, France. He is employed as the head of the Laboratory of Cytogenetics and Molecular Biology and a professor in the Department of Haematology and Blood Transfusion at the National Specialised Hospital for Active Treatment of Haematological Diseases, Sofia, Bulgaria, teaching both undergraduate and graduate studies at the Medical University of Sofia. His major interests are in the field of molecular investigations in leukemias. In regard to his scientific achievements, he worked on the elucidation of the incidence and clinical relevance of molecular biomarkers in chronic and acute leukemias and molecular monitoring of treatment response. Dr. Balatzenko has authored and coauthored many articles in peer-reviewed journals and book chapters. He is a member of several professional societies such as the Bulgarian Society of Hematology and the Bulgarian Society of Genetics, a lifetime member of the UICC, and a referee for international journals.

Contents

Preface

Hematology has constantly been advancing in parallel with technological developments that have expanded our understanding of the phenotypic, genetic, and molecular complexity and extreme clinical and biological heterogeneity of blood diseases. This has in turn allowed for developing more effective and less toxic alternative therapeutic approaches directed against critical molecular pathways. The continuous and rather extensive influx of new information regarding the key features and underlying mechanisms as well as treatment options in hematology requires a frequent update of this topic. The primary objective of this book is to provide the specialists involved in the clinical management and experimental research in hematological diseases with comprehensive and concise information on some important theoretical and practical developments in the biology, clinical assessment, and treatment of patients, as well as on some molecular and pathogenetic mechanisms and the respective translation into novel therapies.

The book comprises two main sections, devoted to hematological malignancies and benign hematological diseases.

Some major biological mechanisms underlying normal and pathological processes in hematopoietic system are comprehensively reviewed, e.g., the current concepts of the role of B-cell receptor (BCR) signaling in normal B-cell biology versus B-cell lymphoma pathogens, as well as the advances in the knowledge about the structure, function, and regulation of the coagulation system and the respective defects resulting in hemorrhagic and thrombotic disorders. The effective implementation of rationally developed therapies requires rapid integration of new biological data.

Specific nosological entities and clinical scenarios such as diffuse large B-cell lymphomas, myeloid sarcoma, or sickle cell nephropathy and idiosyncratic drug-induced neutropenia and agranulocytosis are also within the scope of the book. The rapid pace in understanding biological mechanisms, recent molecular subclassification, and clinical developments has moved into the focus of personalization of therapy.

Innovative laboratory approaches and the rapid transfer from "laboratory to bedside" are the hallmark of hematology. Currently, classical investigations are integrated with extensively developing high-throughput technologies. Digital pathology integrated with advances in machine learning is emerging as a powerful tool to enhance morphology-based decisions. Liquid biopsies emerge as a novel molecular methodology for diagnostics and disease monitoring.

An international panel of experts provides novel insights into various aspects of hematology and contributes their experience to an update of the field. Each chapter is a separate publication that reflects each author's views and concepts. However, the book presents an update and introduces novel insights in novel methodological approaches to study blood, as well as in our current understanding of the biology and clinical presentation, the risk assessment, and therapeutic challenges in patients with hematological diseases.

Prof. Dr. Margarita Guenova, MD, PhD
Laboratory of Haemathopathology and Immunology
National Specialised Hospital for Active Treatment of Haematological Diseases
Sofia, Bulgaria

Prof. Dr. Gueorgui Balatzenko, MD, PhD
Laboratory of Cytogenetics and Molecular Biology
National Specialised Hospital for Active Treatment of Haematological Diseases
Sofia, Bulgaria

Section 1

Introduction

Chapter 1

Introductory Chapter: Hematology in Times of Precision and Innovation

Gueorgui Balatzenko and Margarita Guenova

Additional information is available at the end of the chapter

http://dx.doi.org/10.5772/intechopen.76849

1. Introduction

Hematological diseases are heterogeneous group of benign and malignant, inherited and acquired, acute and chronic disorders of different cell lineages that originate from a cell of the hematopoietic and lymphatic tissue with diverse incidence, etiology, pathogenesis, and prognosis.

During the past two decades, hematological disorders have been extensively studied by means of classical laboratory approaches, for example, microscopy, immunophenotyping, clinical chemistry, genetic diagnostic tests such as conventional cytogenetics, fluorescence in situ hybridization (FISH), and polymerase chain reaction (PCR), as well as by high-throughput technologies, including microarray-based platforms for the global analysis of DNA alterations (single nucleotide polymorphism (SNP); array, comparative genomic hybridization (CGH)), gene expression profiling (GEP), next-generation sequencing (NGS), digitalized imaging, and so on. Systemic application of these techniques has allowed for the refinement of the molecular mechanisms involved in the pathological transformation of hematopoietic stem/progenitor cells and disease progression in a number of hematological disorders. More importantly, they have permitted more precise and reproducible diagnoses of the different entities, risk stratification of patients, and treating them in the most appropriate manner with tailored therapeutic strategies.

2. Hematological malignancies

Hematological malignancies account for around 8–9% of all cancers, being the fourth to fifth most frequently diagnosed cancer in economically developed regions of the world [1]. The estimated deaths from these tumors account for 7% of the cancer-related deaths [2]. The age-standardized incidence rates are 24.5 (per 100,000) for lymphoid malignancies and 7.55 for myeloid malignancies. The most common lymphoid malignancies are plasma cell neoplasms (4.62), small B-cell lymphocytic lymphoma/chronic lymphocytic leukemia (3.79), diffuse large B-cell lymphoma (3.13), and Hodgkin lymphoma (2.41). The commonest myeloid malignancies are acute myeloid leukemia (AML) (2.96), other myeloproliferative neoplasms (MPN) (1.76), and myelodysplastic syndromes (MDS) (1.24) [3].

Hematological malignancies arise through a multistep process of a sequential accumulation of a variety of chromosome aberrations and/or molecular abnormalities in a hematopoietic stem cell or a progenitor cell. These abnormalities affect the normal structure or the function of certain genes resulting in modifications in the genetic programs that control cellular proliferation, differentiation, programmed cellular death (apoptosis), relationships with neighboring cells, and the capacity to escape the immune system [4]. This process leads to the formation of a clone of deregulated cells, which escape the physiological control of normal cell growth and behavior [5].

The spectrum of genetic and epigenetic abnormalities that occur in hematological malignancies is extremely heterogeneous and ranges from single DNA nucleotide changes that affect the coding of a single amino acid to chromosomal gains and losses that disrupt the transcription of hundreds of genes. Frequently, the pattern of genetic defects is highly complex with multiple different abnormalities, such as structural and numerical chromosome aberrations, point mutations, gene amplifications, microdeletions, microinsertions, fusion genes, gene rearrangements, aberrant gene expression, and so on. The diversity in the form of a disease produced results from a combination of factors, particularly the type of cell affected, the nature of the genetic change that precipitates the malignancy, and the point in the cell's maturation process at which the malignant change occurs. Besides, most hematological malignancies are an oligoclonal disease even within a single patient, such that the predominant clone at the initial presentation is not necessarily identical to the clone ultimately responsible for clinical relapse and death. The progression to the overt clinical relapse may be associated (1) with the initial malignant clone that develops chemo-resistance after initial sensitivity to treatment, most frequently due to the acquisition of additional mutations; or (2) with a subclone, which initially presents at low frequency, but given a clonal advantage during treatment, replaces the founder clone and becomes the predominant clone. These add additional biological heterogeneity of the individual patients with one and same diseases.

On the other hand, it is important to specify that the presence of low levels of characteristic "initiating" leukemia- and/or lymphoma-associated molecular abnormalities do not lead directly to disease, even if these abnormalities confer advantages in self-renewal, proliferation or both, resulting in clonal expansion of the affected cells as a "pre-malignant" clone. Using highly sensitive (10^{-6}–10^{-8}) nested primer PCR approaches, a low level of various leukemia- and/or lymphoma-associated molecular abnormalities was detected in a significant proportion of healthy individuals.

Currently, most hematological malignancies are treated with highly cytotoxic drugs, radiation, and/or hematopoietic stem cell transplantation (HSCT), and all these therapeutic approaches are often toxic, elicit incomplete responses, and may have severe long-term negative effects. Besides, despite the improved response and survival rates, drug resistance and relapse remain major problems and several hematological malignancies remain incurable with standard treatments [6].

2.1. The effective implementation of rationally developed therapies requires rapid integration of new biological data

B-cell lymphomas comprise a rapidly developing field of remarkable transfer of knowledge and understanding into precise diagnosis and effective therapeutic approaches. The dissection of B-cell development has been in the focus of tremendous interest in the recent years. The understanding of normal B-cell biology versus B-cell lymphoma pathogenesis leads us inevitably to the B-cell receptor (BCR) signaling. The expression of a functional BCR retains a crucial role for B-cell survival and proliferation. In this regard, BCR activation and signaling pathways can support the growth and evolution of both normal and malignant B-lymphocytes, and as a result, from the functional perspective, it might act as a true oncogene [7]. Julieta Sepulveda et al. review the BCR as a driver of B-cell lymphoma development and evolution in Chapter 2 of this book and discuss the genetic mechanisms that create a functional antigen receptor and their errors leading to oncogenic events, the pathogenic activation of the B-cell receptor signaling cascade, and introduce some novel emerging therapies targeting the B-cell receptor at different levels.

The functional role of the BCR in the pathogenesis and lymphoma progression is particularly well characterized in diffuse large B-cell lymphomas (DLBCL). Gene expression profiling has separated DLBCL into two distinct sub-entities: the germinal center B-cell DLBCL (GCB) and the activated B-cell-like (ABC) DLBCL characterized by ongoing BCR signaling and substantially worse clinical outcomes when treated with standard immunochemotherapy. DLBCL is the most common type of non-Hodgkin lymphoma which accounts for approximately one-third cases of lymphoid malignancies in the Western world. There is a considerable variability in terms of clinical course and therapeutic outcomes due to the unique heterogeneity of biology that exists between and within lymphoma subtypes. In addition to GCB and ABC subtypes, double/triple-hit and double-expressor lymphomas with rearrangements and/or overexpression of MYC, BCL2, and/or BCL6 genes have also been associated with poor prognosis [8]. However, a number of clinical trials have demonstrated the feasibility of novel agents and combinations with encouraging efficacy [9]. The rapid pace in understanding biological mechanisms, recent molecular subclassification, and clinical developments has moved into the focus of personalization of therapy. The third chapter provides an overview of the recent advances in DLBCL presented by Kumar Vivek.

This is yet another demonstration of how hematology has advanced in parallel with technological developments that have expanded our understanding of the phenotypic, genetic, and molecular characteristics of the hematological neoplasms. Dissection of genetic abnormalities critical to leukemia, lymphoma, and myeloma initiation provided insights into the pathogenesis of hematological malignancies, but also identified distinct subsets of patient, predicted prognosis individually, and provided rational therapeutic targets for curative approaches [10].

The molecular characterization of malignant cells is currently regarded as being as important as the traditional morphological and immunological approaches to diagnosis. This trend is being additionally accelerated by the introduction of novel drugs designed to specifically target the molecular abnormalities responsible for the development of the tumor. Such developments are of fundamental clinical importance, as they increasingly define not just the diseases themselves but how an individual patient should be treated.

2.2. Information concerning the tumor genome into the routine clinical management is useful for better treatment strategy selection, delivering "the right treatment to the right patient at the right time"

The best efficacy would be achieved if treatment is directed toward specific genetic lesions within malignant cells, which have a key role in the pathogenesis of the respective disease, while minimizing damage to normal, healthy cells [11]. Unfortunately, several limitations still restrict the widespread application of this personalized approach, such as (1) various technological and methodological diagnostic problems; (2) insufficient level of our knowledge about the molecular mechanisms involved in the pathogenesis of different malignancies and the prognostic significance of individual molecular abnormalities; and (3) relatively low number of available targeted therapeutic agents approved for clinical use. Therefore, in practical terms, the personalized approach in hemato-oncology comprises a personalized risk stratification: refinement of clinical prognostic models for a better risk stratification and identification of biologic subtypes within pathologically similar diseases; identification of patients suitable for targeted treatment and "response-adapted" changes in therapy in individual patients [12].

In several hematological malignancies, such as acute leukemias, MDS, chronic lymphocytic leukemia (CLL), and so on, cytogenetics remains the most important disease-related prognostic factor for predicting remission rate, relapse, and overall survival (OS) [13–15]. In addition, recent genetic studies identified a large number of mutations in most of the hematological malignancies that point to novel pathways involved in the pathogenesis of the respective disease, and some of these molecular abnormalities have allowed substantial improvements in clinical decision making. As a result, the current prognostic models based on genetic abnormalities are nowadays subject to change as new cytogenetic and mutational findings are revealed, contributing to refine better and better these approaches.

Multiple myeloma (MM) is an incurable malignancy characterized by the clonal proliferation of neoplastic plasma cells in the bone marrow that produce monoclonal protein that can be detected in the serum or urine. MM is a highly heterogeneous disease composed of multiple molecularly defined subtypes, each with varying clinico-pathological features and disease outcomes. Cytogenetically, there are two main subtypes: (1) hyperdiploid myeloma—characterized by trisomies of certain odd-numbered chromosomes and generally associated with a better survival; and (2) nonhyperdiploid myeloma—characterized by translocations of the immunoglobulin heavy chain alleles at chromosome 14q32 with various partner chromosomes, the most important of which are 4, 6, 11, 16, and 20. Several abnormalities have been reported to be associated with poor prognosis, such as t(4;14)(p16;q32)/IGH-MMSET, t(14;16)(p32;q23)/

IGG-MAF, t(14;20)(q32;q11)/IGG-MAFB, del(17p), and gains of 1q, despite that the adverse effect of t(4,14) can be partially abrogated by bortezomib-based treatment [16]. Technological development provides various opportunities to evaluate the tumor genome. In this regard, Sridurga Mithraprabhu and Andrew Spencer provide a comprehensive chapter on the possible role of liquid biopsies in multiple myeloma as an innovative methodology for diagnostics and disease monitoring, implementing the analysis of circulating cell-free nucleic acids (CFNAs) and circulating tumor cells (CTCs) as representative of the underlying mutational profile of a cancer as well as of extracellular RNA (exRNA) that can be utilized as a prognostic biomarker. The authors discuss the potential of these noninvasive, repeatable biomarkers to provide additional information as an adjunct to bone marrow biopsies and conventional disease variables in multiple myeloma.

2.3. "Acute leukemia: the challenge of capturing disease variety"

The many levels of morphological, immunophenotypic, clinical, genetic, and epigenetic heterogeneity of acute leukemias represent an extraordinary challenge to our capability to understand and to beat these diseases (Löwenberg modified [17]). Acute leukemias were incurable 50 years ago. Significant progress has been achieved by applying intensive regimes and transplantation programs. The 5-year survival rate of people of all ages with acute lymphoblastic leukemia (ALL) increased from 41% for those diagnosed from 1975 to 1977 to 71% for those diagnosed from 2006 to 2012; however, with considerable variations depending on several factors, including biologic features of the disease and a person's age, the 5-year survival rate for people with acute myeloid leukemia (AML) is still approximately 27% which is fairly unsatisfactory [www.cancer.net]. Many recent biologic insights have shed light on these challenging nosological categories, and attempts have been devoted to develop strategies for improved outcomes.

According to the European LeukemiaNet (ELN) recommendations for the diagnosis and management of acute myeloid leukemia in adults (2017), several genetic abnormalities are associated with the response to therapy and survival, allowing to stratify patients into three genetic risk groups [18]:

Favorable: t(8;21)(q22;q22.1)/*RUNX1-RUNX1T1;* inv(16)(p13.1q22) or t(16;16)(p13.1;q22)/*CBFB-MYH11;* Mutated *NPM1* without *FLT3*-ITD or with *FLT3*-ITD^{low}, Biallelic mutated *CEBPA;*

Intermediate: Mutated *NPM1* and *FLT3*-ITD^{high}, wild-type *NPM1* without *FLT3*-ITD or with *FLT3*-ITD^{low} (without adverse-risk genetic lesions); t(9,11)(p21.3;q23.3)/*MLLT3-KMT2A,* cytogenetic abnormalities not classified as favorable or adverse;

Adverse: t(6;9)(p23;q34.1)/*DEK-NUP214;* t(v;11q23.3)/*KMT2A* rearranged; t(9;22)(q34.1; q11.2) /*BCR-ABL1;* inv(3)(q21.3q26.2) or t(3,3)(q21.3;q26.2)/*GATA2,MECOM (EVI1);* −5/del(5q); −7; −17/abn(17p); complex karyotype, monosomal karyotype; wild-type *NPM1* and *FLT3*-ITD^{high}, mutated *RUNX1,* mutated *ASXL1,* and mutated *TP53.*

AML with t(8;21) or inv(16)/t(16;16) is commonly referred to as core-binding factor (CBF) AML, because in both, the heterodimeric protein complex CBF is affected, which is involved in the transcriptional regulation of normal hematopoiesis. CBF-AMLs in patients treated with cytarabine-anthracycline-based induction and high-dose consolidation are considered to have relatively good prognosis compared to other leukemia subtypes, with 10-year OS, disease-free survival (DFS), and event-free survival (EFS) of 63.9, 54.8, and 49.9%, respectively [19]. Nevertheless, 40–45% of these patients eventually relapse and die of their disease. Integration of cytogenetic results with molecular genetics and epigenetic data refines the risk stratification of CBF AML. Several variables might worse prognosis of these patients, such as the level of the respective fusion transcripts *RUNX1-RUNX1T1* and *CBFB-MYH11* [20]. Some authors even suggested that *FLT3*-ITDs carriers constitute a biologically distinct group of APL patients [21].

Almost half of AML is normal cytogenetically, and this subgroup shows a remarkable heterogeneity in terms of genetic mutations and response to therapy. In patients with normal karyotype, as well as in cases with chromosome abnormalities with intermediate prognosis, the intensity of therapy is driven by the prognostic subgroup. Therefore, the current standard of care combines cytogenetic results with testing for mutations in *FLT3, NPM1, CEBPA,* and *KIT* to precise the risk. The presence of *NPM1* and *CEBPA* gene mutations is associated with a favorable prognosis, however, only in the absence of *FLT3*-ITD [22].

Several other gene alterations (mutations in *WT1, RUNX1, ASXL1, TP53, IDH1, IDH2, DNMT3A* genes, partial tandem duplication of *MLL* gene, overexpression of *BAALC, MN1, EVI1, ERG, WT1*) have also been demonstrated to predict prognosis and probably will play a role in future risk stratification, although some of these have not been confirmed in multiple studies or established as the standard of care [23].

About 30% of AML have an unfavorable karyotype, and if treated with conventional chemotherapy, a complete response rate of about 50% and a 5-year OS of 10–20% are expected. The best chance for patients with an unfavorable karyotype who achieve a complete response is the allogeneic HSCT [24].

A major achievement is the incorporation of genetic and molecular data in the current classification systems. However, the major principle of the World Health Organization (WHO) Classification of tumors of hematopoietic and lymphoid tissues (2016) is to integrate these data with essential clinical features, morphology, and immunophenotyping in order to define distinct disease entities of clinical significance [25]. Morphology is the gold standard, and though it has been the classical tool for diagnosis and classification, it is routinely performed by subjective microscopic evaluation and is strongly dependent on the morphologist's expertise. To extract more accurate and detailed information from patient tissue samples, digital pathology integrated with advances in machine learning is emerging as a powerful tool to enhance morphology-based decisions. In the fifth chapter in this book, Cecilia Lantos et al. provide up to date information about the possibilities that computational histology can provide to improve leukemia diagnosis with an automated biologically meaningful pattern recognition, as well as the additional contribution of deep-learning approach for a higher accuracy. The authors claim that if mathematical pattern recognition methods that recognize cellular phenotypes from microscopic slides and define how morphological features relate to clinical genetic data and protein signatures, this could significantly speed up leukemia diagnosis, reduce the cost of the diagnostic workup, and optimize the assignment of patients to a particular therapy.

Rare conditions pose a number of problems in both theoretical and practical terms. Myeloid sarcoma has been recognized for more than a century; however, owing to the rarity of the entity, most of the study comprises small retrospective studies and case reports. Myeloid sarcoma can occur under different clinical scenarios including an extramedullary leukemic tumor with concurrent AML, preceding the blood and bone marrow involvement or without any history of myeloid neoplasia, as well as an extramedullary AML relapse. These phenomena may not share common mechanisms and outcomes and may need to be treated differently [26]. Kahali Bhaskar presents a review of current published data regarding the incidence, clinical presentation, morphological, cytogenetic and immunophenotypic features, prognosis, and treatment of this rare neoplastic myeloid entity.

3. Benign hematological disorders

"Benign hematology isn't so benign" if we use the words of Prof. Alice Ma in ASH Clinical News (2015). Clotting disorders, anemias, thrombocytopenias, and so on may present as serious as malignant disorders and are a field of significant progress too.

3.1. New therapies improve the outlook of bleeding and clotting disorders

Coagulation is a dynamic process, and the understanding of blood coagulation system and the ways to modulate the process have been evolving significantly. The concept of coagulation originates back to the 1960s when Davie, Ratnoff, and Macfarlane described their cascade theories [27]. Hemostasis is a complex physiological process that maintains the blood flow and is regulated by a delicate balance between procoagulants supporting the formation of hemostatic plugs to prevent the leakage or blood loss and anticoagulants, preventing the formation of unwanted clots. The imbalance between the two components may cause either bleeding or thrombosis. The seventh chapter comprises a review of the defects in the coagulation system and the recent clinical modulators of the coagulation system by Pilli Vijaya.

The different hereditary and acquired defects of the finely regulated coagulation systems might result in severe of even life-threatening bleeding complications or thrombotic events. The recent advances in the knowledge about the structure, function, and regulation of the coagulation system, as well as in the hereditary genetic abnormalities leading to qualitative and/or quantitative defects of the multiple elements of clothing cascade, and acquired disorders of coagulation as a consequence of other underlying conditions, were an important prerequisite of the development of new diagnostic tools and therapeutic strategies based on the product of recombinant technology. The understanding of the physiology of these processes is crucial to identify the pathological scenarios and to predict clinical consequences in order to implement the relevant therapeutic interventions. In combination with the classical laboratory tests and therapeutic blood components, the current management of patients with disorders of hemostasis and thrombosis is based on the individual approach according to the individual patient.

3.2. New sickle cell disease research shows improved patient outcomes

Sickle cell disease (SCD) is one of the most frequent inherited genetic disorders in the world. It predominantly affects people of African descent as well as individuals from the Middle East, India, and Mediterranean regions [28]. It is an autosomal-recessive disease caused by a point mutation in the hemoglobin beta gene found on chromosome 11p15.5, Hb S (HBB: c.20A>T) along with or without any other abnormal Hb gene, and results in a number of health problems, for example, anemia, acute and chronic pain, infection, acute chest syndrome, pulmonary hypertension, cardiac, CNS, gastrointestinal involvement, and so on, leading to significant morbidity and mortality. Significant advances in prophylactics and therapy achieved improved survival among children with sickle cell disease, with the majority of children attaining adulthood [29]. However, the median age at death of 39 years with only 35.0% surviving beyond age 35 years was reported by the Centers for Disease Control (CDC). Sickle cell disease substantially alters renal structure and function leading to nephropathy which is not only a chronic comorbidity but is also one of the leading causes of mortality in patients with sickle cell disease [30]. Knowledge of the natural progression of the disease, as well as identification of persons at risk, allows for timely intervention and improved outcomes. The search for biomarkers for the early diagnosis of the disorder and its outcomes is an area of intense contemporary research [31]. The current understanding of the presentation, diagnostic, and therapeutic challenges in sickle cell nephropathy is presented in detail by Inusa Baba et al. in the chapter 8. Risk factors for renal impairment and acute kidney injury are reviewed in detail. In addition, data coming from established mouse models are invaluable to elucidate the pathogenesis of SCD-associated multiple organ complications and to identify targets for prevention and therapy.

The continuous and rather extensive influx of new information regarding the key features and underlying mechanisms as well as treatment options of blood disorders requires a frequent updating of this topic. The primary objective of this book is to provide the specialists involved in the clinical management and experimental research in hematological diseases with comprehensive and concise information on some important theoretical and practical developments in the biology, clinical assessment, and treatment of patients, as well as on some molecular and pathogenetic mechanisms and the respective translation into novel therapies. Specific clinical scenarios such as myeloid sarcoma or sickle cell nephropathy are also within the scope of this book. An international panel of experts provides novel insights of various aspects of hematology and contributes their experience to an update of the field.

Each chapter is a separate publication that reflects each author's views and concepts. However, this book presents an update and introduces novel insights in our current understanding of the biology and clinical presentation, the risk assessment, and therapeutic challenges in patients with hematological diseases.

Author details

Gueorgui Balatzenko[1] and Margarita Guenova[2]*

*Address all correspondence to: margenova@gmail.com

1 Laboratory of Cytogenetics and Molecular Biology, National Specialized Hospital for Active Treatment of Hematological Diseases, Sofia, Bulgaria

2 Laboratory of Haemathopathology and Immunology, National Specialized Hospital for Active Treatment of Hematological Diseases, Sofia, Bulgaria

References

[1] Smith A, Howell D, Patmore R, Jack A, Roman E. Incidence of haematological malignancy by sub-type: A report from the haematological malignancy research network. British Journal of Cancer. 2011;**105**(11):1684-1692

[2] Rodriguez-Abreu D, Bordoni A, Zucca E. Epidemiology of hematological malignancies. Annals of Oncology. 2007;**18**(Suppl 1):i3-i8

[3] Sant M, Allemani C, Tereanu C, De Angelis R, Capocaccia R, et al. Incidence of hematologic malignancies in Europe by morphologic subtype: Results of the HAEMACARE project. Blood. 2010;**116**(19):3724-3734

[4] Merlo LM, Pepper JW, Reid BJ, et al. Cancer as an evolutionary and ecological process. Nature Reviews Cancer. 2006;**6**:924-935

[5] Boyle P, Levin B. Molecular hallmarks of cancer. In: World Cancer Report 2008. Lyon: World Health Organization; 2008. pp. 190-199

[6] Boehrer S, Nowak D, Hoelzer D, Mitrou PS, Chow KU. Novel agents aiming at specific molecular targets increase chemosensitivity and overcome chemoresistance in hematopoietic malignancies. Current Pharmaceutical Design. 2006;**12**(1):111-128

[7] Wang LD, Clark MR. B-cell antigen-receptor signalling in lymphocyte development. Immunology. 2003;**110**(4):411-420

[8] Riedell PA, Smith SM. Should we use cell of origin and dual-protein expression in treating DLBCL? Clinical Lymphoma, Myeloma & Leukemia. 2018;**18**(2):91-97

[9] Di Rocco A, De Angelis F, Ansuinelli M, Foà R, Martelli M. Is now the time for molecular driven therapy for diffuse large B-cell lymphoma? Expert Review of Hematology. 2017;**10**(9):761-774

[10] Zhou GB, Li G, Chen SJ, Chen Z. From dissection of disease pathogenesis to elucidation of mechanisms of targeted therapies: Leukemia research in the genomic era. Acta Pharmacologica Sinica. 2007;**28**(9):1434-1449

[11] Faulkner E, Annemans L, Garrison L, Helfand M, Holtorf AP, et al. Challenges in the development and reimbursement of personalized medicine-payer and manufacturer perspectives and implications for health economics and outcomes research: A report of the ISPOR personalized medicine special interest group. Value in Health. 2012;**15**(8):1162-1171

[12] Ramsdale E, van Besien K, Smith SM. Personalized treatment of lymphoma: Promise and reality. Seminars in Oncology. 2011;**38**(2):225-235

[13] Grimwade D, Mrózek K. Diagnostic and prognostic value of cytogenetics in acute myeloid leukemia. Hematology/Oncology Clinics of North America. 2011;**25**(6):1135-1161

[14] Giagounidis A, Haase D. Morphology, cytogenetics and classification of MDS. Best Practice & Research Clinical Haematology. 2013;**26**(4):337-353

[15] Puiggros A, Blanco G, Espinet B. Genetic abnormalities in chronic lymphocytic leukemia: Where we are and where we go. BioMed Research International. 2014;**2014**:435983

[16] Prideaux SM, Conway O'Brien E, Chevassut TJ. The genetic architecture of multiple myeloma. Advances in Hematology. 2014;**2014**:864058

[17] Löwenberg B. Acute myeloid leukemia: The challenge of capturing disease variety. Hematology American Society of Hematology Education Program. 2008:1-11

[18] Döhner H, Estey E, Grimwade D, Amadori S, Appelbaum FR, Büchner T, Dombret H, Ebert BL, Fenaux P, Larson RA, Levine RL, Lo-Coco F, Naoe T, Niederwieser D, Ossenkoppele GJ, Sanz M, Sierra J, Tallman MS, Tien HF, Wei AH, Löwenberg B, Bloomfield CD. Diagnosis and management of AML in adults: 2017 ELN recommendations from an international expert panel. Blood. 2017;**129**(4):424-447

[19] Mosna F, Papayannidis C, Martinelli G, Di Bona E, Bonalumi A, Tecchio C, Candoni A, Capelli D, Piccin A, Forghieri F, Bigazzi C, Visani G, Zambello R, Zanatta L, Volpato F, Paolini S, Testoni N, Gherlinzoni F, Gottardi M. Complex karyotype, older age, and reduced first-line dose intensity determine poor survival in core binding factor acute myeloid leukemia patients with long-term follow-up. American Journal of Hematology. 2015;**90**(6):515-523

[20] Schnittger S, Weisser M, Schoch C, Hiddemann W, Haferlach T, Kern W. New score predicting for prognosis in PML-RARA+, AML1-ETO+, or CBFBMYH11+ acute myeloid leukemia based on quantification of fusion transcripts. Blood. 2003;**102**(8):2746-2755

[21] Souza Melo CP, Campos CB, Dutra ÁP, Neto JC, Fenelon AJ, Neto AH, Carbone EK, Pianovski MA, Ferreira AC, Assumpcão JG. Correlation between FLT3-ITD status and clinical, cellular and molecular profiles in promyelocytic acute leukemias. Leukemia Research. 2015;**39**(2):131-137

[22] Helbig G, Wozniczka K, Wieclawek A, Soja A, Bartkowska-Chrobok AK, et al. Clinical relevance of mutant NPM1 and CEBPA in patients with acute myeloid leukaemia—Preliminary report. Contemporary Oncology (Pozn). 2014;**18**(4):241-245

[23] Walker A, Marcucci G. Molecular prognostic factors in cytogenetically normal acute myeloid leukemia. Expert Review of Hematology. 2012;**5**(5):547-558

[24] Orozco JJ, Appelbaum FR. Unfavorable, complex, and monosomal karyotypes: The most challenging forms of acute myeloid leukemia. Oncology (Williston Park, N.Y.). 2012;**26**(8):706-712

[25] Swerdlow SH, Campo E, Harris NL, Jaffe ES, Pileri SA, Stein H, Thiele J, editors. WHO classification of Tumours of Haematopoietic and lymphoid tissues. In: WHO Classification of Tumours. Revised 4th ed. Vol. 2. IARC; ISBN:13 9789283244943

[26] Almond LM, Charalampakis M, Ford SJ, Gourevitch D, Desai A. Myeloid sarcoma: Presentation, diagnosis, and treatment. Clinical Lymphoma, Myeloma & Leukemia. 2017;**17**(5):263-267

[27] Achneck HE, Sileshi B, Parikh A, Milano CA, Welsby IJ, Lawson JH. Pathophysiology of bleeding and clotting in the cardiac surgery patient: From vascular endothelium to circulatory assist device surface. Circulation. 2010;**122**(20):2068-2077

[28] Hassell KL. Population estimates of sickle cell disease in the U.S. American Journal of Preventive Medicine. 2010;**38**(4 Suppl):S512-S521

[29] Quinn CT, Rogers ZR, Buchanan GR. Survival of children with sickle cell disease. Blood. 2004;**103**(11):4023-4027

[30] Hamideh D, Alvarez O. Sickle cell disease related mortality in the United States (1999-2009). Pediatric Blood & Cancer. 2013;**60**(9):1482-1486

[31] McClellan AC, Luthi JC, Lynch JR, Soucie JM, Kulkarni R, Guasch A, Huff ED, Gilbertson D, McClellan WM, DeBaun MR. High one year mortality in adults with sickle cell disease and end-stage renal disease. British Journal of Haematology. 2012;**159**(3):360-367

Section 2

Hematological Malignancies

Chapter 2

The Antigen Receptor as a Driver of B-Cell Lymphoma Development and Evolution

Julieta Sepulveda, Noé Seija, Pablo Oppezzo and Marcelo A. Navarrete

Additional information is available at the end of the chapter

http://dx.doi.org/10.5772/intechopen.72122

Abstract

The expression of a functional antigen receptor is necessary for cell survival of normal B lymphocytes and most B-cell neoplasms alike. When the genetic modifications of the B-cell receptor locus fail to produce a functional antigen receptor or result in deleterious mutations of a previously expressed receptor, the affected B cell will undergo apoptosis. The three physiological mechanisms that generate the B-cell receptor, VDJ recombination, somatic hypermutation, and class switch recombination, can induce double-strand DNA breaks and can specifically contribute to lymphomagenesis. On the other hand, the B-cell receptor activation and signaling pathways, which provide strong survival and proliferation signals to normal B cells, can support the growth and evolution of malignant lymphocytes. As a result, an otherwise structurally normal B-cell receptor can behave, from the functional perspective, as a true oncogene. In this chapter, we provide an in-depth discussion of the most recently discovered recurrent mechanisms involving the B-cell receptor in lymphoma pathogenesis. The discussion is structured around two major topics: (1) the genetic mechanisms that create a functional antigen receptor and their errors leading to oncogenic events, and (2) the pathogenic activation of the B-cell receptor signaling cascade. Finally, we will briefly comment on novel emerging therapies targeting the B-cell receptor at different levels.

Keywords: lymphoma, B-cell receptor, activation-induced deaminase (AID), somatic hypermutation, class switch recombination, lymphomagenesis, pathogenesis, oncogenesis

1. Introduction

The immune system has evolved with the primary purpose of eliminating or at least controlling invading pathogens. In contrast to innate immunity, the adaptive immune system relies for this task on recognition of the pathogen through antigen-specific receptors. In the case of B cells, these receptors are membrane-bound or soluble immunoglobulins that engage soluble or surface-bound antigens.

Hallmarks of the adaptive immune system related to the B-cell receptor are: (1) continuous presence of an extremely broad repertoire of antigen receptors; (2) rapid activation and expansion of cells whose particular receptors recognize a given antigen, and (3) maintenance of a memory of every immune response that has taken place in order to react even more efficaciously upon re-exposure to the evoking antigen [1].

The immune system has, therefore, developed unique molecular mechanisms to generate virtually unlimited numbers of antigen receptors with different specificities. These mechanisms are V, D, and J recombination of immunoglobulin gene segments, class switch recombination, and somatic hypermutation (SHM). Since these events involve genome editing, they entail intrinsic oncogenic risk [2].

The expression of a functional B-cell receptor (BCR) on the cell surface after successful completion of VDJ recombination distinguishes precursor from mature B cells, and correspondingly precursor cell from mature B-cell lymphomas.

Upon antigen recognition, B cells can undergo antibody affinity maturation through SHM, a genetic mechanism that permits antibody diversification. SHM is mediated by activation-induced deaminase (AID), an enzyme physiologically expressed in the germinal center. AID converts C:G base pairs in immunoglobulin genes into U:G mismatches. Repair of these mutations creates almost random point mutations [2–4].

Signals generated by the BCR govern the development, function, and survival of normal B cells. However, its ability to efficiently activate anti-apoptotic and proliferation pathways can be adopted by malignant B-cell, and even become essential for their survival [5].

In the current chapter, the discussion is structured around two major pathogenic mechanisms: (1) genetic mechanisms that create a functional antigen receptor and their errors leading to oncogenic events, and (2) pathogenic activation of the B-cell receptor signaling cascade.

2. Major B-cell receptor–related lymphomagenic mechanisms

2.1. Genetic mechanisms that create a functional antigen receptor and their errors leading to oncogenic events

Three unique genetic mechanisms operate sequentially in various stages of B-cell development to generate a functional antigen receptor: VDJ recombination, class switch recombination (CSR), and somatic hypermutation (SHM). Errors during these events may lead to lymphomagenesis.

2.1.1. V(D)J recombination

In the germ line DNA configuration, the antigen receptor gene loci contain discontinuous, non-functional V, D, and J segments. Committed B lymphocyte precursor cells create functional immunoglobulin heavy and light chain genes through VDJ recombination and VJ recombination, respectively [6]. The V(D)J recombination starts at the pro-B cell stage by activation of recombination-activating genes (RAG) 1 and 2. The first step is the DJ joining in the IgH locus followed by the joining of V segments to DJ, resulting in the rearrangement of the μ-chain (μH). The μH paired with a surrogate light chain (SLC) is expressed on the cell membrane as a part of a structure known as pre–B-cell receptor.

In pre-B cells, RAG1/2 expression results in the recombination of the kappa light chain. A successful rearrangement will induce RAG downregulation; otherwise, RAG will start a second rearrangement of the light chain [7].

During V(D)J recombination, a successful rearrangement of the heavy chain will suppress the rearrangement of the second allele, a process known as allelic exclusion. In the case of Ig-Kappa chains, if neither of both alleles generates a productive receptor the process will continue with the rearrangement of the Ig-Lambda locus [8].

V(D)J recombination can be divided into two phases: the cleavage phase and the joining phase. In the cleavage phase, RAG1/2 creates double-strand breaks (DSB) at recombination signal sequences (RSS), which are located at the start of each antigen receptor gene segment. RSS is composed by a heptamer, a spacer sequence (12–23 nucleotides) and a nonamer sequence. RAG acts on RSS by introducing a nick between the coding sequence and the heptamer [9]. At each of the two remaining ends, called the coding ends, the two strands of DNA are joined to form a hairpin structure. The Artemis nuclease nicks the hairpin, whose ends are then joined by non-homologous end joining (NHEJ) [10]. The recombination process activates the DNA damage response (DDR), a system that detects any signal of DNA damage. The action of DDR may result in DNA repair or induction of apoptosis [11].

2.1.2. Class switch recombination

Class switch recombination (CSR) is a process that replaces the default Cμ exons with exons from a downstream constant chain (Cα, Cϵ, or Cγ), resulting in a change from IgM expressed by naïve B cells to expression of one of the downstream isotypes IgA, IgG, IgE.

CSR occurs by intrachromosomal deletion and recombination events between two different switch (S) regions localized upstream of each constant region in the IgH locus. S regions are GC-rich with a high frequency of the WGCW (A/T-G-G-A/T) motif, which is a target of activation-induced deaminase (AID) activity. CSR has two phases: (1) the break at the donor and acceptor S regions, and (2) the ligation process between distal breaks [12].

The recombination is initiated by AID, an enzyme that deaminates cytosines into uracil at the donor and acceptor S regions. Subsequently, the base excision repair (BER) pathway creates a single strand break (SSB) that is processed to double strand breaks (DSB) by mismatch repair

(MMR). After the formation of DSBs in the S regions (donor and acceptor), these S regions are recombined by non-homologous end joining (NHEJ) [13].

During normal B-cell development, the DNA repair pathways (BER and MMR) reduce the effect of off-target AID activity. However, several external factors like cellular stress, hypoxia, and viral infections; or intrinsic factors such as alterations in repair pathways may change the outcome of AID-induced lesions [14].

2.1.3. V(D)J recombination, class switch recombination, and neoplastic transformation

One evident deviation of the normal V(D)J recombination and CSR processes is the possibility of rearrangements between segments belonging to different genes. In fact, reciprocal chromosomal translocations are the most common recurrent genetic anomalies in lymphoid malignancies and the newly formed junctions generated in most human lymphoid translocations have the canonical features of NHEJ [15].

One paradigmatic example is follicular (FL), a lymphoid neoplasm characterized by the t(14;18)(q32;q21) translocation that juxtaposes the anti-apoptotic proto-oncogene BCL2 to the immunoglobulin heavy chain locus [16]. The functional result of this translocation is constitutive transcriptional upregulation of BCL2. Although this translocation is considered the founding event in FL pathogenesis, t(14;18)-positive B cells can be detected in many healthy individuals [17]. Therefore, this genetic event alone seems insufficient to cause lymphoma.

The t(11;14)(q13;q32) translocation, a hallmark of mantle cell lymphoma (MCL), results in the overexpression of cyclin D1 and also appears to be a V(D)J-mediated translocation [18]. As in FL, the sole constitutive overexpression of this cell cycle regulator is insufficient to explain malignant transformation.

Whereas the t(14;18) or t(11;14) translocations result from a mistake during V(D)J recombination, some translocations involve the IgH class switch regions in a failed CSR event. Translocations at the IgH class switch regions seem to depend on AID activity and commonly involve c-MYC and BCL-6 [19]. BCL6 is the most commonly rearranged gene in activated B cell (ABC) diffuse large B-cell lymphoma (DLBCL) and c-MYC rearrangements can be observed in Burkitt lymphoma (BL) and DLBCL.

BCL6 is a proto-oncogene encoding a transcriptional repressor expressed during B cell differentiation in germinal centers. A block in the normal downregulation of BCL6, through its translocation with more than 20 possible partner genes, might favor differentiation arrest, continuous cell proliferation, survival, and genetic instability [20]. BCL6 also suppresses the activity of the tumor suppressor gene TP53, which allows BCL6-expressing cells to escape apoptosis [21].

The c-MYC gene at 8q24 is involved in three translocations observed in DLBCL, most commonly t(8;14) (q24;q32), and less often t(2;8) (p12;q24) and t(8;22) (q24;q11) [21]. In the t(8;14) (q24;q32) translocation, also observed in BL, the gene segments from the IgH locus are joined with various regions around and within the c-MYC proto-oncogene [22]. As a result, IgH regulatory elements are misplaced upstream, of the c-MYC proto-oncogene [23].

Four recurrent translocations, t(1;14)(p22;q32), t(3;14)(p14.1;q32), t(11;18)(q21;q21), and t(14;18)(q32;q21), have been described in marginal zone B-cell lymphomas of MALT type. The two latter translocations involve the MALT1 gene. These translocations seem to occur as a result of illegitimate V(D)J-mediated recombination [22, 24].

2.1.4. Somatic hypermutation (SHM)

Somatic hypermutation (SHM) is the biological underlying mechanism for the generation of the secondary antibody repertoire. AID is the single enzyme that is responsible for the initiation of this process [25].

SHM is a post-rearrangement diversification process that introduces point mutations in the variable regions of the Ig loci, which can alter the antibody binding to its cognate antigen. AID acts enzymatically as a cytosine deaminase that converts cytosine to uracil. Uracil is mutagenic when paired with guanosine, this U:G mismatch triggers error-prone DNA repair in B cells. SHM results in a mutation rate of circa 1 mutation/1000 bp per cell generation. This mutation frequency is a million-fold higher than spontaneous mutation rate in somatic cells [26]. Highly selected antibodies with neutralizing activity against influenza virus can accumulate 30–40 mutations, and broadly neutralizing antibodies against HIV more than 100 mutations [27, 28].

AID acts on a single strand, thus its activity is probably generated during at transcription bubbles (**Figure 1**). Once AID produced deamination of dC to dU the error-prone processing begins. First AID-catalyzed uracils in the DNA are recognized by either the uracil-DNA glycosylase (UNG)—triggering the base excision repair (BER) pathway—or by the mismatch recognition heterodimer MutSα—initiating the mismatch repair (MMR) pathway. In BER, UNG binds to the U:G mispair and produces an abasic site, then this site is cleaved by the apurinic/apyrimidinic endonuclease (APE1), which removes the abasic site nucleotide and the DNA polymerase Polβ resynthesizes the DNA strand [29]. In the MMR pathway, the proteins MSH2 and MSH6 bind to the U:G mismatch and recruit DNA Polη, a low fidelity polymerase, that introduces error during nucleotide synthesis [30].

The processing of uracils by BER and MMR may result in different outcomes. The introduced uracils may (1) be replaced by another nucleotide, (2) expose DNA to further mutations in its vicinity like mutations at A:T pairs or (3) can be converted into DNA DSBs. The latter seems to be necessary for CSR.

Because of its mutagenic potential, SHM has multiple layers of regulation and competition between alternative pathways that define the level of SHM [31]. There is also increasing evidence that epigenetic factors, such as DNA methylation and post-translational histone modifications play major roles in regulating SHM [32]. Its implications in lymphoma development remain elusive.

When SHM affect off-target genes, it is referred to as aberrant SHM. Aberrant SHM can be mainly detected in FL, BL, DLBCL, and CLL [33–35]. This topic has been extensively reviewed elsewhere [36–39].

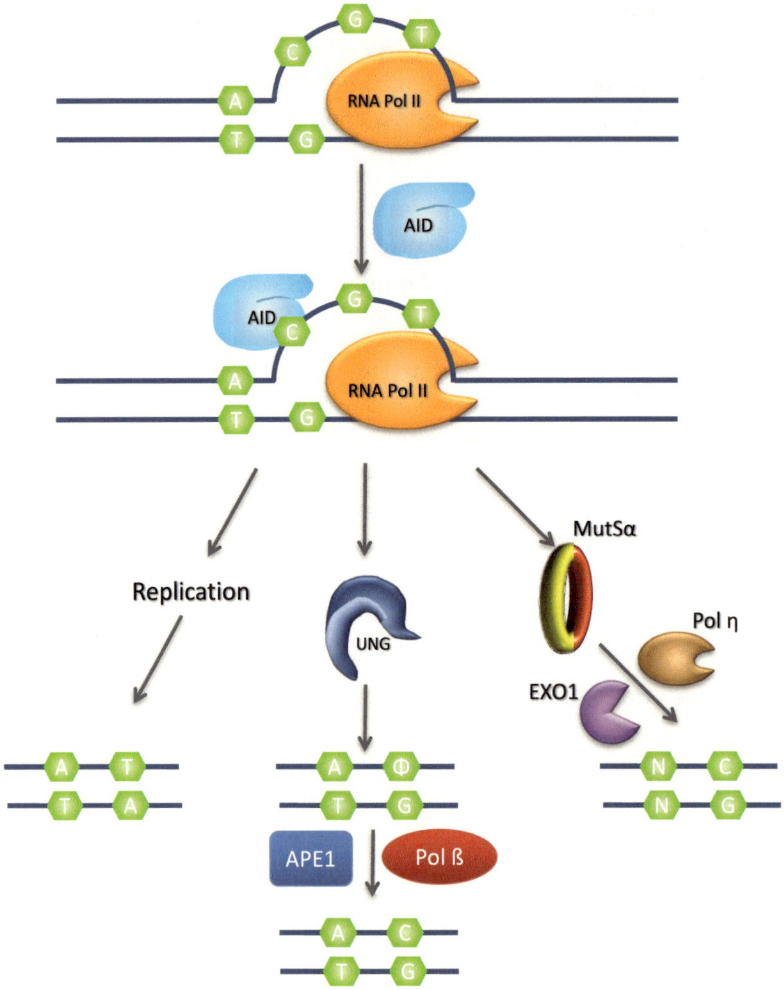

Figure 1. Molecular mechanism of somatic hypermutation (SHM). AID requires a single strand to initiate the SHM process. Transcription by RNA polymerase II (RNA Pol II) exposes the single-stranded DNA template for AID. AID deaminates a cytosine to create an uracil, which can then be processed by different pathways. Replication over the uracil results in C to T or G to A transition mutations. Processing by uracil DNA glycosylase (UNG) generates an abasic site (Φ) that is cleaved by the apurinic/apyrimidinic endonuclease (APE1), which removes this site and then Polβ resynthesizes the DNA. Recognition of the U-G mismatch by MutSα (represented by a torus shape) followed by the action of Exo1 and Polη spreads mutations (indicated as "N") to surrounding A-T nucleotides. UNG and Msh2/Msh6 can also act in the context of high fidelity base excision repair (BER) and mismatch repair (MMR) pathways, which results in error-free repair.

We have recently described that, in IgM expressing FL, the mutation load of the Ig genes can be described as a function of the AID expression level. In contrast, in FL cases that underwent class switch recombination (i.e., IgG expressing lymphomas) AID expression and SHM of immunoglobulin genes are dissociated [40, 41]. The distinctive patterns induced by SHM may also have implications for the clinical evolution of the disease [42].

AID expression is detected in a tumor subset in the peripheral blood of CLL patients [43, 44]. These cases display the dissociation between CSR and SHM, an observation that resembles our findings in FL. Our data also suggest that functional AID expression in CLL correlates with a distinctive genomic landscape and disease evolution [45].

Analysis of whole genome and whole exome sequencing data classified by the trinucleotide context of single nucleotide variants in so-called mutation signatures can help to elucidate underlying mutagenic mechanisms in tumor samples [46]. Our data indicate that the mutational landscape of both CLL and FL seems to be strongly shaped by AID activity. In FL, AID-induced mutations are mainly restricted to canonical AID hotspots and CpG methylation-dependent mutagenesis sites. In strong contrast, both canonical and non-canonical AID motifs seem to contribute to the mutational landscape of CLL [47].

SHM may not only contribute to lymphomagenesis by acting on oncogenes and proto-oncogenes, but also may provide adaptive advantages. As suggested by our data, BCR editing through SHM may allow FL cells to escape from immunosurveillance [48–50].

2.2. Pathogenic activation of the B-cell receptor signaling cascade

Antibody molecules, when expressed on the cell surface, constitute the binding moiety of a molecular complex known as B-cell antigen receptor (BCR). Signals from the BCR regulate the development and function of B cells. However, the ability of the BCR signaling pathway to induce cell survival and proliferation could be adopted and distorted by malignant cells.

The BCR immunoglobulin consists of a heavy chain and a light chain, whereas its precursor, the pre-BCR, consists of a heavy chain and a surrogate light chain. The transmembrane domain of the heavy chains anchors the BCR to the cell membrane, where each BCR molecule associates with the signaling subunit. The signaling subunit is constituted by a heterodimer of Igα (CD79A) and Igβ (CD79B) [51]. Within their cytoplasmic tails, Igα and Igβ harbor 2 conserved tyrosine residues as part of a 26 amino acid-long sequence, also referred to as an immunoreceptor tyrosine-based activation motif (ITAM) [52]. Phosphorylation of ITAM through kinases, such as Lck/Yes-related novel protein tyrosine kinase (LYN), B-lymphoid kinase (BLK), or spleen tyrosine kinase (SYK), marks the first step in signal transduction from the BCR to the nucleus [53]. SYK in conjunction with PI3K recruits Burton's tyrosine kinase (BTK). Upon activation of the BCR pathway, BTK binds to PIP3 and attaches to the plasma membrane [54]. These events contribute to BCR-induced calcium release, cell proliferation, and activation of the NF-κB pathway (**Figure 2A**) [55].

In pre-B cells, the BCR signaling cascade is activated through autonomous signaling, a mechanism that relies on the structural conformation of the pre-BCR which is constituted by a heavy chain and a surrogate light chain [56, 57]. While pre-B cells rely on autonomous BCR signaling, immature and mature B-cells receive two types of signals from their BCRs: the antigen-dependent, and the antigen-independent "tonic" signals. The antigen-dependent signal is generated by binding of an external antigen to the BCR and results in the clustering and

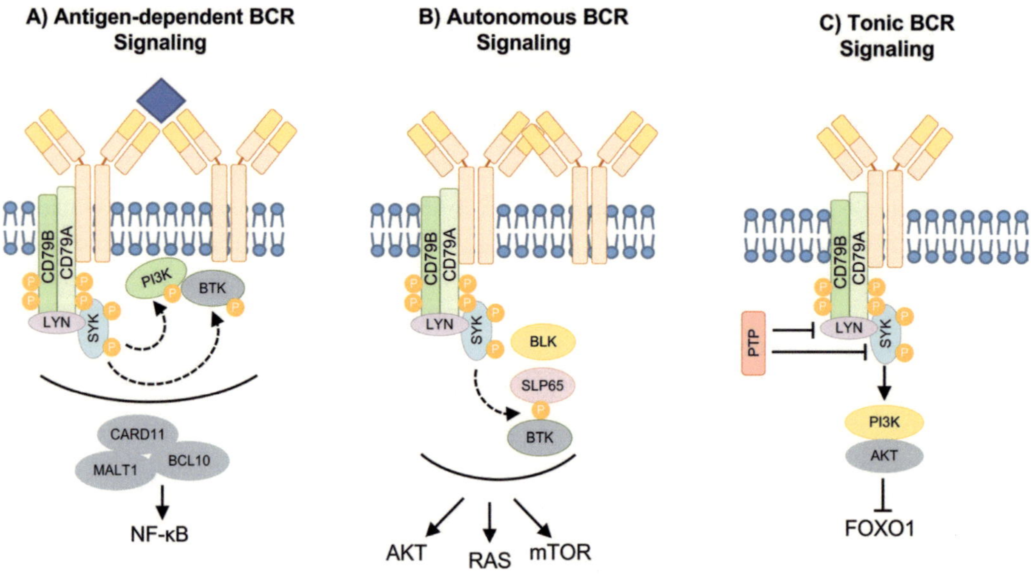

Figure 2. BCR signals generated in malignant and normal B cells. (A) Tonic signaling: random and transient disruptions in the equilibrium between positive regulators of BCR signaling, such as the CD79a/CD79b heterodimer, LYN and SYK, and negative regulators, such as the various phosphatases (PTP), could generate a tonic antigen-independent BCR signal characterized by increased activity of the PI3K/AKT pathway. (B) Aggregation of neighboring BCRs in polyreactive receptors initiates a cell-autonomous BCR signal in the absence of an external antigen. (C) The binding of the cognate antigen induces aggregation of neighboring BCRs that initiate the classical antigen-dependent BCR signal (see text for details).

activation of a signaling complex that transmits the signal inside the cell. In contrast, the tonic signal occurs in the absence of external ligands (**Figure 2**) [58, 59].

Current evidence indicates that all three, tonic, autonomous, as well as antigen-dependent BCR signaling, are used by different B-cell lymphoid neoplasms. Activation may occur through physiological mechanisms such as antigen interaction or by pathological mechanisms such as mutations in genes acting downstream the signaling cascade. The relative contribution of these types of signals varies across different B-cell neoplasms and is currently subject to debate.

2.2.1. Antigen-driven BCR activation and lymphomagenesis

The hypothesis that antigenic stimulation can contribute to the development of B-cell malignancies was proposed over half a century ago [60]. There is growing indirect and direct evidence suggesting that antigen recognition may have a role in the pathogenesis of chronic lymphocytic leukemia (CLL), follicular lymphoma (FL), marginal zone lymphoma (MZL) of the spleen, and MZL of mucosa-associated lymphoid tissue (MALT)-type.

Indirect evidence for the role of antigen stimulation includes the association between certain lymphoma subtypes and specific infections and autoimmune diseases, as well as the identification of an antigen selection footprint in the BCR; i.e., a bias in gene usage and positive selection of somatic mutations in the complementarity determining regions [40, 42, 50, 61, 62]. More direct evidence for the role of antigen stimulation and BCR activation in lymphomagenesis is based on the identification of BCR reactivity toward foreign or auto-antigens, and the induction of intracellular BCR signaling in primary lymphoma cells in response to specific antigens [63–65].

Although several bacterial and viral infections have been associated with the development different lymphoma types, direct demonstration of lymphoma development due to infectious agent-derived antigenic stimulation remains limited.

Helicobacter pylori infection is associated with gastric MZL of MALT-type. This association relies on epidemiological, biological, molecular, and clinical data [41, 66–70]. Indeed, since the initial evidence of the association between *H. pylori* infection with the development of gastric MALT lymphoma [67], *H. pylori* eradication has established as the first-line therapy for this lymphoma [71, 72]. It has been demonstrated that MALT lymphoma B cells exhibit polyreactive surface BCR immunoglobulins. Direct stimulation by specific alloantigens (including *H. pylori* sonicate) and autoantigens recognized by these surface antibodies leads to the proliferation of tumor cells [73]. *H. pylori* infection may also induce aberrant AID expression followed by accumulation of mutations in tumor-related genes, suggesting a link between BCR activation and AID expression [74]. Nevertheless, a direct link to the activation of the BCR signaling pathway remains elusive.

Chlamydia psittaci infection is associated with ocular adnexal extranodal marginal zone lymphomas (OAEMZLs) [75]. These neoplasms express a biased repertoire of mutated surface immunoglobulins suggesting, which suggests that antigen receptors have been subject to clonal selection. In OAEMZL patients, local monocytes and macrophages are the carriers of *Chlamydia psittaci*, and lymphomas seem to preferentially arise in organs primarily exposed to antigens [76].

Certain lymphomas, such as splenic marginal zone lymphoma (SMZL), are associated with *hepatitis C virus* (HCV) infection. Current evidence suggests that a subset of HCV-associated lymphomas originate from B cells that were initially activated by the HCV-E2 protein, suggesting that this subgroup of lymphomas arise as an expansion of HCV-reactive B cells [77]. Consistently, antiviral treatment results in complete responses in about 75% of HCV positive lymphoma patients, whereas no responses are seen in HCV negative patients [78]. Altogether, this data suggest that antigen-dependent BCR activation may be the driver of lymphomagenesis for some SMZL cases; and removal of the antigen can lead to clinical remission in these patients.

Several viral, bacterial, and fungal antigens may bind specific BCRs on chronic lymphocytic leukemia (CLL) cells [79–81]. Moreover, CLL cells in the lymph node contain increased levels of activated SYK and express genes upregulated in response to BCR activation [82]. In addition, the observation of a reversible down-modulation of surface IgM expression on CLL cells also supports the idea of chronic antigen stimulation [83].

In follicular lymphoma (FL), the BCR is characterized by abnormal N-linked glycosylation. The mannosylated variable regions of FL immunoglobulins bind to recombinant lectin domains of the mannose receptor and dendritic-cell-specific intercellular adhesion molecule-3-grabbing nonintegrin (DC-SIGN), which results in stimulation of FL cells [84]. It has also been demonstrated that V-region mannosylation conferred the ability of B cells to be activated by soluble bacterial lectins from common opportunistic pathogens such as *Pseudomonas aeruginosa* or *Burkholderia cenocepacia* while disrupting the initial receptor specificity for potential autoantigens [64].

The source of the antigen is not necessarily derived from an external pathogen as it has also been shown to derive from self-antigens. CLL BCRs can react with many different self-antigens, including antigens released by apoptotic cells [85, 86]. In addition, BCR derived from CLL patients can bind to a conserved epitope within the second framework region (FR2) of their own BCR [87]. About 26% of FL cases recognize autoantigens, and the interaction with certain self-antigens such as myoferlin can induce BCR-mediated signaling *in vitro* [65]. It has also been demonstrated that interaction of the BCR of ABC DLBCL with a self-antigen is essential for the survival of these lymphoma cells. This interaction may explain the microclusters observed in the plasma membrane of ABC DLBCL cells [5, 88].

2.2.2. Tonic B-cell receptor signaling and lymphomagenesis

The tonic B-cell receptor signaling (BCR) is thought to provide an antigen-independent constitutive baseline signal essential for B cell survival and development [58, 89]. Although the detailed molecular mechanisms regulating tonic signaling remain to be defined, current evidence highlights the central role of the SYK tyrosine kinase and the balance between BCR-associated SYK activation and protein tyrosine phosphatase (PTP)-mediated SYK inhibition [53, 90]. The tonic signaling transmitted via SYK appears to activate the phosphatidylinositol 3-kinase (PI3K)/AKT/mTOR pathway [91]. The inhibition of the tonic BCR signal results in increased activation of FOXO1 and increased expression of its target genes, including the pro-apoptotic BCL2 family member, BCL2L11, and the cell-cycle inhibitor p27 [92].

Evidence about the use of tonic antigen-independent type of BCR signaling by malignant B cells is reported for Burkitt lymphoma (BL) and germinal center B diffuse large B-cell lymphoma (GCB-DLBCL) [93, 94].

In BL, PI3K signals promote the survival and proliferation of BL cells [95]. One study demonstrated by quantitative phosphoproteomics, in which phosphorylation events in tonic BCR signaling differ from those induced by BCR engagement in BL cells [96].

In DLBCL, BCR signaling differs between the germinal center B-cell (GCB) subtype, which is insensitive to Bruton's tyrosine kinase inhibition by ibrutinib, and the activated B-cell (ABC) subtype [97]. As recently reported, the replacement of antigen-binding regions of the BCR has no effect on BCR signaling in GCB-DLBCL cell lines, which supports the hypothesis of the use of tonic BCR signaling by this DLBCL subtype [94]. Unlike antigen-driven BCR signaling, tonic BCR signaling requires specific phosphorylation of CD79A. This finding provides a rationale for the development of novel molecular targeted drugs for the treatment of DLBCL [94].

2.2.3. *Autonomous signaling and lymphomagenesis*

Autonomous antigen-independent, BCR signaling is a survival mechanism characteristic of the pre–B-cell receptor [57, 98]. However, immature and mature B cells with BCRs, that recognize multiple self-antigens, may also induce autonomous signaling and selective expansion of B cell in a manner comparable to the pre-BCR [56]. This functional similarity between autoreactive BCRs and the pre-BCR suggests that recognition of self-antigens might not only play a role in the positive selection of early B cells, but also could contribute to lymphomagenesis [87, 99–101].

Autonomous signaling has been proposed as a novel oncogenic mechanism in chronic lymphocytic leukemia (CLL) and diffuses large B-cell lymphoma (DLBCL) [87, 100, 101]. BCR, derived from both mutated and unmutated CLL cases, expressed in a cellular system designed to measure BCR signaling cascade activation, show signaling properties that are equivalent to those of the pre-BCR [87]. This striking signaling property is dependent on the antigen-binding site of the clonal BCR and an internal motif in framework region 2, a part of the structural BCR backbone [102].

The gene expression profile of activated B-cell (ABC) type of DLBCL resembles that of mature B cells upon stimulation via their B-cell receptor (BCR). In up to 30% of ABC DLBCL cases, this signature can be explained by gain-of-function mutations in CD79A, CD79B, or CARD11 [103]. However, in patients without CARD11 mutations activation of the BCR may occur through autonomous signaling. We have recently demonstrated the presence of autonomous BCR activity in 72% of non-GCB DLBCL, including primary mediastinal DLBCL [100, 101]. This finding may provide a complementary or alternative explanation to the characteristic gene expression signature of ABC DLBCL.

These findings in CLL and DLBCL support the concept of the BCR acting as a true oncogene, despite being structurally normal and solely characterized by this autonomous signaling property.

2.2.4. *Mutations in the BCR signaling cascade*

In addition to the natural activation, BCR signaling can be induced by acquired mutations.

Different ABC DLBCL cases carry diverse activating mutations in the BCR pathway (**Table 1**). Mutations of a critical tyrosine residue in the ITAM of CD79B increase the signaling response by interfering with activation of LYN. In this subset of ABC DLBCL cells, PI3K and BTK signaling remain essential for NF-κB activation [104]. About 10% of ABC DBCL cases show activating mutations of CARD11, a key protein that connects BCR activation to NF-κB signaling. This mutation is sufficient to intrinsically activate survival signaling in the malignant B cells and obviates the need for upstream BCR signaling [103]. Loss of function mutations in the tumor suppressor A20 contributes to NF-κB pro-survival signaling have also been described in ABC DLBCL and CLL cases [105, 106].

	Errors in VDJ recombination	Errors in class switch recombination	Resulting event
Mantle cell lymphoma	t(11;14)(q13;q32)		Cyclin D1 overexpression
Follicular lymphoma	t(14;18)(q32;q21)		BCL2 overexpression
Marginal zone lymphoma of MALT type	t(11;18)(q21;q21), t(14;18)(q32;q21)		MALT1 dysregulation
GCB-diffuse large B-cell lymphoma		t(8;14) (q24;q32), t(2;8) (p12;q24), t(8;22) (q24;q11	c-MYC overexpression
ABC-diffuse large B-cell lymphoma		BCL6 rearrangement—multiple partner genes	BCL6 dysregulation
Burkitt lymphoma		t(8;14)(q24;q32)	c-MYC overexpression

Table 1. Recurrent translocations and their link to V(D)J recombination or class switch recombination in mature B-cell neoplasms.

Although germinal center B (GCB) DLBCL seems independent of BCR signaling, still may require intrinsic activation of the PI3K pathway (**Table 1**). Some germinal center B (GCB) DLBCLs display activating mutations in the PIK3CA domain of PI3K [107].

Another example of a transition from a dependence on extrinsic BCR activation to intrinsic activation has been described in MALT lymphomas (**Table 2**). In advanced cases, the t(11;18) chromosomal results in a fusion transcript of API2-MALT1 and the t(1;14) leads to overexpression of BCL10 under the control of the Ig heavy chain locus. Consequently, MALT1/BCL10/CARD11 complex activates the classical NF-κB pathway (**Figure 2A**) [108].

Burkitt lymphoma (BL) seems dependent upon tonic BCR survival signaling through PI3K but not upon the NF-κB pathway. The hallmark of BL is a translocation of MYC to the Ig heavy chain locus. However, MYC has strong pro-apoptotic effects and requires activation of pro-survival signaling through the PI3K pathway. In BL activation of PI3K resembles the tonic signaling in normal resting B cells [95, 96]. Consistently, BL cells are sensitive to genetic knockdown of CD79A or SYK and pharmacologic inhibition of PI3K, however, are not affected by knockdown of BTK [95].

In follicular lymphoma, at least half of the patients show evidence of mutations in the interconnected BCR and CXCR4 signaling pathways such as mutations in CD79B, CARD11, CXCR4, SYK, BTK, and HVCN1 [3, 109]. Considering the unique characteristics of the BCR in this lymphoma type, such as high hypermutation rates, distinctive selection patterns, mannosylation of the antigen binding site and autoantigen binding, the understanding of the precise interplay between the tumor dependence on a functional BCR and the presence of this recurrent mutation requires further investigation [3, 40, 42, 48].

In CLL there is evidence for mutations in BTK and PLCγ2 that may confer resistance to BTK inhibition [110]. Despite the general consensus on the absence of somatic mutation on both CD79A and CD79B in CLL, one study has reported mutations in CD79B [111].

	Antigen-dependent BCR signaling	Tonic BCR signaling	Autonomous BCR signaling	Recurrent mutations in the signaling pathway
Chronic lymphocytic leukemia	++	+	+++	BTK, PLCγ2
Follicular lymphoma	+	–	–	CD79B, CARD11, CXCR4, SYK, BTK
Marginal zone lymphoma of MALT type	++	–	–	MALT1
GCB-diffuse large B-cell lymphoma	–	++	–	PI3K, PTEN
ABC-diffuse large B-cell lymphoma	–	+	++	ITAM, CARD11, NF-kB dependent
Burkitt lymphoma	–	++	–	NF-kB independent

The estimated relative contribution of antigen-dependent, tonic, and autonomous BCR signaling to the pathogenesis is represented as follows: [++] = major contribution, [+] = potential contribution, [–] = no evidence of contribution or minor contribution to pathogenesis.

Table 2. Pathogenic activation of the B-cell receptor signaling cascade.

3. Therapeutic implications

In malignancies, in which chromosomal translocations result in the constitutive overexpression of oncogenes, the use of targeted therapy in these oncogenes represents a very attractive concept. One example is venetoclax, a highly potent and selective oral BCL-2 antagonist. Venetoclax has proven to be highly active in patients with CLL, FL, and MCL [112].

The link between antigen-driven BCR activation and lymphomagenesis immediately suggest that the identification and elimination of the putative antigen could result in tumor regression. The induction of complete remission of gastric MZL by antibiotic therapy aimed to eradicate *H. pylori* represents a paradigmatic example of this idea [70]. However, the identification of cognate foreign antigens has been extremely difficult. Another therapeutic concept is the idea of disrupting the interaction of the BCR with its antigen by the generation of anti-idiotype antibodies. Despite promising results in early phase clinical trials, phase III studies failed to show a substantial benefit of this approach when used as consolidation therapy [49, 113].

The evident dependence of B-cell lymphomas on the BCR signaling pathway establishes BCR signaling blockade as a rational and disease-specific therapeutic approach. This strategy has the potential to block all three BCR signaling mechanisms: antigen-dependent signaling, tonic signaling, and autonomous signaling.

The BCR signal can be blocked by specific inhibitors of essential tyrosine kinases of the signaling cascade such as BTK [114] or SYK [115, 116], or by blocking integration point of signals originating from cell surface receptors. PI3Kδ represents one of this integration points and idelalisib, a small molecular PI3Kδ inhibitor has shown clinical efficacy in CLL and FL [117, 118].

Ibrutinib, a BTK inhibitor has demonstrated durable clinical responses in relapsed/refractory CLL patients, including those with the high-risk del(17p) cytogenetic abnormality. Durable clinical responses have also been demonstrated MCL and DLBCL [97, 114]. Several oral SYK inhibitors, including fostamatinib, entospletinib, and cerdulatinib, are being assessed in clinical trials [119].

All these new drugs share a pattern of response resulting in nodal reduction and increased lymphocytosis. This phenomenon may reflect unique properties such as micro-environment modulation, and activity on the proliferative pools existing in the bone marrow and lymph nodes [74, 120].

4. Conclusion and perspective

The understanding of lymphomagenesis remains essential for the development of novel therapeutic strategies. Both the errors in the genetic mechanisms that create a functional BCR and the pathogenic activation of the BCR signaling cascade have a clearly established role in B-cell lymphoma pathogenesis.

AID, an essential enzyme for the generation of the BCR, seems to play an important role in origin and progression of B-cell neoplasms. AID may also be involved in both mechanisms: the BCR origin and the BCR activation. Its study as a therapeutic target certainly deserves further research.

Novel technologies, such as next-generation sequencing, are helping to depict the complex genomic landscape of lymphoid malignancies. Recent developments, not only are enabling the identification of the underlying mutagenic mechanisms, but also the ongoing determination of "targetable" genetic aberrations is currently pushing forward the development of molecularly driven targeted therapeutics.

Current developments may change the natural history of this group of diseases in the near future. Nevertheless, further progress still depends on our ability to understand and integrate knowledge on the B-cell biology, the evolving tumor dynamics, clonal heterogeneity, and microenvironment interaction.

Author details

Julieta Sepulveda[1,2], Noé Seija[3], Pablo Oppezzo[3] and Marcelo A. Navarrete[4*]

*Address all correspondence to: m.a.navarrete@me.com

1 Department of Hematology, Leiden University Medical Center, Leiden, The Netherlands

2 Faculty of Health Sciences, University of Magallanes, Punta Arenas, Chile

3 Institut Pasteur Montevideo, Montevideo, Uruguay

4 School of Medicine, University of Magallanes, Punta Arenas, Chile

References

[1] Iwasaki A, Medzhitov R. Control of adaptive immunity by the innate immune system. Nature Immunology. 2015;**16**(4):343-353

[2] Gazumyan A et al. Activation-induced cytidine deaminase in antibody diversification and chromosome translocation. Advances in Cancer Research. 2012;**113**:167-190

[3] Navarrete MA, Oppezzo P. The pathogenesis of follicular lymphoma, beyond apoptosis resistance. Translational Cancer Research. 2017;**6**:S529-S532

[4] Kenter AL et al. AID hits the jackpot when missing the target. Current Opinion in Immunology. 2016;**39**:96-102

[5] Young RM et al. Survival of human lymphoma cells requires B-cell receptor engagement by self-antigens. Proceedings of the National Academy of Sciences of the United States of America. 2015;**112**(44):13447-13454

[6] Carsetti R. The development of B cells in the bone marrow is controlled by the balance between cell-autonomous mechanisms and signals from the microenvironment. The Journal of Experimental Medicine. 2000;**191**(1):5-8

[7] Tiegs SL, Russell DM, Nemazee D. Receptor editing in self-reactive bone marrow B cells. The Journal of Experimental Medicine. 1993;**177**(4):1009-1020

[8] Vettermann C, Schlissel MS. Allelic exclusion of immunoglobulin genes: Models and mechanisms. Immunological Reviews. 2010;**237**(1):22-42

[9] van Gent DC, Ramsden DA, Gellert M. The RAG1 and RAG2 proteins establish the 12/23 rule in V(D)J recombination. Cell. 1996;**85**(1):107-113

[10] Ma Y et al. Hairpin opening and overhang processing by an Artemis/DNA-dependent protein kinase complex in nonhomologous end joining and V(D)J recombination. Cell. 2002;**108**(6):781-794

[11] Bredemeyer AL et al. ATM stabilizes DNA double-strand-break complexes during V(D)J recombination. Nature. 2006;**442**(7101):466-470

[12] Stavnezer J, Guikema JE, Schrader CE. Mechanism and regulation of class switch recombination. Annual Review of Immunology. 2008;**26**:261-292

[13] Petersen S et al. AID is required to initiate Nbs1/gamma-H2AX focus formation and mutations at sites of class switching. Nature. 2001;**414**(6864):660-665

[14] Liu M et al. Two levels of protection for the B cell genome during somatic hypermutation. Nature. 2008;**451**(7180):841-845

[15] Lieber MR. Mechanisms of human lymphoid chromosomal translocations. Nature Reviews. Cancer. 2016;**16**(6):387-398

[16] Tsujimoto Y et al. The t(14;18) chromosome translocations involved in B-cell neoplasms result from mistakes in VDJ joining. Science. 1985;**229**(4720):1390-1393

[17] Tellier J et al. Human t(14;18)positive germinal center B cells: A new step in follicular lymphoma pathogenesis? Blood. 2014;**123**(22):3462-3465

[18] Vogt N et al. The molecular pathogenesis of mantle cell lymphoma. Leukemia & Lymphoma. 2017;**58**(7):1530-1537

[19] Lu Z et al. BCL6 breaks occur at different AID sequence motifs in Ig-BCL6 and non-Ig-BCL6 rearrangements. Blood. 2013;**121**(22):4551-4554

[20] Lenz G. Insights into the molecular pathogenesis of activated B-cell-like diffuse large B-cell lymphoma and its therapeutic implications. Cancers (Basel). 2015;**7**(2):811-822

[21] Lossos IS. Molecular pathogenesis of diffuse large B-cell lymphoma. Journal of Clinical Oncology. 2005;**23**(26):6351-6357

[22] Du MQ. MALT lymphoma: Genetic abnormalities, immunological stimulation and molecular mechanism. Best Practice & Research. Clinical Haematology. 2017;**30**(1-2):13-23

[23] Neri A et al. Different regions of the immunoglobulin heavy-chain locus are involved in chromosomal translocations in distinct pathogenetic forms of Burkitt lymphoma. Proceedings of the National Academy of Sciences of the United States of America. 1988;**85**(8):2748-2752

[24] Murga Penas EM et al. The t(14;18)(q32;q21)/IGH-MALT1 translocation in MALT lymphomas contains templated nucleotide insertions and a major breakpoint region similar to follicular and mantle cell lymphoma. Blood. 2010;**115**(11):2214-2219

[25] Methot SP, Di Noia JM. Molecular mechanisms of somatic hypermutation and class switch recombination. Advances in Immunology. 2017;**133**:37-87

[26] Tiller T et al. Autoreactivity in human IgG+ memory B cells. Immunity. 2007;**26**(2):205-213

[27] Klein F et al. Somatic mutations of the immunoglobulin framework are generally required for broad and potent HIV-1 neutralization. Cell. 2013;**153**(1):126-138

[28] Wrammert J et al. Rapid cloning of high-affinity human monoclonal antibodies against influenza virus. Nature. 2008;**453**(7195):667-671

[29] Wu X, Stavnezer J. DNA polymerase beta is able to repair breaks in switch regions and plays an inhibitory role during immunoglobulin class switch recombination. The Journal of Experimental Medicine. 2007;**204**(7):1677-1689

[30] Delbos F et al. Contribution of DNA polymerase eta to immunoglobulin gene hypermutation in the mouse. The Journal of Experimental Medicine. 2005;**201**(8):1191-1196

[31] Maul RW, Gearhart PJ. AID and somatic hypermutation. Advances in Immunology. 2010;**105**:159-191

[32] Klymenko T et al. Lamin B1 regulates somatic mutations and progression of B-cell malignancies. Leukemia. 2017;**8**(14):online

[33] Pasqualucci L et al. Expression of the AID protein in normal and neoplastic B cells. Blood. 2004;**104**(10):3318-3325

[34] Koning MT et al. Template-switching anchored polymerase chain reaction reliably amplifies functional lambda light chain transcripts of malignant lymphoma. Leukemia & Lymphoma. 2014;**55**(5):1212-1214

[35] Koning MT et al. ARTISAN PCR: Rapid identification of full-length immunoglobulin rearrangements without primer binding bias. British Journal of Haematology. 2017 Sep;**178**(6):983-986

[36] Green MR et al. Hierarchy in somatic mutations arising during genomic evolution and progression of follicular lymphoma. Blood. 2013;**121**(9):1604-1611

[37] Lossos IS, Levy R. Mutation analysis of the 5′ noncoding regulatory region of the BCL-6 gene in non-Hodgkin lymphoma: Evidence for recurrent mutations and intraclonal heterogeneity. Blood. 2000;**95**(4):1400-1405

[38] Pasqualucci L et al. AID is required for germinal center-derived lymphomagenesis. Nature Genetics. 2008;**40**(1):108-112

[39] Pasqualucci L et al. Hypermutation of multiple proto-oncogenes in B-cell diffuse large-cell lymphomas. Nature. 2001;**412**(6844):341-346

[40] Scherer F et al. Isotype-switched follicular lymphoma displays dissociation between activation-induced cytidine deaminase expression and somatic hypermutation. Leukemia & Lymphoma. 2016;**57**(1):151-160

[41] Hu Q et al. Gastric mucosa-associated lymphoid tissue lymphoma and *Helicobacter pylori* infection: A review of current diagnosis and management. Biomarker Research. 2016;**4**:15

[42] Scherer F et al. Selection patterns of B-cell receptors and the natural history of follicular lymphoma. British Journal of Haematology. 2016;**175**(5):972-975

[43] Oppezzo P et al. Chronic lymphocytic leukemia B cells expressing AID display dissociation between class switch recombination and somatic hypermutation. Blood. 2003; **101**(10):4029-4032

[44] Palacios F et al. High expression of AID and active class switch recombination might account for a more aggressive disease in unmutated CLL patients: Link with an activated microenvironment in CLL disease. Blood. 2010;**115**(22):4488-4496

[45] Seija N, Uriepero A, Navarrete MA, Oppezzo P. Unraveling CLL progression in unmutated patients: Linking functional AID expression with disease evolution. In: XVII International Workshop on Chronic Lymphocytic Leukemia; New York. 2017

[46] Alexandrov LB et al. Signatures of mutational processes in human cancer. Nature. 2013; **500**(7463):415-421

[47] Sepulveda J et al. The mutation landscape of follicular lymphoma and chronic lymphocytic leukemia reveals a distinctive frequency and composition of AID-related mutation signatures. In: American Society of Hematology 59th Annual Meeting and Exposition. Atlanta, USA. 2017. p. 621

[48] Strothmeyer AM et al. Comparative analysis of predicted HLA binding of immunoglobulin idiotype sequences indicates T cell-mediated immunosurveillance in follicular lymphoma. Blood. 2010;**116**(10):1734-1736

[49] Navarrete MA et al. Upfront immunization with autologous recombinant idiotype Fab fragment without prior cytoreduction in indolent B-cell lymphoma. Blood. 2011;**117**(5):1483-1491

[50] Papaioannou D et al. Evidence for idiotype-directed immunosurveillance is restricted to follicular lymphoma and attributable to somatic hypermutation. Haematologica. 2015;**100**(4):e143-e146

[51] Schamel WW, Reth M. Monomeric and oligomeric complexes of the B cell antigen receptor. Immunity. 2000;**13**(1):5-14

[52] Reth M. Pillars article: Antigen receptor tail clue. Nature. 1989. 338: 383-384. Journal of Immunology. 2014;**192**(9):4015-4016

[53] Rolli V et al. Amplification of B cell antigen receptor signaling by a Syk/ITAM positive feedback loop. Molecular Cell. 2002;**10**(5):1057-1069

[54] Murayama K et al. Crystal structure of the Bruton's tyrosine kinase PH domain with phosphatidylinositol. Biochemical and Biophysical Research Communications. 2008;**377**(1): 23-28

[55] Niemann CU, Wiestner A. B-cell receptor signaling as a driver of lymphoma development and evolution. Seminars in Cancer Biology. 2013;**23**(6):410-421

[56] Kohler F et al. Autoreactive B cell receptors mimic autonomous pre-B cell receptor signaling and induce proliferation of early B cells. Immunity. 2008;**29**(6):912-921

[57] Meixlsperger S et al. Conventional light chains inhibit the autonomous signaling capacity of the B cell receptor. Immunity. 2007;**26**(3):323-333

[58] Monroe JG. ITAM-mediated tonic signalling through pre-BCR and BCR complexes. Nature Reviews. Immunology. 2006;**6**(4):283-294

[59] Rickert RC. New insights into pre-BCR and BCR signalling with relevance to B cell malignancies. Nature Reviews. Immunology. 2013;**13**(8):578-591

[60] Dameshek W, Schwartz RS. Leukemia and auto-immunization—Some possible relationships. Blood. 1959;**14**:1151-1158

[61] Agathangelidis A et al. Stereotyped B-cell receptors in one-third of chronic lymphocytic leukemia: A molecular classification with implications for targeted therapies. Blood. 2012;**119**(19):4467-4475

[62] Ottensmeier CH et al. Analysis of VH genes in follicular and diffuse lymphoma shows ongoing somatic mutation and multiple isotype transcripts in early disease with changes during disease progression. Blood. 1998;**91**(11):4292-4299

[63] Krysov S et al. Surface IgM of CLL cells displays unusual glycans indicative of engagement of antigen *in vivo*. Blood. 2010;**115**(21):4198-4205

[64] Schneider D et al. Lectins from opportunistic bacteria interact with acquired variable-region glycans of surface immunoglobulin in follicular lymphoma. Blood. 2015;**125**(21): 3287-3296

[65] Sachen KL et al. Self-antigen recognition by follicular lymphoma B-cell receptors. Blood. 2012;**120**(20):4182-4190

[66] Doglioni C et al. High incidence of primary gastric lymphoma in northeastern Italy. Lancet. 1992;**339**(8797):834-835

[67] Parsonnet J et al. *Helicobacter pylori* infection and gastric lymphoma. The New England Journal of Medicine. 1994;**330**(18):1267-1271

[68] Wundisch T et al. Long-term follow-up of gastric MALT lymphoma after *Helicobacter pylori* eradication. Journal of Clinical Oncology: Official Journal of the American Society of Clinical Oncology. 2005;**23**(31):8018-8024

[69] Sena Teixeira Mendes L, Attygalle DA, Wotherspoon CA. *Helicobacter pylori* infection in gastric extranodal marginal zone lymphoma of mucosa-associated lymphoid tissue (MALT) lymphoma: A re-evaluation. Gut. 2014;**63**(9):1526-1527

[70] Cheung DY. *Helicobacter pylori* eradication therapy, the reasonable first line therapy for gastric mucosa-associated lymphoid tissue lymphoma irrespective of infection status and disease stages. Gut Liver. 2016;**10**(5):659-660

[71] Zucca E et al. Gastric marginal zone lymphoma of MALT type: ESMO clinical practice guidelines for diagnosis, treatment and follow-up. Annals of Oncology. 2013;**24**(Suppl 6): vi144-vi148

[72] Szanto I et al. Regression of gastric MALT lymphoma after eradication of *Helicobacter pylori* infection followed by endoscopic ultrasound. Orvosi Hetilap. 2000;**141**(26):1455-1458

[73] Craig VJ et al. Gastric MALT lymphoma B cells express polyreactive, somatically mutated immunoglobulins. Blood. 2010;**115**(3):581-591

[74] Matsumoto Y et al. *Helicobacter pylori* infection triggers aberrant expression of activation-induced cytidine deaminase in gastric epithelium. Nature Medicine. 2007;**13**(4):470-476

[75] Ferreri AJ et al. Evidence for an association between *Chlamydia psittaci* and ocular adnexal lymphomas. Journal of the National Cancer Institute. 2004;**96**(8):586-594

[76] Ponzoni M et al. Chlamydia infection and lymphomas: Association beyond ocular adnexal lymphomas highlighted by multiple detection methods. Clinical Cancer Research. 2008;**14**(18):5794-5800

[77] Quinn ER et al. The B-cell receptor of a hepatitis C virus (HCV)-associated non-Hodgkin lymphoma binds the viral E2 envelope protein, implicating HCV in lymphomagenesis. Blood. 2001;**98**(13):3745-3749

[78] Gisbert JP et al. Systematic review: Regression of lymphoproliferative disorders after treatment for hepatitis C infection. Alimentary Pharmacology & Therapeutics. 2005;**21**(6): 653-662

[79] Steininger C et al. Recombinant antibodies encoded by IGHV1-69 react with pUL32, a phosphoprotein of cytomegalovirus and B-cell superantigen. Blood. 2012;**119**(10):2293-2301

[80] Hoogeboom R et al. A mutated B cell chronic lymphocytic leukemia subset that recognizes and responds to fungi. The Journal of Experimental Medicine. 2013;**210**(1):59-70

[81] Lanemo Myhrinder A et al. A new perspective: Molecular motifs on oxidized LDL, apoptotic cells, and bacteria are targets for chronic lymphocytic leukemia antibodies. Blood. 2008;**111**(7):3838-3848

[82] Hoellenriegel J et al. The phosphoinositide 3′-kinase delta inhibitor, CAL-101, inhibits B-cell receptor signaling and chemokine networks in chronic lymphocytic leukemia. Blood. 2011;**118**(13):3603-3612

[83] Mockridge CI et al. Reversible anergy of sIgM-mediated signaling in the two subsets of CLL defined by VH-gene mutational status. Blood. 2007;**109**(10):4424-4431

[84] Coelho V et al. Glycosylation of surface Ig creates a functional bridge between human follicular lymphoma and microenvironmental lectins. Proceedings of the National Academy of Sciences of the United States of America. 2010;**107**(43):18587-18592

[85] Herve M et al. Unmutated and mutated chronic lymphocytic leukemias derive from self-reactive B cell precursors despite expressing different antibody reactivity. The Journal of Clinical Investigation. 2005;**115**(6):1636-1643

[86] Chu CC et al. Many chronic lymphocytic leukemia antibodies recognize apoptotic cells with exposed nonmuscle myosin heavy chain IIA: Implications for patient outcome and cell of origin. Blood. 2010;**115**(19):3907-3915

[87] Duhren-von Minden M et al. Chronic lymphocytic leukaemia is driven by antigen-independent cell-autonomous signalling. Nature. 2012;**489**(7415):309-312

[88] Davis RE et al. Chronic active B-cell-receptor signalling in diffuse large B-cell lymphoma. Nature. 2010;**463**(7277):88-92

[89] Monroe JG. Ligand-independent tonic signaling in B-cell receptor function. Current Opinion in Immunology. 2004;**16**(3):288-295

[90] Chen L et al. Protein tyrosine phosphatase receptor-type O truncated (PTPROt) regulates SYK phosphorylation, proximal B-cell-receptor signaling, and cellular proliferation. Blood. 2006;**108**(10):3428-3433

[91] Srinivasan L et al. PI3 kinase signals BCR-dependent mature B cell survival. Cell. 2009;**139**(3):573-586

[92] Szydlowski M et al. FOXO1 activation is an effector of SYK and AKT inhibition in tonic BCR signal-dependent diffuse large B-cell lymphomas. Blood. 2016;**127**(6):739-748

[93] Walter R et al. HSP90 promotes Burkitt lymphoma cell survival by maintaining tonic B-cell receptor signaling. Blood. 2017;**129**(5):598-608

[94] Havranek O et al. Tonic B-cell receptor signaling in diffuse large B-cell lymphoma. Blood. 2017;**130**(8):995-1006

[95] Schmitz R et al. Burkitt lymphoma pathogenesis and therapeutic targets from structural and functional genomics. Nature. 2012;**490**(7418):116-120

[96] Corso J et al. Elucidation of tonic and activated B-cell receptor signaling in Burkitt's lymphoma provides insights into regulation of cell survival. Proceedings of the National Academy of Sciences of the United States of America. 2016;**113**(20):5688-5693

[97] Wilson WH et al. Targeting B cell receptor signaling with ibrutinib in diffuse large B cell lymphoma. Nature Medicine. 2015;**21**(8):922-926

[98] Ohnishi K, Melchers F. The nonimmunoglobulin portion of lambda5 mediates cell-autonomous pre-B cell receptor signaling. Nature Immunology. 2003;**4**(9):849-856

[99] Koning MT et al. Autonomous, antigen-independent B-cell receptor signalling as a novel pathogenetic mechanism in non-GCB DLBCL. Cancer Research. 2016;**76**(14 Suppl): Abstract nr LB-012

[100] Koning MT et al. Antigen-independent, autonomous B-cell receptor signaling as a dominant candidate oncogenic mechanism in ABC DLBCL. Blood. 2016;**128**(22):778

[101] Koning MT et al. Primary mediastinal large B-cell lymphoma exhibits autonomous BCR signaling and responds to the second generation BTK inhibitor Acalabrutinib. Blood. 2016;**128**(22):4171

[102] Binder M et al. CLL B-cell receptors can recognize themselves: Alternative epitopes and structural clues for autostimulatory mechanisms in CLL. Blood. 2013;**121**(1):239-241

[103] Lenz G et al. Oncogenic CARD11 mutations in human diffuse large B cell lymphoma. Science. 2008;**319**(5870):1676-1679

[104] Kloo B et al. Critical role of PI3K signaling for NF-kappaB-dependent survival in a subset of activated B-cell-like diffuse large B-cell lymphoma cells. Proceedings of the National Academy of Sciences of the United States of America. 2011;**108**(1):272-277

[105] Philipp C et al. Mutation analysis of the TNFAIP3 (A20) tumor suppressor gene in CLL. International Journal of Cancer. 2010;**128**(7):1747-1750

[106] Wenzl K et al. Higher incidence of the SNP Met 788 Ile in the coding region of A20 in diffuse large B cell lymphomas. Tumour Biology. 2016;**37**(4):4785-4789

[107] Abubaker J et al. PIK3CA mutations are mutually exclusive with PTEN loss in diffuse large B-cell lymphoma. Leukemia. 2007;**21**(11):2368-2370

[108] Akyuz N et al. MALT1 sequencing analyses in marginal zone B-cell lymphomas reveal mutations in the translocated MALT1 allele in an IGH-MALT1-positive MALT lymphoma. Leukemia & Lymphoma. 2017;**58**(10):2480-2484

[109] Krysiak K et al. Recurrent somatic mutations affecting B-cell receptor signaling pathway genes in follicular lymphoma. Blood. 2017;**129**(4):473-483

[110] Woyach JA et al. Resistance mechanisms for the Bruton's tyrosine kinase inhibitor ibrutinib. The New England Journal of Medicine. 2014;**370**(24):2286-2294

[111] Payelle-Brogard B et al. Analysis of the B-cell receptor B29 (CD79b) gene in familial chronic lymphocytic leukemia. Blood. 1999;**94**(10):3516-3522

[112] Davids MS. Targeting BCL-2 in B-cell lymphomas. Blood. 2017;**130**(9):1081-1088

[113] Schuster SJ, Neelapu SS, Gause BL, Muggia FM, Gockerman JP, Sotomayor EM, Winter JN, Flowers CR, Stergiou AM, Kwak LW. Idiotype vaccine therapy (BiovaxID) in follicular lymphoma in first complete remission: Phase III clinical trial results. Journal of Clinical Oncology. 2009;**27**(18s)

[114] Byrd JC et al. Targeting BTK with ibrutinib in relapsed chronic lymphocytic leukemia. The New England Journal of Medicine. 2013;**369**(1):32-42

[115] Friedberg JW et al. Inhibition of Syk with fostamatinib disodium has significant clinical activity in non-Hodgkin lymphoma and chronic lymphocytic leukemia. Blood. 2010;**115**(13):2578-2585

[116] Chen L et al. SYK inhibition modulates distinct PI3K/AKT-dependent survival pathways and cholesterol biosynthesis in diffuse large B cell lymphomas. Cancer Cell. 2013;**23**(6):826-838

[117] Furman RR et al. Idelalisib and rituximab in relapsed chronic lymphocytic leukemia. The New England Journal of Medicine. 2014;**370**(11):997-1007

[118] Barrientos JC. Idelalisib for the treatment of indolent non-Hodgkin lymphoma: A review of its clinical potential. OncoTargets and Therapy. 2016;**9**:2945-2953

[119] Liu D, Mamorska-Dyga A. Syk inhibitors in clinical development for hematological malignancies. Journal of Hematology & Oncology. 2017;**10**(1):145

[120] Oppezzo P, Dighiero G. Role of the B-cell receptor and the microenvironment in chronic lymphocytic leukemia. Blood Cancer Journal. 2013;**3**:e149

Chapter 3

Recent Advances in Diffuse Large B Cell Lymphoma

Vivek Kumar, Sarvadaman Makardhwaj Shrivastava,
Trishala Meghal and Binod Abhinav Chandra

Additional information is available at the end of the chapter

http://dx.doi.org/10.5772/intechopen.74263

Abstract

More recently, DLBCL has witnessed advances in the molecular profiling and treatment of patients with refractory and relapsed disease. DLBCL is biologically and clinically a heterogeneous disease. Despite its aggressive behavior, DLBCL is a potentially curable disease with overall survival of 94 and 55% in patients with low and high rIPI scores, respectively. The combination of anti-CD 20 monoclonal antibody rituximab and cyclophosphamide, doxorubicin, oncovin (vincristine) and prednisone (R-CHOP) chemotherapy every 3 weeks is the first line treatment. Radiotherapy is reserved for the patients with bulky disease who fail to achieve complete remission after first line treatment. CNS prophylaxis is reserved for the patients with high lactate dehydrogenase (LDH) levels and involvement of more than one extranodal sites and for the patients with involvement of selective extranodal sites like testes and orbits (the sanctuary sites). Patients who suffer relapse after first line treatment receive high-dose chemotherapy supported by autologous stem cell transplantation (HDC/ASCT). Variants of DLBCL like double-hit (presence of MYC and BCL2/BCL6) and triple-hit (presence of MYC, BCL2 and BCL6) lymphomas are treated differently and these patients have worse outcome. Several novel immunotherapeutic agents like checkpoint inhibitors and chimeric antigen receptor T cell (CART) are being investigated in randomized trials on patients with DLBCL.

Keywords: diffuse large B cell lymphoma, double-hit lymphoma, update, triple-hit lymphoma, R CHOP, DA-R EPOCH

1. General information

1.1. Epidemiology

Diffuse large B cell lymphoma (DLBCL) is the most common histologic subtype of non-Hodgkin lymphoma (NHL). It constitutes for approximately 25% of patients with NHL [1].

The incidence of NHL is 19.5 per 100,000 men and women per year. Approximately 2.1% of men and women will be diagnosed with NHL at some point based on 2012–2014 SEER database [2] (SEER data). The incidence of DLBCL is approximately 7 cases per 100,000 persons per year. Males have a higher incidence with (M/F) incidence ratio of 1.5–1.6. Incidence is higher among whites than blacks or Asians and increases steeply with age. The overall incidence of DLBCL has declined 0.5% per year during 1992–2001 [2]. This decline was observed predominantly in men aged 25–54, on contrary in the elderly, the incidence of DLBCL increased 1.4% per year during the same time-period.

1.2. Etiology and risk factors

DLBCL is a mature B cell neoplasm arising from germinal center and post germinal center B cells. Etiology of DLBCL is complex and multifactorial. DLBCL can arise de-novo or from transformation of indolent diseases like chronic lymphocytic lymphoma/small lymphocytic lymphoma (so-called Richter's transformation), follicular lymphoma, and marginal zone lymphoma. Those that originate from previous hematological malignancies are generally more aggressive and carry a poor prognosis. Chemical substances such as pesticides, herbicides, alkylating agents, ionizing radiation have been implicated as risk factors. An association has been found between inherited immune deficiency disorders such as ataxia-telangiectasia, Wiskott-Aldrich syndrome, common variable immunodeficiency, severe combined immunodeficiency, X-linked lymphoproliferative disorder [3]. Patients with acquired immunodeficiency states such as AIDS, organ or stem cell transplantation, autoimmune or rheumatologic diseases also have a higher incidence of DLBCL [4].

2. Pathology and biology

2.1. Pathogenesis

DLBCL is composed of large B cells with a diffuse growth pattern arising from mature B cells at different stages of differentiation. Normal B cell development takes place in the bone marrow and results in the transformation of a B-progenitor cell into mature B cell. Mature B cells have undergone immunoglobulin VDJ gene rearrangement and express a complete IgM antibody molecule on the cell surface [4]. After release from the bone marrow, antigen naïve mature B cells are exposed to antigen in the interfollicular area of the secondary lymphoid tissues. Majority then migrate into the germinal center. Mature antigen exposed B cells proliferate in the center of a primary follicle to form the germinal center. The centroblasts mature into centrocytes as they transition into light zone of the germinal center. In the germinal center, B cell undergoes class-switch recombination and somatic hypermutation. Centroblasts are thought to give rise to germinal center B cell (GCB) DLBCL. After transition through the germinal center, B cells can become memory cells or plasmablasts which undergo further development to become plasma cells. Plasmablasts are thought to give rise to activated B cell like (ABC) DLBCL [4].

2.2. Cell of origin

The cell of origin classification (COO) has been the most significant development in the understanding of DLBCL biology. The gold standard test to identify COO is Gene expression profiling (GEP). GEP divides DLBCL into germinal center B cell (GCB), activated B cell (ABC) or unclassifiable (Type 3) types. GCB DLBCL is derived from normal GC centroblasts. Various mechanisms have been elucidated that drives pathogenesis of these subclasses based on COO [5]. GCB like tumors contain the (14;18) translocation (IgH/BCL-2 fusion gene) typical of follicular lymphoma and amplifications of the locus on chromosome 2 which codes for the c-Rel oncogene. BCL2 is dysregulated by t (14;18), PTEN deletions and amplification of miR-17-92 leading to deregulation of PI3K/mTOR pathway which are activated further promoting cell survival, proliferation and growth. GCB is further characterized by gain or amplification of MDM2, a negative regulator of the tumor suppressor p53 as well as deletions of the known tumor suppressor genes TP73 and ING1 that lead to genomic stability. The GEP of ABC DLBCL suggests that it is derived from B cells that are in the process of differentiating into plasma cells. Most of the genes expressed by normal GCB cells are down regulated in ABC DLBCL. There is upregulation of many genes normally expressed by plasma cells including XBP-1, amplification of BCL2, CD79A/CD79B ITAM mutation/deletion leading to chronic active BCR signaling, CARD11/A20 mutation, MYD88 mutation, STAT3 activation which lead to NFkB activation, FOXP1 activation. ABC-like DLBCL is associated with loss of 6q21, trisomy 3, and gains of 3q and 18q21–22. This locus on 6q encodes suppressor gene PRDM1 (Blimp-1) which is a master regulator in the differentiation of mature B lymphocytes to plasma cells, loss of which may lead to inhibition of terminal differentiation. ABC DLBCL has high expression and constitutive activity of the nuclear factor kappa B (NF-κB) complex involved in the B cell receptor signaling pathway. This classification not only defined subgroups with distinct biology and pathogenesis but also identified groups of patients with different outcomes after treatment [4]. In a study done at British Columbia looking at outcomes in patients treated with R-CHOP, there were 56% patients with GCB subtype and 32% with ABC subtype. The ABC group experienced significantly inferior outcomes as compared to the GCB group [6]. A third type, type III DLBCL (Unclassifiable as per GEP profiling) is also identified in which tumor cells have gene expression profiles that do not resemble either germinal center or post germinal center B cells [4, 7].

2.3. Double-hit lymphomas/double expressor

DLBCL with MYC gene rearrangement in addition to BCL2 and/or BCL6 gene rearrangements by Fluorescent in Situ Hybridization (FISH) or standard cytogenetics are known as double-hit lymphomas. MYC is rearranged in 5–15% of DLBCL and is frequently associated with BCL2 or to a lesser extent, BCL6 translocation. They are more aggressive and have a much poorer prognosis. Double-hit lymphomas are now recognized as a distinct entity in the 2016 WHO classification [8]. MYC and BCL2 are the key regulators of cellular proliferation and apoptosis, respectively. Dysregulation of MYC and BCL2 can cause chromosomal translocation or gene amplification but it may also occur by transcriptional upregulation downstream of NFkB pathway signaling [9]. This leads to a highly aggressive clinical behavior with very high Ki67 and overlapping pathologic features with Burkitt's lymphoma. These patients have an inferior prognosis compared to those with DLBCL without these mutations. FISH for MYC, BCL2 and BCL6 gene rearrangements should be tested for patients with expression of MYC and either BCL2 or BCL6 by IHC and a GCB like immunophenotype to identify these double- (or triple-hit) lymphomas [10]. They have very poor outcomes with standard R-CHOP-based chemotherapy [11]. While the cases identified by FISH positive results are called double- (or triple-hit) lymphomas, those patients with high expression of MYC and BCL2 protein by Immunohistochemistry (IHC) alone in the absence of gene rearrangements by FISH are labeled as double expressor and they seem to have an intermediate prognosis.

In a study on 193 patients who were double expressor the 3 year OS rate was 46 vs. 75% and the 3 year PFS rate was 46 vs. 65% [11].

2.4. Morphology

Under light microscopy, the normal architecture of lymph nodes is completely effaced by the sheets of atypical lymphoid cells. The tumor cells resemble normal centroblasts or immunoblasts with nuclei size at least twice the size of a small lymphocyte. While the centroblasts are large,

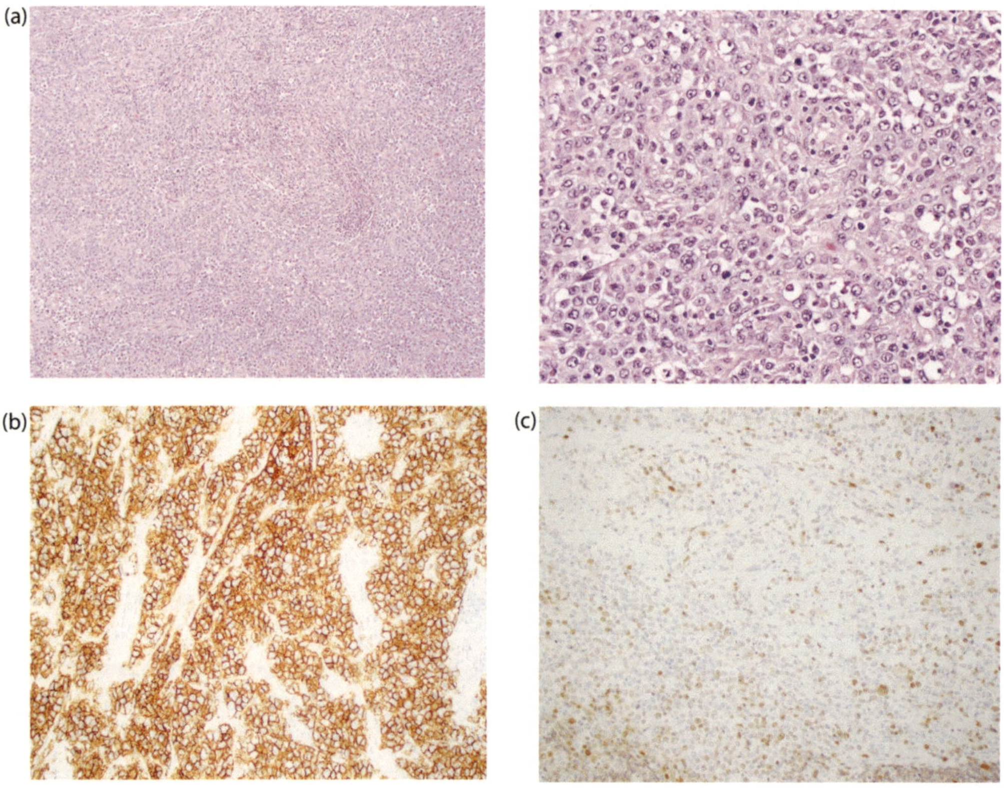

Figure 1. Lymph node sections showing GC type DLBCL (a) The H&E stained sections of lymph node showing diffuse infiltration of atypical lymphoid cells that are large in size with irregular nuclear contours, vesicular chromatin, and some with prominent nucleoli (X10 and X40 magnification). (b) On immunohistochemistry, CD20 highlights the infiltrating cells (X20 magnification) (c) cells are negative for MUM1 (major subset) (X20 magnification).

noncleaved cells, with round to oval nuclei with multiple nucleoli and thin rim of basophilic cytoplasm, the immunoblasts are larger cells with more prominent nucleoli and abundant cytoplasm. Other less common cytological variants include multilobated and anaplastic forms. However the clinical significance of less common forms is debatable. Due to inter- and intra-observer variability in the characterization of DLBCL based on the appearance of tumor cells, all the morphological subtypes are grouped as one category in the current WHO classification except for plasmablastic lymphoma. The plasmablastic lymphoma displays immunophenotype characteristics which allows its distinction from other morphological subtypes of DLBCL (**Figures 1–3**).

Histopathological and immunohistochemistry slides of diffuse large B cell Lymphoma showing characteristics of DLBCL of germinal center origin (GC) in **Figure 1** and activated B cell origin (ABC) in **Figure 2**.

2.5. WHO classification

The revised WHO classification 2016 [8] classifies DLBCL NOS into GCB and ABC/non-GC subtypes based on cell of origin. The use of IHC algorithm is accepted [8]. We also now have a

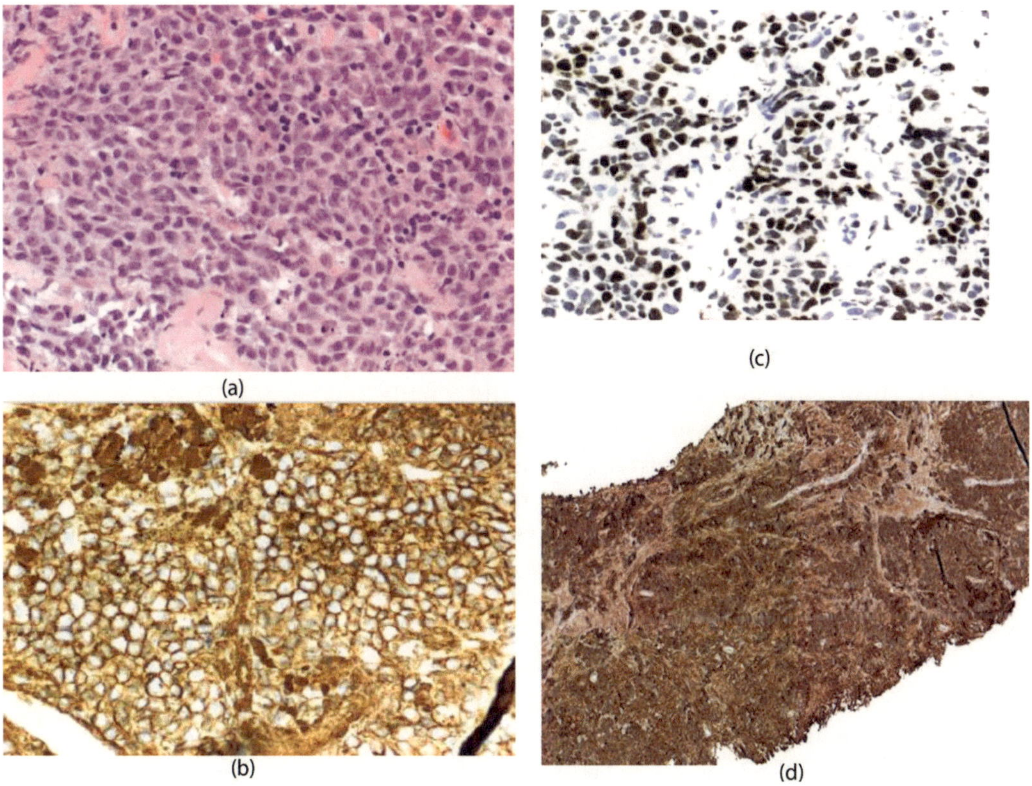

Figure 2. Lymph node sections showing ABC type DLBCL (a) The H&E stained sections showing diffuse infiltration of large atypical lymphoid cells with irregular nuclear contours and vesicular chromatin (X40 magnification). On immunohistochemistry cells are (b) CD20 positive (X20 magnification) (c) MUM1 positive (X20 magnification) (d) CD 79A positive (X20 magnification).

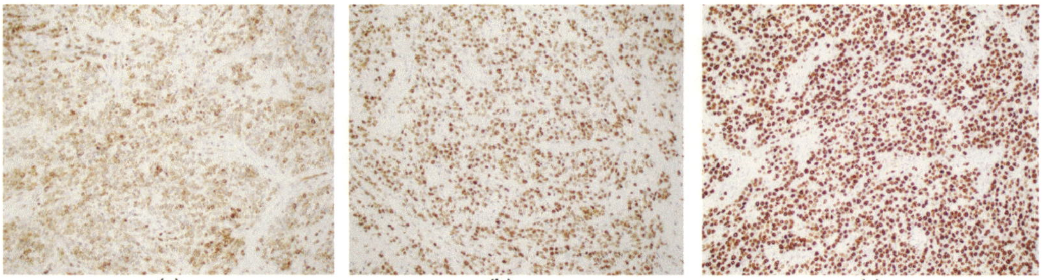

Figure 3. Lymph node sections showing very aggressive DLBCL on immunohistochemistry. (a) bcl-2 positive (X20 magnification) (b) bcl-6 positive (X20 magnification) (c) ki 67 proliferation index is approximately 70-80% positive (X20 magnification).

better understanding of MYC alterations in DLBCL. These are included in a new category of "High grade B cell lymphoma with MYC and BCL2 and/or BCL6 translocations". Co-expression of MYC and BCL2 is considered a new prognostic marker (double-expressor lymphoma). High grade lymphoma, NOS replaces B cell lymphoma unclassifiable (BCLU) category. It includes blastoid appearing large B cell lymphomas and cases lacking MYC and BCL2 or BCL6 that would formerly have been called BCLU.

2.6. Other distinctive clinicopathological subtypes of DLBCL

2.6.1. T cell histiocyte-rich large B cell lymphoma

As the name suggests this variant is characterized by the predominance of infiltrating reactive T cells and macrophages (histiocytes). Presence of <10% cellularity, has been suggested to label this diagnosis. This pathological subtype does not appear to affect the outcome when adjusted for IPI. In a study of 40 patients comprising of predominantly middle-aged males, splenomegaly, bone marrow involvement, and hepatomegaly were present in 60, 43, and 40%, respectively [12]. The International Prognostic Index (IPI) (**Table 3**) was ≥2 in 77% of the patients. Tumor cells were uniformly positive for CD20 and negative for CD5, CD10, CD15, and CD138. Although these patients were relatively young, the use of combination chemotherapy, led to complete remission in only 40%, with an overall survival of 50% at 3 years. On multivariate analysis, only the IPI and deletions or point mutations in p53 were predictive of survival. In another study, the 5-year overall or event-free survival between this variant and DLBCL was not different among the IPI matched patients [13].

2.6.2. Plasmablastic lymphoma

The tumor cells in plasmablastic lymphoma have large eccentrically placed nuclei, usually with single placed nucleoli and abundant basophilic cytoplasm. However these cells are distinct immunophenotypically. Instead of pan B cell markers which are present in typical DLBCL (CD 20, CD 79a), these tumors comprise of late B cell and express plasma cell markers like CD 138. MYC rearrangement is present in up to 50% of cases and 70% of these patients are Epstein-Barr virus (EBV) positive. Some tumors in this subtype are distinct genetically and clinically. For example oropharyngeal plasmablastic lymphomas occur most frequently in HIV-patients and are positive for EBV. Another rare variant of plasmablastic lymphoma is characterized by rearrangements of the ALK tyrosine kinase gene [7].

2.6.3. *Primary mediastinal large B cell lymphoma*

Primary large B cell lymphoma of the mediastinum is a distinct clinicopathological entity that arises from the thymic (medullary) B cell. It has clinical and pathologic features that differ from DLBCL.

2.6.4. *Intravascular large B cell lymphoma*

This is variously known as intravascular lymphomatosis, angiotropic large cell lymphoma, and malignant angioendotheliomatosis. It usually presents with disseminated intravascular proliferation of large lymphoid cells involving small blood vessels without an obvious extra-vascular tumor mass or leukemia. It commonly affects central nervous system, kidneys, lungs, and skin, but virtually any site may be involved.

2.6.5. *Diffuse large B cell lymphoma, leg type*

It manifests as red or bluish (violaceous) nodules or tumors on one or both legs, usually below the knee; 10–15% develop outside of the lower extremities. Contrary to other cutaneous B cell lymphomas, these tumors frequently disseminate to extracutaneous sites and pursue an aggressive course. MYD88 L265P mutations are seen in ~50% of cases.

2.6.6. *Diffuse large B cell lymphoma associated with chronic inflammation*

Also known as pyothorax-associated DLBCL, it usually develops in patients with a long standing history of pyothorax; however it may also arise at other sites with chronic inflammation [14]. It is seen worldwide but is more common in Japan and China. Clinically, it is an aggressive tumor. These tumors are almost always EBV-positive and are believed to arise from EBV-infected post germinal center B cells. The pattern of EBV gene expression present in this type of lymphoma (LMPI and EBNA2 positivity) suggests the role of local immunosuppression within the sites of chronic inflammation.

2.6.7. *Lymphomatoid granulomatosis*

This is also an EBV-positive large B cell lymphoma with a T cell-rich background which is clinically and pathologically distinct from DLBCL [15]. The usual manifestations are cough and fever (60%), rash/nodules (40%), malaise and weight loss (35%), neurological abnormalities and dyspnea (30%), or chest pain (15%) [16]. Extranodal involvement is common. The lungs are commonly affected. Other commonly involved sites include kidney, liver, brain, and skin. Lymph nodes and splenic involvement is rare. Histologically, the infiltrates are either angiocentric or angioinvasive. Often extensive necrosis is present with only a few atypical large B cells in a pleomorphic background of lymphocytes, plasma cells, and histiocytes. The large atypical B cells represent the neoplastic component and show evidence of EBV infection with in situ hybridization. Pulmonary nodules exhibit central necrosis and cavitation.

2.6.8. EBV-positive DLBCL, NOS

EBV-positive DLBCL, NOS is a variant of DLBCL that replaced the entity, EBV-positive DLBCL of the elderly and was added in the 2016 WHO classification. It may affect persons of all ages [17–21]. This is seen in patients without known immunodeficiency or prior lymphoma. It is seen most commonly in Asian countries where it accounts for 8–10% of DLBCL among patients without a known immunodeficiency. The majority of patients present with extranodal disease, with or without nodal involvement. While the initial reports were in adults >50 years old, this entity has been increasingly recognized in younger patients [17, 22].

2.6.9. EBV-positive mucocutaneous ulcer

It is considered a provisional entity in the 2016 revision of the WHO classification. This is characterized by the presence of isolated circumscribed ulcerative lesions, typically affecting elderly individuals [23, 24]. Its association with immunosuppression is not clear. Usually, the oropharynx is affected but lesions may also occur in the skin or in the gastrointestinal tract. Histologically, a polymorphous inflammatory infiltrate mixed with scattered EBV-infected B cells is seen in the lesions, which frequently include cells resembling Hodgkin/Reed-Sternberg cells both morphologically and immunophenotypically. This entity is distinguished from Hodgkin lymphoma by its extranodal presentation and has a benign disease course which is characterized by frequent spontaneous regressions and its excellent response to conservative treatment.

2.7. Molecular subtypes

As noted above, the classification of DLBCL NOS, into GCB vs. ABC subtypes is important for the prognostication. The prognosis of GCB-type DLBCL is considered to be better than ABC-type DLBCL. In the rituximab era the 5-year survival of GC type DLBCL is 87–92% as compared to 44% in the ABC-type DLBCL [7, 25]. Moreover, response to novel therapies may be different for the two subtypes. The classification into GCB- vs. ABC-type is best conducted by genomic expression profiling [26]. The DNA microarray is an effective tool to characterize the molecular features of DLBCL and specific genes associated with response to therapy. Though microarray GEP are gold standard for profiling of DLBCL to determine COO, they are expensive and not readily available. Moreover, they have poor flexibility and reproducibility in evaluating low quality RNA samples from formalin-fixed paraffin-embedded (FFPE) tissues and for high quality data, they require RNA extraction from the frozen tissues [27]. Thus their implementation in the routine clinical practice is limited [28]. IHC-based methods are rapid, cost effective and thus are widely used in the clinical practices. Different algorithms have been developed to improve the accuracy. These algorithms use different combinations of antibodies to identify germinal center or activated B cell-related proteins [4, 7, 29]. The relatively simple and most well-known is the Hans algorithm which is based upon the application of 3 antibodies, CD10, BCL6, IRF4/MUM1 and has a reasonable correlation with the GEP [30]. Cases are considered positive if 30% or more of the tumor cells are stained with an antibody (CD10, BCL6, and MUM1). The overall concordance with gene expression array is 80%. The Choi algorithm added FOXP1 and GCET 1 to Hans algorithm and showed 93% concordance with GEP [25, 31]. A Tally classifier substituted BCL6 for the LMO2 antibody which predicted COO better than rest of the IHC algorithms [32].

http://dx.doi.org/10.5772/intechopen.74263

However, it was not superior in predicting the outcome. In a study on 108 patients, it was shown that Hans and Choi algorithms predicted OS and PFS significantly better than the Tally method [33]. Other algorithms use combinations of other markers (Muris et al.: BCL2, CD10, MUM1 [34]), (Natkunam et al.: LMO2 [35]), (Nyman et al. 50: MUM1, CD10, GCET1, MUM1, FOXP1, LMO2 [36]) and have been described in detail in **Figure 4**.

However, the utility of IHC methodology is also limited by its poor concordance to GEP, inferior accuracy and reproducibility and a lack of prognostic utility. IHC algorithms do not recognize the 10–15% of tumors and are not always reproducible [37]. Lymph2Cx is a 20-gene version of a Nanostring code set for a COO typing assay of DLBCL. This represents GEP like

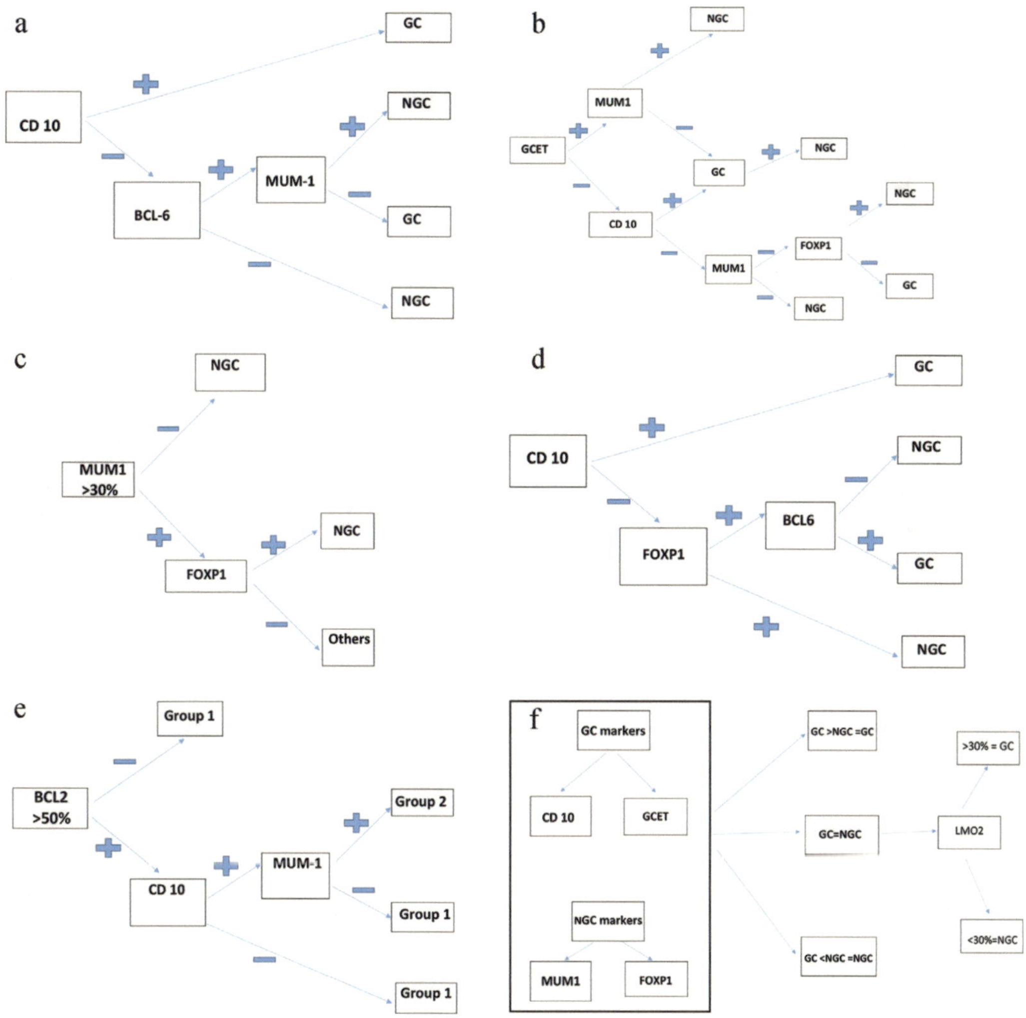

Figure 4. Immunohistochemistry algorithms for the characterization of diffuse large B-cell lymphoma on the basis of cell of origin. (a) Hans algorithm; (b) Choi algorithm; (c) Nyman algorithm; (d) Visco-young algorithm; (e) Muris algorithm; and (f) Tally algorithm.

platform that can run on FFPE tissue. Twenty genes have been selected out of 93 candidate genes [38, 39] to identify COO using this platform. In NanoString technology, digitally colored code sets are attached to the sequence-specific probes to directly measure mRNA [28, 40]. This technique offers highly sensitive, quantitative and reproducible results on FFPE and frozen tissue samples. This requires a very small amount of RNA and covers a large number of genes enabling complex genetic analysis. Studies have demonstrated strong concordance between patient-matched frozen and FFPE materials. It showed 98% concordance for ABC/GCB and 95% in the unclassifiable cases when compared with GEP [38]. In a study on 82 patients, who were treated with R-CHOP the concordance rate between Lymph2Cx assay and Hans algorithm was 73.6%. The outcome of Lymph2Cx-defined ABC (77.1%) was significantly poor as compared to the GCB type (96.6%). On contrary, there was no difference in the outcome of two groups classified by the Hans algorithm [41].

3. Clinical presentation, diagnosis and staging

3.1. Clinical presentation

Patients typically present with a rapidly enlarging single or multiple masses. In case of lymph nodes, enlargement usually involves cervical or the abdominal lymph nodes. The primary mediastinal DLBCL presents as a mediastinal mass. Patients with early stage (I/II) disease often presents with extranodal involvement. These comprise of about 40% of cases [42], while remainder 60% present with stages III/IV disease [43]. Extranodal disease is often seen in elderly patients with poor performance status and lower disease burden [42]. In a series published by Guillermo et al. extranodal gastrointestinal tract involvement was noted to be the most frequent in 12% of all cases, with majority of the lesions being in stomach; other regions included 4.5% soft tissue, 2.5% central nervous system (CNS), 2% each of liver and bone, 1% of skin, breast, kidney, testis/ovaries, and the remainder <1% each of thyroid, bone marrow, lung, prostate, uterus and pericardium [44]. Presenting symptoms may be related to the rapidly enlarging mass depending upon the site of the mass; B symptoms such as fever, night sweats, weight loss may be seen in about 30% of patients [43]. Some may present with hypercalcemia of unknown origin with imaging work up leading to diagnosis of lymphoma. Others may present with oncologic emergencies such as spinal cord compression, superior vena cava syndrome, acute airway obstruction, CNS mass lesions, renal failure due to hydronephrosis and liver failure.

3.2. Diagnosis

Diagnosis of DLBCL needs an expert hematopathologist with expertise in hematologic malignancies. An incisional or excisional lymph node biopsy is recommended when possible, to establish the diagnosis. This allows evaluation of the lymph node architectural details. Core needle biopsy is not encouraged. FNA is not suitable for the initial diagnosis although it may be sufficient to establish the relapse.

3.3. Immunophenotype

It is essential for the differentiation of various subtypes of DLBCL. This is established either by flow cytometry or IHC. Flow cytometry can be employed in determining bone marrow involvement [45] when PET/CT is not readily available for staging and in determining CNS involvement by CSF flow cytometry [46]. Immunophenotype findings are usually combined with morphologic findings to arrive at a diagnosis. Tumor cells in DLBCL generally express pan B cell antigens (CD19, CD20, CD22, and CD79a) as well as CD45. The typical immunophenotype is CD20+, CD45+, and CD3−. The panel should include CD20, CD3, CD5, CD10, CD45, BCL2, BCL6, Ki-67, IRF4/MUM1, and MYC. 50–75% of tumors express surface and cytoplasmic monoclonal immunoglobulin (Ig). The proliferative fraction of cells is usually higher than 40% and may occasionally be >90%. CD5 positive tumors are associated with a more aggressive disease and a higher incidence of CNS involvement and a worse prognosis. CD10+ and BCL6+ indicates GCB lymphoma while MUM1+ indicates ABC lymphoma. The three most common translocations noted in DLBCL include MYC, BCL2 and BCL6. MYC is an oncogene involved in pathogenesis of aggressive lymphomas based on partner gene translocation. MYC protein is a transcription regulator for cellular proliferation acting on metabolic and angiogenic mechanism. Genetic translocation involving MYC are considered primary events in 5–15% of DLBCL [47] and in around 20% on first relapse [48]. In DLBCL frequently the partner gene is BCL-2 or to a lesser extent BCL-6 or both, in the so-called double-hit or triple-hit lymphomas. Overexpression of MYC protein can be tested with IHC which can occur independent of translocation in 30% of cases; however for confirmation of specific translocation FISH studies are required [49]. Both, overexpression and translocation confer adverse outcome as documented in different studies [50]. More information on this translocation and their effect on outcome is detailed in Sections 2.3 and 6.2.

3.4. Workup

Initial work up includes thorough physical examination with special attention to node bearing areas and evaluation of performance status (PS) and constitutional symptoms. Appropriate site for excisional/incisional biopsy should be earmarked as stated above. Laboratory assessments include complete blood count (CBC) with differential, complete metabolic profile (CMP), lactate dehydrogenase (LDH) and Beta-2 microglobulin. Additional tests including uric acid and phosphorus, in patients with high tumor burden. Hepatitis B virus (HBV) testing is also warranted as there is an increased risk of HBV reactivation in patients who may require Rituximab. Positron emission tomography (PET)/computed tomography (CT) scan is recommended for initial staging as upstaging can result in altered therapy. Also baseline PET/CT is necessary to confirm the response on the post treatment PET scans. A systematic review and meta-analysis by Adams et al. showed that sensitivity and specificity of PET/CT for detection of bone marrow involvement ranged from 70.8 to 95.8% and from 99.0 to 100%, respectively [51]. There were 3.1% patients who were PET negative but had bone marrow involvement on bone marrow biopsy. On contrary 12.5% patients with negative bone marrow biopsies had marrow involvement on PET scan and PET/CT [51]. Bone marrow biopsy is not needed if the PET/CT is negative unless finding another concomitant lymphoma is important in treatment decision. Another study showed that the incidence of bone marrow involvement was 3.6% in 192 patients with stage I and II DLBCL [52]. Echocardiogram or multigated acquisition (MUGA) scan if required if anthracycline-based regimen is being considered. In selected cases discussion of fertility issues and sperm banking should be considered. Consider lumbar puncture if there is suspicion of CNS disease or if patient is at high risk of CNS involvement such in patients with testicular lymphoma, aggressive histology, human immunodeficiency virus (HIV) lymphoma, double-expressor lymphoma and in patients with 4–6 factors on the prognostic score which is discussed in the section on CNS prophylaxis. The role of various imaging modalities has been reviewed in detail elsewhere [53].

3.5. Staging

Ann Arbor staging system was originally introduced for Hodgkin's lymphoma and was later adopted for NHL. Lister et al. classified patients with NHL into stages I (localized) to IV (extensive) disease [54]. Patients are classified into A or B depending on the absence or presence of B symptoms, respectively. B symptoms mainly include fevers, drenching night sweats or weight loss of 10% or more within 6 months of diagnosis. DLBCL is a non-contiguous disease while Hodgkin's lymphoma involves contiguous sites hence the Ann Arbor staging has limited utility in DLBCL. In 2014, the Lugano classification was proposed (**Table 1**) [55]. According to this classification, patients with stage I or II disease can be grouped and considered as having limited disease while patients with Ann Arbor stage III or IV disease can be grouped as advanced stage disease. The suffix A and B is only reserved for Hodgkin's lymphoma. The X for bulky disease is now replaced with the recording of the largest nodal diameter by CT scan. Limited evidence suggests that 6–10 cm should be considered as bulky disease in the rituximab era for DLBCL. National comprehensive cancer network (NCCN)

Stage	Involvement	Extranodal (E) status
Limited		
I	Single lymph node or a group of adjacent nodes	One extranodal lesion without nodal involvement
II	Two or more lymph nodal groups on the same side of the diaphragm	Stage I or II by nodal involvement with limited contiguous extranodal extension
II bulky[1]	II as above with "bulky" disease	Not applicable
Advanced		
III	Lymph nodes on both sides of the diaphragm or lymph nodes above the diaphragm with splenic involvement	Not applicable
IV	Wide spread extralymphatic involvement	Not applicable

Note: Extent of disease in DLBCL is determined by PET-CT or CECT if former is not available. Tonsils, Waldeyer's ring, and spleen are considered nodal tissue.
[1]The decision to treat stage II bulky disease as limited or advanced disease is determined by the histology and IPI.

Table 1. Revised staging system for primary nodal lymphomas.

considers more than or equal to 7.5 cm as bulky disease. A single nodal mass of 10 cm or greater than third of the transthoracic diameter is the definition of bulky disease only for Hodgkin's lymphoma.

Staging has limited prognostic value due to the heterogeneity of the disease. To fully incorporate prognostic information several models have been developed to predict survival. The staging should generally be used with these prognostic models for accurate information.

3.6. Role of PET/CT in management of DLBCL

In oncology, the focus of imaging modalities is drifting from morphological to functional imaging and combined PET/CT is making its foray in each step of DLBCL management. Bone marrow evaluation is a part of staging that upstages DLBCL to stage IV if positive. Focal positivity on PET/CT scan can obviate the need for bone marrow biopsy in staging these patients. In a study where it was compared to standard bone marrow biopsy, PET/CT showed higher sensitivity, accuracy and negative predictive value (94, 98 and 98%, respectively, for PET/CT vs. 24, 80 and 81% for bone marrow examination) [56]. Similarly PET/CT has established its role in response assessment (see Section 7.6). Interim PET/CT can be used as a predictive marker for prognosis with PET response in the interim denoting better outcomes. In a study [57] negative PET/CT after 2 cycles when compared to those who had positive scans, showed significantly higher CR (97.3 vs. 33.3%), 3-year PFS (75.8 vs. 38.2%) and 3-year OS rates (93.5 vs. 55.6%). This advantage was also seen in those patients whose PET/CT was negative after 4 cycles and showed higher CR (96.9 vs. 16.2%), 3-year PFS (75.3 vs. 24.7%) and 3-year OS rate (91.6 vs. 49.4%).

4. Differential diagnosis

Includes wide range of pathologies that cause lymphadenopathy such as infectious mononucleosis, Carcinoma, anaplastic large cell lymphoma, gray zone lymphoma, Burkitt's lymphoma, rarely pathologies that cause small blue round cells such as Ewing's sarcoma may be in the differential diagnosis.

5. Subtypes

Several distinct subtypes of large B cell lymphoma need to be distinguished from DLBCL, NOS (see sec 2.6 above) [8].

1. Primary mediastinal (thymic) B cell lymphoma
2. Gray zone lymphoma.
3. T cell/histiocytes rich large B cell lymphoma.
4. DLBCL associated with chronic inflammation.

5. Primary cutaneous lymphomas, leg type.

6. ALK positive large B cell lymphoma.

7. EBV-positive DLBCL NOS.

8. Primary cutaneous B cell lymphomas.

9. Primary DLBCL of the CNS.

10. Lymphomatoid granulomatosis.

11. Intravascular large B cell lymphoma.

6. Prognosis

6.1. International Prognostic Index (IPI)

Staging in DLBCL has a limited value. The original IPI was developed to identify variables that could predict OS and PFS (**Table 2**). The factors included were age >60 years, elevated serum lactate dehydrogenase (LDH), Eastern Cooperative group (ECOG) performance status ≥2, clinical stage III or IV, more than 1 involved extranodal disease sites. One point was given for each of the characteristics ranging from zero to five. Five-year survival rates worsened as the scores increased. Five-year overall survival rates for patients with scores of zero to one, two,

Original IPI (1 point to each)	Age adjusted IPI (1 point to each)	NCCN IPI
Stage III or IV disease	Stage III or IV disease	Stage III or IV disease—1 point
Elevated serum LDH	Elevated serum LDH	[1]LDH ratio > 1–3—1 point LDH ratio > 3—2 points
PS of 2, 3, or 4	PS of 2, 3, or 4	PS of 2 or more—2 points
Age greater than 60 years		Age 41–60 years—1 point 61–75 years—2 points >75 years—3 points
More than 1 extranodal site		Extranodal sites involving bone marrow, CNS, liver/GI tract or lung—1 point
Low risk—0–1	Low risk—0	Low risk—0–1
Low-intermediate risk—2	Low-intermediate risk—1	Low-intermediate risk—2–3
High-intermediate risk—3	High-intermediate risk—2	High-intermediate risk—4–5
High risk—4 or 5	High risk—3	High risk—6 or above

[1]Ratio of patient's LDH level to the labs upper limit of normal.

Table 2. Original and modified International Prognostic Index.

three, four to five were 73, 51, 43, 26%, respectively [58] (project TIN-HsLPF). This was before the rituximab era. The utility of IPI was reassessed in a retrospective analysis of patients with DLBCL treated with R-CHOP in the province of British Columbia to assess the value of IPI [5]. They redistributed the IPI into revised IPI which identified 3 distinct prognostic groups of very good (score-0), good (scores 1, 2) and poor (scores 3, 4, 5) with a 4 year OS of 94, 79 and 55%, respectively. The NCCN incorporated detailed information about the variables in the original IPI and the location of extranodal disease is used rather than the number of extranodal disease as the lymphomatous involvement in major organs (bone marrow, CNS, liver/GI tract or lung) appeared to be a stronger predictor for a worse prognosis. It stratifies patients into four risk groups low—0–1 points, low-intermediate risk—2–3 points, high-intermediate risk—4–5 points and high risk—≥6 points with OS of 94, 72, 54, 35%, respectively. Both the R-IPI and the NCCN-IPI predict clinical outcome with accuracy and the use of R-IPI or the NCCN-IPI routinely to better understand the prognosis of these patients is recommended [59].

6.2. Double-/triple-hit lymphoma

Several strategies with intense regimens have been tried to mitigate this risk. **Table 3** illustrates the studies of these regimens. Additional randomized control trials are needed to evaluate the efficacy of intense regimens. Based on these small data sets, R-CHOP is associated with inferior outcome. Current literature indicates better outcomes when treated with DA-EPOCH-R in this group of patients [60]. The regimen is a dose adjusted regimen combining etoposide, prednisone, vincristine, cyclophosphamide and doxorubicin in an infusional manner targeting prolonged drug exposure to reduce resistance and dynamic dose adjustments allowing for highest acceptable doses.

Study	Number of patients	Treatment	PFS	OS
Petrich et al. [44] Induction therapy with HDSCT	311	R-CHOP (32%) Hyper CVAD/MA (2%) R-EPOCH (21%) R-CODOX-M/IVAC (14%)	10.9 months PFS (R-CHOP): 7.8 months vs. 26.6 months (intensive regimen p = 0.001)	21.9 months (p = 0.14)
Oki et al. [43]	129	R-CHOP R-Hyper CVAD/MA R-EPOCH	25% 32% 67%	OS with R-EPOCH vs. R-CHOP (p = 0.057)
Dunleavy et al. [45]	52	DA-REPOCH	79% (14 months follow up)	77%
Howlett et al. [46]	394	R-CHOP R-EPOCH R-Hyper-CVAD/MC R-CODOX-M/R-IVAC	12.1 months **22.2 months*** 18.9 months 18.9 month	I

*$p = 0.032$ (significant at $p < 0.05$).

Table 3. Intense regimen studies for MYC rearranged with/without BCL2 rearrangement.

7. Treatment

Treatment for DLBCL includes chemo-immunotherapy with an anthracycline backbone. Options differ for patients with limited vs. advanced disease.

7.1. Initial treatment of limited stage DLBCL

Limited stage DLBCL which is usually Ann Arbor stage I or II (usually non-bulky stage II which may be included in one irradiation field) accounts for 30-40% of patients with DLBCL. Combined modality therapy is considered the standard of care for these patients. This was initially established by a large randomized SWOG 8736 trial which was conducted in the pre-rituximab era. The trial compared 3 cycles of CHOP plus RT (radiotherapy) vs. 8 cycles of CHOP alone in localized stage IE, non-bulky stage IIE aggressive lymphoma. The PFS for patients receiving CHOP plus RT and for patients receiving CHOP alone were 77 and 64%, $p = 0.03$, respectively. The 5 year OS for patients receiving CHOP plus RT vs. CHOP alone were 82 and 72%, $p = 0.02$, respectively [61]. However, further follow up showed that the advantage negated. Patients with RT had more late relapses while patients with CHOP alone had increased toxicity. Addition of rituximab to combination chemo showed improved responses in patients with early stage disease. In a multicenter randomized clinical trial, MInT, which comprised of atleast 2/3rd early stage patients, 3-year event-free survival (EFS) in R-Chemo arm (79% [95% CI 75–83]) was higher as compared to chemo alone arm (59% [54–64]) and 3-year overall survival (OS) in R-chemo arm was also higher than the chemo alone arm (93 vs. 84%) [62]. The SWOG S0014 study [63] was a phase II study where patients with limited stage disease and at least 1 adverse feature, based on stage modified-IPI were given rituximab with 3 cycles of CHOP followed by involved field radiation therapy (IFRT). The study showed 2-year PFS of 93% and 4 years PFS of 88%. OS was 95% at 2 years and 93% at 4 years. These results were better than SWOG 8736 trial where CHOP+ RT without rituximab was given. R-CHOP × 3 followed by RT remains the standard of care for patients with limited stage non-bulky disease while R-CHOP × 6 cycles with or without RT remains the standard for patients with limited stage bulky disease (NCCN guidelines).

7.2. Initial treatment of advanced stage DLBCL

60–70% of patients present with advanced disease. R-CHOP every 21 days is the standard of care for this group of patients. About 60% of patients are cured with this approach. The beginnings of modern chemotherapy dates back to the use of nitrogen mustard with remarkable tumor response in a patient at Yale in 1942. The initial use of Adriamycin containing drug combinations (CHOP) was reported in 1979 by Miller et al. in 45 patients with localized NHL [61]. In Phase III trials, a complete remission (CR) rate was 53% and the survival rate was 30% after 12 years of follow up [64]. Several intense regimens such as m-BACOD; proMACe-CytaBOM and MACOP-B were investigated to improve on the results of CHOP. SWOG and ECOG did a prospective randomized phase III trial to compare these with CHOP and found no difference between these regimens but higher toxicity with the intense regimens [65]. It remained the standard of care for two decades until the introduction of first monoclonal antibody Rituximab which improved the OS by 10–15%. In the landmark GELA trial, 399 DLBCL patients 60–80 years old were randomly assigned to receive either 8 cycles of CHOP every 3 weeks vs. 8 cycles of CHOP plus rituximab every 3 weeks. There was an improvement in all endpoints including complete response rate, event-free and overall survival without significant increase in toxicity. R-CHOP became the standard of care [66]. (**Table 4**). Recent follow up of the study reported 10 year OS of 43.5%. The Mabthera International trial (MlnT) studied R-CHOP for 6 cycles vs. CHOP for 6 cycles in young patients 18–60 years who had IPI score of 0 or 1, advanced disease or stage I bulky disease. The EFS was 79 vs. 58% and OS of 93 vs. 84% which established 6 cycles of R-CHOP as the standard of care in advanced stage disease. Eight cycles of R-CHOP 21 has not been compared with 6 cycles of R-CHOP 21, 6 cycles is recommended in most patients (NCCN guidelines).

An attempt to intensify R-CHOP-21 by giving it every 14 days in a dose dense manner has been tried in several trials. The first trial by Cunningham et al. assigned 1080 patients to R-CHOP 21 × 8 or R-CHOP 14 × 6 along with two more infusions of rituximab along with G-CSF support. There was no significant improvement in OS and PFS [67]. Another study, LNH03-6B also showed no difference in EFS in elderly patients treated with R-CHOP-14. R-CHOP-21 has thus remained the standard of care.

Maintenance Rituximab has shown some benefit in some subtypes of lymphoma. This was tested in ECOG intergroup 4494 study comparing CHOP vs. R-CHOP in elderly patients. Patient who had a CR had a second randomization to maintenance rituximab every 6 months for 2 years vs. no maintenance. There was no difference in OS or PFS. The maintenance was only useful in patients who did not receive it during induction. Based on these results, there is no role for maintenance Rituximab in DLBCL therapy [68].

7.3. Role of transplant

High-dose therapy with autologous stem cell rescue (HDT/ASCR) has shown significant improvement in OS and PFS in pre-rituximab era [69, 70]. However in the era of chemo-immunotherapy with addition of rituximab to chemotherapy, the indication for HDT/ASCR has significantly become limited with many studies showing no statistical significant advantage of proceeding to transplant in first remission except may be in patients with high risk score [71, 72].

7.4. Treatment in the elderly

Conventionally, very elderly patients are not considered candidates for aggressive therapy for various reasons. This population is not represented well in the clinical trials that form the basis for standard treatment. To address this issue GELA study group undertook a phase II study where 149 patients age 80 years and above were administered reduced dose CHOP with conventional dose rituximab (so-called R-mini-CHOP). The extended follow up from this study revealed 4-year OS and PFS rates of 49 and 41% with neutropenia being most frequent

Initial evaluation

History

- Demographics including age and gender
- Clinical including fever (>38.3°C or 101°F), night sweats, significant weight loss (>10% in 6 months) of unknown etiology and swelling.
- Assessment of comorbidities which could affect the lymphoma management and outcome.

Physical examination

- Specifically assessment of nodal regions and size of spleen and liver. CT imaging is more accurate for organomegaly.

Diagnosis

- FNAC is inadequate for initial diagnosis. Incisional and excisional biopsy is the standard if feasible core needle biopsy is acceptable if excisional biopsy cannot be done.
- Morphology, IHC and flow cytometry in most of the cases and molecular studies in selected cases.
- Additional tissue or cell suspension should be preserved for future research.

Staging

- PET-CT is the preferred imaging modality over CT scan wherever available. Chest X-ray is not required.
- CECT should be included in selected cases for more precise measurement of lymph nodes, to distinguish bowel from lymph nodes, in cases with compression or thrombosis of mediastinal or central vessels and for planning of radiation.
- If CT is used for imaging, up to 6 of the largest lymph node masses or other lesions should be measured (largest diameter LDi] and smallest diameter) as marker of disease burden. It should include mediastinal and retroperitoneal regions, if affected. Significant lesions are lymph node with LDi > 1.5 cm and extranodal masses with LDi >1 cm
- Instead of classical, modified Ann Arbor staging is used in which bulky stage II is a separate stage.

Bulky disease

- Exact size for bulky tumor is not clear for DLBCL. 6–10 cm is reported as bulky in various studies in the rituximab era.

Splenic involvement-

- The exact cut off is affected by ethnicity, body size and height. No consensus. More than 10–12 cm has been used in various studies. Current recommendations are >13 cm.
- Normal size does not rule out lymphomatous involvement. PET-CT is the best modality which could show homogenous splenomegaly, diffuse infiltration, miliary lesions, nodular or solitary mass.

Hepatic involvement

- Size is not a reliable marker of lymphomatous involvement. Presence of focal or diffuse uptake, with/without focal or disseminated nodules support involvement.

Bone marrow involvement

- Routine bone marrow biopsy is not required in DLBCL.
- Involvement of BM on DLBCL is sufficient to label advanced stage disease. In patients with negative PET
- CT, BM may be required to r/o simultaneous presence of other histologies or when malignant transformation is suspected.

Response assessment

- Should be done with PET-CT wherever available.
- 5-point scale should be used both for interim analysis (for early treatment response) and end of treatment assessment (to establish the remission).
- Score of 1 (no uptake) and 2 (uptake < mediastinum) = complete metabolic response at interim or end of treatment
- Score of 3 (uptake > mediastinum but < liver) = good response in real practice but in clinical trials should be considered as inadequate response.
- Score of 4 (uptake moderately > liver) and 5 (uptake markedly > liver) = in interim analysis, if uptake is decreased from baseline, is considered as chemosensitive disease. However, if it persists till end of treatment, it is considered as treatment failure. New foci of lymphoma at any time is also considered treatment failure.

	• In Waldeyer's ring uptake may be more than mediastinum with complete response but should not be higher than the uptake in surrounding normal tissues.
Follow up evaluation	
	• Every 3 months for first 2 years, then every 6 months for 3 years followed by annually afterwards. • Physical assessment and lab investigations including CBC, metabolic panel and LDH should be checked. • No role of imaging and it should be discouraged.

Table 4. Summary of updated recommendations for the initial evaluation, staging, response assessment and follow up evaluation of patients with DLBCL as suggested in Lugano classification.

high grade toxicity [73]. Comprehensive geriatric assessment may help in identifying patients suitable for chemotherapy [74].

7.5. Supportive care

Supportive care is imperative to mitigate the toxic effects of the chemotherapy. Care must be taken during initial cycles of chemotherapy and patients should have prophylactic allopurinol to prevent tumor lysis syndrome with highly effective regimens used currently. Patients should be screened for and appropriately treated for underlying hepatitis B infection if rituximab use is contemplated [75].

7.6. Assessment of therapeutic response

Assessment of response to therapy is accomplished by PET scans. Interim PET scans after 2 cycles may have prognostic significance. In a study 2-year PFS and OS were shown to be significantly better for the patients with PET negative disease after 2 cycles of therapy than those with positive scans [69]. Interpretation of PET scans should be done according to 5-point scoring system—Deauville criteria [76]. As per Deauville criteria score of 1, 2 or 3 with or without residual mass is considered a complete response, while a score of 4 or 5 with reduced uptake from baseline, represents responding disease when PET-CT is performed in the interim or residual disease if the PET-CT is performed at the end of the treatment. A score of 4 or 5 with no significant change in FDG uptake from baseline at interim or end of treatment is regarded as no response or stable disease. New lesions or a score of 4 and 5 with increase in intensity of uptake from baseline at interim or end of treatment, signify disease progression [77]. There is not enough evidence that this can be used to change the therapy when performed in the interim. Re-biopsy should be performed if contemplating change of therapy due to positive scans, since false positive scans may be encountered [78]. Additional imaging with MRI or biopsy is also recommended when bone marrow only findings are evident on PET-CT.

7.7. Surveillance and follow up

Routine imaging in patients after complete remission (CR) without any symptoms can safely be deterred, in a study by Guppy et al. only 6% relapses were noted in asymptomatic patients as against 86% in those who had symptoms [79]. However, imaging can also pick up changes early on when disease recurs. Although imaging can diagnose recurrence earlier, it has not been shown to alter the outcomes. The current work up and follow up recommendations for DLBCL are summarized in **Table 4**.

7.8. CNS prophylaxis

The rate of secondary CNS involvement is 3–5% but it is much higher with certain risk factors. Risk factors for CNS involvement include [80] elevated LDH, >1 extranodal site, involvement of testis, renal, breast, epidural space or adrenal gland, high CNS-IPI or MYC + BCL2/BCL6 gene rearrangement. Patients with 3 or more of these risk factors have a risk of CNS recurrence of as high as 25%. Prognosis is very poor with CNS recurrence and death is inevitable with median overall survival of 2–5 months. Hence patients at high risk of CNS recurrence should be considered for intrathecal chemotherapy with methotrexate or ara-C or high-dose IV methotrexate with leucovorin rescue. The intrathecal chemotherapy can be incorporated once in each cycle; alternatively, IV high-dose methotrexate can be given on Day 15 of 21-day R-CHOP. CNS prophylaxis has been reviewed elsewhere in detail [81].

8. Therapy of relapsed refractory DLBCL

Patients with relapsed/refractory disease have traditionally been treated with HDT/ASCR as per PARMA trial in the pre-rituximab era [82]. However, many chemotherapy regimen combinations with rituximab have since been shown to be active. For instance, R-ICE (rituximab, ifosfamide, carboplatin and etoposide) when given in out-patient setting has shown ORR of 71% with an estimated 1-year EFS rate and OS rate of 60 and 72%, respectively [83]. More recently lenalidomide monotherapy in a phase II trial in patients not eligible for transplant, showed improvement in RR, PFS and OS in non-GCB subtype DLBCL [84]. Brentuximab vedotin, a CD30-directed antibody-drug conjugate has shown ORR of 44% (CR17%) in a planned subset analysis in a phase II study [85]. Bruton's tyrosine kinase (BTK) inhibitor ibrutinib is proposed to be active in DLBCL and is being tried in combination with R-ICE in relapsed patients [86] (clinical trials.gov-NCT02955628).

8.1. Novel therapies and future directions

Many novel targeted agents are under trial and have been reviewed elsewhere [5]. A brief description of novel immune and cellular therapies has been presented below and in **Table 5**. Some novel therapeutic strategies being tested in double-hit lymphoma include the BCL2 inhibitor, PI3K inhibitor and mTOR inhibitor. The INKa/ARF deletion cause genomic instability. Constitutive activation of NFkB is being targeted in several trials of proteasome inhibitors, immunomodulatory agents, and B cell receptor signaling pathway inhibitors.

Drug	MOA (target)	Eligibility (and design)	Phase	Subjects (N)	Results
Chemotherapeutic agents					
Pixantrone [95]	Aza-anthracenedione	Ist line CHOP-R vs. CPOP-R	II	N = 124	ORR 82% for the CPOP-R arm vs. 90% for the CHOP-R arm, and median PFS not reached in the CPOP-R arm and was 40 months in the CHOP-R arm; median OS not reached in either arm. OS inferior for CPOP-R (hazard ratio 2.37, p = 0.029), with more deaths occurring in the CPOP-R arm (30% vs. 14%)
Liposomal vincristine [96]	Chemotherapy	Refractory/relapsed	II	N = 60	ORR: 95%; (CR/CRu: 92%, PR: 3%) 5 years OS 87% and PFS 81%
Monoclonal antibodies					
Obintuzumab Plus Lenalidomide plus CHOP [97]	Anti-CD 20	Refractory/relapsed	I	N = 6	CR 100%; neutropenia (grade 3: 50%, grade 4: 33%), thrombocytopenia (grade 3: 17%), and Rash (grade 2: 17%).
Veltuzumab plus Milatuzumab [98]	Anti-CD20 plus anti-CD74	Heavily pretreated NHL	II	N = 7	PD in all DLBCL: 100%
Blinatumomab [99]	Single chain bispecific T cell engaging antibody anti-CD19 and anti-CD3 mAb	Refractory/relapsed	II	N = 25 stepwise (9–28–112 μg/d with weekly dose increases; n = 23) or flat (112 μg/d; n = 2)	ORR 43%, CR 19%. Three patients had late CR in follow up without other treatment
Antibody drugs conjugates					
I-131 tositumomab [100]	Anti-CD20 radio-immunotherapy	Previously untreated DLBCL (with R-CHOP)		15	CR rate increased from 60% post-CHOP to 80% post TST/I-131 TST. At 120.0 months, median DOR was 58.4 months. PFS and time to treatment failure were 63.0 months. OS was not reached. Grade 3/4 hematologic adverse events were decreased absolute neutrophil count (47%), white blood cell count (40%), platelet count (27%), and hemoglobin (20%)
		Consolidation therapy after first line R-CHOP	II	71	2 year event-free survival was 75%; grade 3–4

Drug	MOA (target)	Eligibility (and design)	Phase	Subjects (N)	Results
^{90}Y-epratuzumab tetraxetan [101]	Radiolabeled humanized anti-CD22 mAb	in DLBCL in untreated patients aged 60–80 years			thrombocytopenia in 84% and neutropenia in 79%
Brentuximab vedotin (SGN-35) [102]	Antitubulin monomethyl auristatin E (MMAE) anti-CD30 mAb conjugate	Refractory/relapsed	II	49 DLBCL	ORR 49% for DLBCL, including 17% CR with a DOR of 16.6 months
Immunomodulatory agents					
Lenalidomide [103]	Immunomodulator	Lenalidomide as maintenance therapy vs. placebo in elderly patients with DLBCL who achieved a complete response (CR) or partial response (PR) to R-CHOP induction	III	650	At 39 months median PFS was not reached for lenalidomide maintenance vs. 58.9 months for placebo. At 52 months OS was similar between the two arms. Most common grade 3 or 4 adverse events associated with lenalidomide vs. placebo maintenance were neutropenia (56 vs. 22%) and cutaneous reactions (5 vs. 1%), respectively
Targeted therapies					
Bortezomib [104]	Proteasome inhibitor	Previously untreated non-GCB DLBCL (R-CHOP vs. VR-CHOP)	II	206	PFS 25% with R-CHOP and 18% with VR-CHOP. 2-year PFS rates were 77.6% with R-CHOP and 82.0% with VR-CHOP; ORR with R-CHOP and VR-CHOP was 98% and 96%, respectively. 2-year OS was 88.4 and 93.0%
Panobinostat [105]	Deacetylase inhibitor	Refractory/relapsed	II	40	28% response. DOR 14.5 months. MEF2B positive were significantly associated with response
Immune checkpoint inhibitors					
Ipilimumab [106]	CTLA-4 inhibitor	Refractory/relapsed	I	18	2 patients had clinical responses, 1 CR at 31+ months
Nivolumab [93]	PD-1 inhibitor	Refractory/relapsed	I	11	ORRs 36% (CR, 18%; PR, 18%)
Pembrolizumab [107]	PD-L1 inhibitor	PMBCL	Ib	19	ORR 41% (12% CR and 29% PR). 35% SD. DOR not reached

Drug	MOA (target)	Eligibility (and design)	Phase	Subjects (N)	Results
Kinase inhibitors					
Fostamatinib [108]	Spleen oral tyrosine kinase (Syk) inhibitor	Refractory/relapsed	II	68	The most common treatment-related adverse events of all patients were diarrhea (21% total, 6% grade 3/4), nausea (19% total, 3% grade 3/4), and, fatigue (18% total, 9% grade 3/4). The ORR rate was 3% across both arms and clinical benefit (≥stable disease) was achieved for 13% of all patients
Enzastaurin [109]	Protein kinase beta inhibitor	For maintenance among high risk patients after CR to first line therapy	III	758	At 48 months, DFS hazard ratio for Enzastaurin vs. placebo was 70 vs. 71%, respectively

Table 5. Novel therapies undergoing clinical trials for the treatment of DLBCL.

8.2. CAR T cells

Chimeric antigen receptor (CAR) confers antigen specificity to T cells for antigens expressed by lymphoma cells in a non-MHC restricted fashion. The typical CAR T cell in clinical practice has an antigen binding pocket or single chain variable fragment (scFv) derived from an immunoglobulin molecule and a spacer or a hinge region and a range of different co-stimulatory molecules (CD 28, OX 40, 4-1BB). CD19 is expressed during all stages of B cell differentiation and is absent in any other cell types. Kochenderfer et al. reported the initial results on 15 patients with advanced B cell malignancies of which 8 achieved complete remissions (CR), 4 achieved partial remissions (PR) [87]. Some of the patients had a durable response. This led to the single arm, phase II JULIET study of CTL09 in adult patients with relapsed or refractory DLBCL. The overall response rate (ORR) was 45 with 37% achieved a complete response, and 80% achieving a partial response (PR), respectively [88]. This overall response rate was impressive in this heavily pretreated population. 57% of all treated patients experienced cytokine release syndrome (CRS) and 26% experienced grade 3, 4 CRS. The CAR T cell therapy received FDA breakthrough designation for treatment for relapsed refractory lymphoma in the United States based on the interim results of the JULIET trial. United States FDA finally approved axicabtagene ciloleucel for DLBCL following 2 prior therapies based on phase II Zuma-1 study [89] that showed 82% ORR and 54% CR rate. Development of the CAR T cells takes time and that becomes a limitation of this therapy in patients with rapidly progressive disease. Also cytokine release syndrome (CRS) and neurotoxicity (grade 3 or more CRS in Zuma-1 in 13% and neurotoxicity in 28% patients) can be life threatening and requires considerable expertise and critical care support which may be a limitation to the wide use of CAR T cells in the community hospital setting [90]. The use of humanized anti IL-6 receptor antibody tocilizumab have been successfully used to manage these toxicities. Pretreating these patients with lymphotoxic agents such as cyclophosphamide or fludarabine is helpful for the survival of the infused T cells. Targeting of normal B cells results in B cell aplasia which may require intermittent infusion of immunoglobulin as prophylaxis from infectious complications. Upregulation of PD-1 expression has been shown among responders to CD19 CAR T cells. This may be vital in developing further strategies including combination therapies [91].

8.3. Immune checkpoint inhibitors

Checkpoint proteins such as PD-1 on T cells and PD-L1 on tumor cells help keep immune responses in check. The binding of PD-L1 to PD 1 keeps T cells from killing tumor cells in the body. Blocking the binding of PD-L1 to PD-1 with an immune checkpoint inhibitor allows T cell to kill tumor cells. PD L-1 expression has been variable in different subsets of lymphomas. PD-L1 expression in follicular lymphomas is seen but the role in DLBCL is not that clear [92]. Lesokhin et al. did a phase 1b study of Nivolumab every 2 weeks in patients with relapsed refractory B cell, T cell, Multiple myeloma patients. 11 patients had DLBCL. ORR were 36% in the DLBCL patients [93]. Genetic alterations in 9p24.1 are known to upregulate PD-L1 and PD-L2 expression. This is seen in Hodgkin's lymphoma and also in patients with primary mediastinal B cell lymphoma. This was studied in a phase 1b trial of pembrolizumab in relapsed refractory primary mediastinal B cell lymphoma. ORR of 41% was seen among the 18 patients enrolled with 35% of patients had stable disease [94]. Patients with EBV-associated DLBCL and T cell rich B cell lymphomas express high levels of PD-L1 and warrant further studies with checkpoint inhibitors.

Author details

Vivek Kumar[1*†], Sarvadaman Makardhwaj Shrivastava[2†], Trishala Meghal[2†] and Binod Abhinav Chandra[3†]

*Address all correspondence to: 77.viveck@gmail.com

1 Brigham and Women's Hospital, Harvard Medical School, Boston, MA, USA

2 Maimonides Cancer Center, Brooklyn, New York, USA

3 Yuma Regional Medical Center, Cancer Center, Yuma, AZ, USA

† These authors contributed equally

References

[1] Morton LM, Wang SS, Devesa SS, Hartge P, Weisenburger DD, Linet MS. Lymphoma incidence patterns by WHO subtype in the United States, 1992–2001. Blood. 2005;**107**(1): 265-276

[2] Non-Hodgkin Lymphoma— Cancer Stat Facts. 2017. Available from: https://seer.cancer.gov/statfacts/html/nhl.html

[3] Leeksma OC, de Miranda NF, Veelken H. Germline mutations predisposing to diffuse large B-cell lymphoma. Blood Cancer Journal. 2017;**7**(3):e541

[4] Alizadeh AA, Elsen MB, Davis RE, Ma C. Distinct types of diffuse large B-cell lymphoma identified by gene expression profiling. Nature. 2000;**403**(6769):503

[5] Sehn LH, Gascoyne RD. Diffuse large B-cell lymphoma: Optimizing outcome in the context of clinical and biologic heterogeneity. Blood. 2015;**125**(1):22-32

[6] Scott DW, Mottok A, Ennishi D, Wright GW, Farinha P, Ben-Neriah S, et al. Prognostic significance of diffuse large B-cell lymphoma cell of origin determined by digital gene expression in formalin-fixed paraffin-embedded tissue biopsies. Journal of Clinical Oncology. 2015;**33**(26):2848-2856

[7] Rosenwald A, Wright G, Chan WC, Connors JM, Campo E, Fisher RI, et al. The use of molecular profiling to predict survival after chemotherapy for diffuse large-B-cell lymphoma. New England Journal of Medicine. 2002;**346**(25):1937-1947

[8] Swerdlow SH, Campo E, Pileri SA, Harris NL, Stein H, Siebert R, et al. The 2016 revision of the World Health Organization classification of lymphoid neoplasms. Blood. 2016; **127**(20):2375-2390

[9] Adams J, Harris A, Pinkert C, Corcoran L, Alexander W, Cory S, et al. The c-myc oncogene driven by immunoglobulin enhancers induces lymphoid malignancy in transgenic mice. Nature. 1985;**318**(6046):533-538

[10] Johnson NA, Slack GW, Savage KJ, Connors JM, Ben-Neriah S, Rogic S, et al. Concurrent expression of MYC and BCL2 in diffuse large B-cell lymphoma treated with rituximab plus cyclophosphamide, doxorubicin, vincristine, and prednisone. Journal of Clinical Oncology. 2012;**30**(28):3452-3459

[11] Green TM, Young KH, Visco C, Xu-Monette ZY, Orazi A, Go RS, et al. Immunohistochemical double-hit score is a strong predictor of outcome in patients with diffuse large B-cell lymphoma treated with rituximab plus cyclophosphamide, doxorubicin, vincristine, and prednisone. Journal of Clinical Oncology. 2012;**30**(28):3460-3467

[12] Achten R, Verhoef G, Vanuytsel L, De Wolf-Peeters C. T-cell/histiocyte–rich large B-cell lymphoma: A distinct clinicopathologic entity. Journal of Clinical Oncology. 2002;**20**(5): 1269-1277

[13] Bouabdallah R, Mounier N, Guettier C, Molina T, Ribrag V, Thieblemont C, et al. T-cell/histiocyte-rich large B-cell lymphomas and classical diffuse large B-cell lymphomas have similar outcome after chemotherapy: A matched-control analysis. Journal of Clinical Oncology. 2003;**21**(7):1271-1277

[14] S-I N, Yao M, Hoshida Y, Yamamoto S, Iuchi K, Aozasa K. Pyothorax-associated lymphoma: A review of 106 cases. Journal of Clinical Oncology. 2002;**20**(20):4255-4260

[15] Colby TV. Current histological diagnosis of lymphomatoid granulomatosis. Modern Pathology. 2012;**25**(S1):S39

[16] Katzenstein ALA, Carrington CB, Liebow AA. Lymphomatoid granulomatosis. A clinicopathologic study of 152 cases. Cancer. 1979;**43**(1):360-373

[17] Nicolae A, Pittaluga S, Abdullah S, Steinberg SM, Pham TA, Davies-Hill T, et al. EBV-positive large B-cell lymphomas in young patients: A nodal lymphoma with evidence for a tolerogenic immune environment. Blood. 2015;**126**(7):863-872

[18] Hong J, Yoon D, Suh C, Huh J, Do I-G, Sohn I, et al. EBV-positive diffuse large B-cell lymphoma in young adults: Is this a distinct disease entity? Annals of Oncology. 2014; **26**(3):548-555

[19] Dojcinov SD, Venkataraman G, Pittaluga S, Wlodarska I, Schrager JA, Raffeld M, et al. Age-related EBV-associated lymphoproliferative disorders in the Western population: A spectrum of reactive lymphoid hyperplasia and lymphoma. Blood. 2011;**117**(18):4726-4735

[20] Castillo JJ, Beltran BE, Miranda RN, Paydas S, Winer ES, Butera JN. Epstein-Barr virus–positive diffuse large B-cell lymphoma of the elderly: What we know so far. The Oncologist. 2011;**16**(1):87-96

[21] Adam P, Bonzheim I, Fend F, Quintanilla-Martínez L. Epstein-Barr virus-positive diffuse large B-cell lymphomas of the elderly. Advances in Anatomic Pathology. 2011;**18**(5):349-355

[22] Said J. The expanding spectrum of EBV+ lymphomas. Blood. 2015;**126**(7):827-828

[23] Hart M, Thakral B, Yohe S, Balfour HH Jr, Singh C, Spears M, et al. EBV-positive mucocutaneous ulcer in organ transplant recipients: A localized indolent posttransplant lymphoproliferative disorder. The American Journal of Surgical Pathology. 2014;**38**(11):1522-1529

[24] Dojcinov SD, Venkataraman G, Raffeld M, Pittaluga S, Jaffe ES. EBV positive mucocutaneous ulcer—A study of 26 cases associated with various sources of immunosuppression. The American Journal of Surgical Pathology. 2010;**34**(3):405-417

[25] Choi WW, Weisenburger DD, Greiner TC, Piris MA, Banham AH, Delabie J, et al. A new immunostain algorithm classifies diffuse large B-cell lymphoma into molecular subtypes with high accuracy. Clinical Cancer Research. 2009;**15**(17):5494-5502

[26] O'Malley DP, Auerbach A, Weiss LM. Practical applications in immunohistochemistry: Evaluation of diffuse large B-cell lymphoma and related large B-cell lymphomas. Archives of Pathology and Laboratory Medicine. 2015;**139**(9):1094-1107

[27] Barton S, Hawkes EA, Wotherspoon A, Cunningham D. Are we ready to stratify treatment for diffuse large B-cell lymphoma using molecular hallmarks? The Oncologist. 2012;**17**(12):1562-1573

[28] Veldman-Jones MH, Brant R, Rooney C, Geh C, Emery H, Harbron CG, et al. Evaluating robustness and sensitivity of the NanoString technologies nCounter platform to enable multiplexed gene expression analysis of clinical samples. Cancer Research. 2015;**75**(13):2587-2593

[29] Wright G, Tan B, Rosenwald A, Hurt EH, Wiestner A, Staudt LM. A gene expression-based method to diagnose clinically distinct subgroups of diffuse large B cell lymphoma. Proceedings of the National Academy of Sciences. 2003;**100**(17):9991-9996

[30] Hans CP, Weisenburger DD, Greiner TC, Gascoyne RD, Delabie J, Ott G, et al. Confirmation of the molecular classification of diffuse large B-cell lymphoma by immunohistochemistry using a tissue microarray. Blood. 2004;**103**(1):275-282

[31] Rimsza LM, Wright G, Schwartz M, Chan WC, Jaffe ES, Gascoyne RD, et al. Accurate classification of diffuse large B-cell lymphoma into germinal center and activated B-cell subtypes using a nuclease protection assay on formalin-fixed, paraffin-embedded tissues. Clinical Cancer Research. 2011;**17**(11):3727-3732

[32] Meyer PN, Fu K, Greiner TC, Smith LM, Delabie J, Gascoyne RD, et al. Immunohistochemical methods for predicting cell of origin and survival in patients with diffuse large B-cell lymphoma treated with rituximab. Journal of Clinical Oncology. 2010;**29**(2): 200-207

[33] Hill BT, Collie AM, Radivoyevitch T, Hsi ED, Sweetenham J. Cell of origin determination in diffuse large b-cell lymphoma: Performance of immunohistochemical (IHC) algorithms and ability to predict outcome. Blood. 2011;**118**(21):950

[34] Muris J, Meijer C, Vos W, van Krieken J, Jiwa N, Ossenkoppele G, et al. Immunohistochemical profiling based on Bcl-2, CD10 and MUM1 expression improves risk stratification in patients with primary nodal diffuse large B cell lymphoma. The Journal of Pathology. 2006; **208**(5):714-723

[35] Natkunam Y, Farinha P, Hsi ED, Hans CP, Tibshirani R, Sehn LH, et al. LMO2 protein expression predicts survival in patients with diffuse large B-cell lymphoma treated with anthracycline-based chemotherapy with and without rituximab. Journal of Clinical Oncology. 2008;**26**(3):447-454

[36] Nyman H, Adde M, Karjalainen-Lindsberg M-L, Taskinen M, Berglund M, Amini R-M, et al. Prognostic impact of immunohistochemically defined germinal center phenotype in diffuse large B-cell lymphoma patients treated with immunochemotherapy. Blood. 2007; **109**(11):4930-4935

[37] Gleeson M, Hawkes EA, Cunningham D, Jack A, Linch D. Caution in the use of immunohistochemistry for determination of cell of origin in diffuse large B-cell lymphoma. Journal of Clinical Oncology. 2015;**33**(28):3215-3216

[38] Scott DW, Wright GW, Williams PM, Lih C-J, Walsh W, Jaffe ES, et al. Determining cell-of-origin subtypes of diffuse large B-cell lymphoma using gene expression in formalin-fixed paraffin-embedded tissue. Blood. 2014;**123**(8):1214-1217

[39] Lenz G, Wright G, Dave S, Xiao W, Powell J, Zhao H, et al. Stromal gene signatures in large-B-cell lymphomas. New England Journal of Medicine. 2008;**359**(22):2313-2323

[40] Reis PP, Waldron L, Goswami RS, Xu W, Xuan Y, Perez-Ordonez B, et al. mRNA transcript quantification in archival samples using multiplexed, color-coded probes. BMC Biotechnology. 2011;**11**(1):46

[41] Yoon N, Ahn S, Yoo HY, Kim SJ, Kim WS, Ko YH. Cell-of-origin of diffuse large B-cell lymphomas determined by the Lymph2Cx assay: Better prognostic indicator than Hans algorithm. Oncotarget. 2017;**8**(13):22014

[42] Moller MB, Pedersen NT, Christensen BE. Diffuse large B-cell lymphoma: Clinical implications of extranodal versus nodal presentation—A population-based study of 1575 cases. British Journal of Haematology. 2004;**124**(2):151-159

[43] Armitage JO, Weisenburger DD. New approach to classifying non-Hodgkin's lymphomas: Clinical features of the major histologic subtypes. Non-Hodgkin's Lymphoma Classification Project. Journal of Clinical Oncology. 1998;**16**(8):2780-2795

[44] Lopez-Guillermo A, Colomo L, Jimenez M, Bosch F, Villamor N, Arenillas L, et al. Diffuse large B-cell lymphoma: Clinical and biological characterization and outcome according to the nodal or extranodal primary origin. Journal of Clinical Oncology. 2005; **23**(12):2797-2804

[45] Talaulikar D, Dahlstrom JE. Staging bone marrow in diffuse large B-cell lymphoma: The role of ancillary investigations. Pathology. 2009;**41**(3):214-222

[46] Alvarez R, Dupuis J, Plonquet A, Christov C, Copie-Bergman C, Hemery F, et al. Clinical relevance of flow cytometric immunophenotyping of the cerebrospinal fluid in patients with diffuse large B-cell lymphoma. Annals of Oncology: Official Journal of the European Society for Medical Oncology. 2012;**23**(5):1274-1279

[47] Ott G, Rosenwald A, Campo E. Understanding MYC-driven aggressive B-cell lymphomas: Pathogenesis and classification. Blood. 2013;**122**(24):3884-3891

[48] Cuccuini W, Briere J, Mounier N, Voelker HU, Rosenwald A, Sundstrom C, et al. MYC+ diffuse large B-cell lymphoma is not salvaged by classical R-ICE or R-DHAP followed by BEAM plus autologous stem cell transplantation. Blood. 2012;**119**(20):4619-4624

[49] Horn H, Ziepert M, Becher C, Barth TF, Bernd HW, Feller AC, et al. MYC status in concert with BCL2 and BCL6 expression predicts outcome in diffuse large B-cell lymphoma. Blood. 2013;**121**(12):2253-2263

[50] Thieblemont C, Briere J. MYC, BCL2, BCL6 in DLBCL: Impact for clinics in the future? Blood. 2013;**121**(12):2165-2166

[51] Adams HJ, Kwee TC, de Keizer B, Fijnheer R, de Klerk JM, Nievelstein RA. FDG PET/CT for the detection of bone marrow involvement in diffuse large B-cell lymphoma: Systematic review and meta-analysis. European Journal of Nuclear Medicine and Molecular Imaging. 2014;**41**(3):565-574

[52] Lim S, Tao M, Cheung Y, Rajan S, Mann B. Can patients with early-stage diffuse large B-cell lymphoma be treated without bone marrow biopsy? Annals of Oncology. 2005;**16**(2): 215-218

[53] Shah HJ, Keraliya AR, Jagannathan JP, Tirumani SH, Lele VR, DiPiro PJ. Diffuse large B-cell lymphoma in the era of precision oncology: How imaging is helpful. Korean Journal of Radiology. 2017;**18**(1):54-70

[54] Lister T, Crowther D, Sutcliffe S, Glatstein E, Canellos G, Young R, et al. Report of a committee convened to discuss the evaluation and staging of patients with Hodgkin's disease: Cotswolds meeting. Journal of Clinical Oncology. 1989;**7**(11):1630-1636

[55] Cheson BD, Fisher RI, Barrington SF, Cavalli F, Schwartz LH, Zucca E, et al. Recommendations for initial evaluation, staging, and response assessment of Hodgkin and non-Hodgkin lymphoma: The Lugano classification. Journal of Clinical Oncology. 2014; **32**(27):3059-3067

[56] Berthet L, Cochet A, Kanoun S, Berriolo-Riedinger A, Humbert O, Toubeau M, et al. In newly diagnosed diffuse large B-cell lymphoma, determination of bone marrow involvement with 18F-FDG PET/CT provides better diagnostic performance and prognostic stratification than does biopsy. Journal of Nuclear Medicine. 2013;**54**(8):1244-1250

[57] Zhang X, Fan W, Xia ZJ, Hu YY, Lin XP, Zhang YR, et al. Use of subsequent PET/CT in diffuse large B-cell lymphoma patients in complete remission following primary therapy. Chinese Journal of Cancer. 2015;**34**(2):70-78

[58] Shipp M, Harrington D, Anderson J, Armitage J, Bonadonna G, Brittinger G, et al. A predictive model for aggressive non-Hodgkin's lymphoma. New England Journal of Medicine. 1993;**329**(14):987-994

[59] Zhou Z, Sehn LH, Rademaker AW, Gordon LI, LaCasce AS, Crosby-Thompson A, et al. An enhanced International Prognostic Index (NCCN-IPI) for patients with diffuse large B-cell lymphoma treated in the rituximab era. Blood. 2014;**123**(6):837-842

[60] Dunleavy K, Wilson WH. Primary mediastinal B-cell lymphoma and mediastinal gray zone lymphoma: Do they require a unique therapeutic approach? Blood. 2015;**125**(1):33-39

[61] Miller TP, Jones SE. Initial chemotherapy for clinically localized lymphomas of unfavorable histology. Blood. 1983;**62**(2):413-418

[62] Pfreundschuh M, Trumper L, Osterborg A, Pettengell R, Trneny M, Imrie K, et al. CHOP-like chemotherapy plus rituximab versus CHOP-like chemotherapy alone in young patients with good-prognosis diffuse large-B-cell lymphoma: A randomised controlled trial by the MabThera International Trial (MInT) Group. The Lancet Oncology. 2006;**7**(5): 379-391

[63] Persky DO, Unger JM, Spier CM, Stea B, LeBlanc M, McCarty MJ, et al. Phase II study of rituximab plus three cycles of CHOP and involved-field radiotherapy for patients with

limited-stage aggressive B-cell lymphoma: Southwest Oncology Group study 0014. Journal of Clinical Oncology. 2008;**26**(14):2258-2263

[64] Coltman C, Dahlberg S, Jones SE, Miller TP, Dana BW, Weick JK, et al. Southwest Oncology Group Studies in Diffuse Large Cell Lymphoma: A Subset Analysis. Cancer Chemotherapy: Challenges for the Future. Tokyo, Japan: Excerpta Medica; 1988. pp. 194-202

[65] Fisher RI, Gaynor ER, Dahlberg S, Oken MM, Grogan TM, Mize EM, et al. Comparison of a standard regimen (CHOP) with three intensive chemotherapy regimens for advanced non-Hodgkin's lymphoma. New England Journal of Medicine. 1993;**328**(14):1002-1006

[66] Coiffier B, Lepage E, Brière J, Herbrecht R, Tilly H, Bouabdallah R, et al. CHOP chemotherapy plus rituximab compared with CHOP alone in elderly patients with diffuse large-B-cell lymphoma. New England Journal of Medicine. 2002;**346**(4):235-242

[67] Cunningham D, Hawkes EA, Jack A, Qian W, Smith P, Mouncey P, et al. Rituximab plus cyclophosphamide, doxorubicin, vincristine, and prednisolone in patients with newly diagnosed diffuse large B-cell non-Hodgkin lymphoma: A phase 3 comparison of dose intensification with 14-day versus 21-day cycles. Lancet. 2013;**381**(9880):1817-1826

[68] Habermann TM, Weller EA, Morrison VA, Gascoyne RD, Cassileth PA, Cohn JB, et al. Rituximab-CHOP versus CHOP alone or with maintenance rituximab in older patients with diffuse large B-cell lymphoma. Journal of Clinical Oncology. 2006;**24**(19):3121-3127

[69] Haioun C, Itti E, Rahmouni A, Brice P, Rain JD, Belhadj K, et al. [18F]fluoro-2-deoxy-D-glucose positron emission tomography (FDG-PET) in aggressive lymphoma: An early prognostic tool for predicting patient outcome. Blood. 2005;**106**(4):1376-1381

[70] Haioun C, Lepage E, Gisselbrecht C, Salles G, Coiffier B, Brice P, et al. Survival benefit of high-dose therapy in poor-risk aggressive non-Hodgkin's lymphoma: Final analysis of the prospective LNH87–2 protocol—A groupe d'Etude des lymphomes de l'Adulte study. Journal of Clinical Oncology. 2000;**18**(16):3025-3030

[71] Vitolo U, Chiappella A, Brusamolino E, Angelucci E, Rossi G, Carella AM, et al. Rituximab dose-dense chemotherapy followed by intensified high-dose chemotherapy and autologous stem cell transplantation (HDC+ ASCT) significantly reduces the risk of progression compared to standard rituximab dose-dense chemotherapy as first line treatment in young patients with high-risk (aa-IPI 2–3) diffuse large B-cell lymphoma (DLBCL): Final results of phase III randomized trial DLCL04 of the Fondazione Italiana Linfomi (FIL). Blood. 2012;**120**(21):688

[72] Le Gouill S, Milpied N, Lamy T, Delwail V, Gressin R, Guyotat D, et al. First-line rituximab (R) high-dose therapy (R-HDT) versus R-CHOP14 for young adults with diffuse large B-cell lymphoma: Preliminary results of the GOELAMS 075 prospective multicenter randomized trial. Journal of Clinical Oncology. 2011;**29**(15_suppl):8003

[73] Peyrade F, Fain O, Fabiani B, Bauduer F, Van Den Neste E, Macro M, et al. Long-term follow-up of the GELA LNH 03-7B study: A prospective phase II study of 150 patients over 80 years with diffuse large B-cell lymphoma (DLBCL) treated with RminiCHOP.

Journal of Clinical Oncology. May 2013;**31**(15_suppl):8536-8536. DOI: 10.1200/jco.2013.31.15_suppl.8536

[74] Owusu C, Berger NA. Comprehensive geriatric assessment in the older cancer patient: Coming of age in clinical cancer care. Clinical Practice (London, England). 2014;**11**(6): 749-762

[75] NCCN. Clinical Practice Guidelines in Oncology. 2017. Available from: https://www.nccn.org/professionals/physician_gls/f_guidelines.asp#supportive

[76] Barrington SF, Mikhaeel NG, Kostakoglu L, Meignan M, Hutchings M, Müeller SP, et al. Role of imaging in the staging and response assessment of lymphoma: Consensus of the international conference on malignant lymphomas imaging working group. Journal of Clinical Oncology. 2014;**32**(27):3048-3058

[77] Cheson BD, Fisher RI, Barrington SF, Cavalli F, Schwartz LH, Zucca E, et al. Recommendations for initial evaluation, staging, and response assessment of Hodgkin and non-Hodgkin lymphoma: The Lugano classification. Journal of Clinical Oncology. 2014;**32**(27):3059-3068

[78] Moskowitz CH, Schoder H, Teruya-Feldstein J, Sima C, Iasonos A, Portlock CS, et al. Risk-adapted dose-dense immunochemotherapy determined by interim FDG-PET in advanced-stage diffuse large B-cell lymphoma. Journal of Clinical Oncology. 2010;**28**(11):1896-1903

[79] Guppy AE, Tebbutt NC, Norman A, Cunningham D. The role of surveillance CT scans in patients with diffuse large B-cell non-Hodgkin's lymphoma. Leukemia & lymphoma. 2003;**44**(1):123-125

[80] Penalver FJ, Sancho JM, de la Fuente A, Olave MT, Martin A, Panizo C, et al. Guidelines for diagnosis, prevention and management of central nervous system involvement in diffuse large B-cell lymphoma patients by the Spanish Lymphoma Group (GELTAMO). Haematologica. 2016;**102**(2):235-245

[81] Cheah CY, Collin KC. How I treat patients with aggressive lymphoma at high risk of CNS relapse. Blood. 2017;**130**(7):867-874

[82] Thierry P, Guglielmi C, Hagenbeek A, Somers R, Lelie HVD, Bron D, Sonneveld P, et al. Autologous bone marrow transplantation as compared with salvage chemotherapy in relapses of chemotherapy-sensitive non-Hodgkin's lymphoma. New England Journal of Medicine. 1995;**333**(23):1540-1545

[83] Vose J, Sneller V. Outpatient regimen rituximab plus ifosfamide, carboplatin and etoposide (R-ICE) for relapsed non-Hodgkin's lymphoma. Annals of Oncology: Official Journal of the European Society for Medical Oncology. 2003;**14**(Suppl 1):i17-i20

[84] Czuczman MS, Trneny M, Davies A, Rule S, Linton KM, Wagner-Johnston N, et al. A phase 2/3 multicenter, randomized, open-label study to compare the efficacy and safety of Lenalidomide versus Investigator's choice in patients with relapsed or refractory diffuse large B-cell lymphoma. Clinical Cancer Research: An Official Journal of the American Association for Cancer Research. 2017;**23**(15):4127-4137

[85] Jacobsen ED, Sharman JP, Oki Y, Advani RH, Winter JN, Bello CM, et al. Brentuximab vedotin demonstrates objective responses in a phase 2 study of relapsed/refractory DLBCL with variable CD30 expression. Blood. 2015;**125**(9):1394-1402

[86] Wilson WH, Young RM, Schmitz R, Yang Y, Pittaluga S, Wright G, et al. Targeting B cell receptor signaling with ibrutinib in diffuse large B cell lymphoma. Nature Medicine. 2015;**21**(8):922

[87] Kochenderfer JN, Wilson WH, Janik JE, Dudley ME, Stetler-Stevenson M, Feldman SA, et al. Eradication of B-lineage cells and regression of lymphoma in a patient treated with autologous T cells genetically engineered to recognize CD19. Blood. 2010;**116**(20):4099-4102

[88] Novartis interim results from global, pivotal CTL019 trial show durable complete responses in adults with r/r DLBCL | Novartis: @novartis; 2017 Available from: https://www.novartis.com/news/media-releases/novartis-interim-results-global-pivotal-ctl019-trial-show-durable-complete

[89] Neelapu SS, Locke FL, Bartlett NL, Lekakis LJ, Miklos DB, Jacobson CA, et al. Axicabtagene Ciloleucel CAR T-cell therapy in refractory large B-cell lymphoma. The New England Journal of Medicine. 2017;**377**(26):2531-2544

[90] Bonifant CL, Jackson HJ, Brentjens RJ, Curran KJ. Toxicity and management in CAR T-cell therapy. Molecular Therapy—Oncolytics. 2016;**3**:16011

[91] Lulla P, Heslop HE. Checkpoint inhibition and cellular immunotherapy in lymphoma. ASH Education Program Book. 2016;**2016**(1):390-396

[92] Chen BJ, Chapuy B, Ouyang J, Sun HH, Roemer MG, Xu ML, et al. PD-L1 expression is characteristic of a subset of aggressive B-cell lymphomas and virus-associated malignancies. Clinical Cancer Research. 2013;**19**(13):3462-3473

[93] Lesokhin AM, Ansell SM, Armand P, Scott EC, Halwani A, Gutierrez M, et al. Nivolumab in patients with relapsed or refractory hematologic malignancy: Preliminary results of a phase Ib study. Journal of Clinical Oncology. 2016;**34**(23):2698-2704

[94] Zinzani PL, Ribrag V, Moskowitz CH, Michot J-M, Kuruvilla J, Balakumaran A, et al. Safety & tolerability of pembrolizumab in patients with relapsed/refractory primary mediastinal large B-cell lymphoma. Blood. 2017;**130**:267-270. DOI: 10.1182/blood-2016-12-758383

[95] Herbrecht R, Cernohous P, Engert A, Le Gouill S, Macdonald D, Machida C, et al. Comparison of pixantrone-based regimen (CPOP-R) with doxorubicin-based therapy (CHOP-R) for treatment of diffuse large B-cell lymphoma. Annals of Oncology. 2013; **24**(10):2618-2623

[96] Hagemeister F, Rodriguez MA, Deitcher SR, Younes A, Fayad L, Goy A, et al. Long term results of a phase 2 study of vincristine sulfate liposome injection (Marqibo®) substituted for non-liposomal vincristine in cyclophosphamide, doxorubicin, vincristine, prednisone with or without rituximab for patients with untreated aggressive non-Hodgkin lymphomas. British Journal of Haematology. 2013;**162**(5):631-638

[97] Westin JR, Sathyanarayanan V, Fayad LE, Nastoupil LJ, Turturro F, Hagemeister FB, et al. Lenalidomide and obinutuzumab with CHOP for Newly Diagnosed diffuse large B-cell lymphoma: Phase I results. American Society of Hematology. 2016

[98] Christian BA, Poi M, Jones JA, Porcu P, Maddocks K, Flynn JM, et al. The combination of milatuzumab, a humanized anti-CD74 antibody, and veltuzumab, a humanized anti-CD20 antibody, demonstrates activity in patients with relapsed and refractory B-cell non-Hodgkin lymphoma. British Journal of Haematology. 2015;**169**(5):701-710

[99] Viardot A, Goebeler M-E, Hess G, Neumann S, Pfreundschuh M, Adrian N, et al. Phase 2 study of the bispecific T-cell engager (BiTE) antibody blinatumomab in relapsed/refractory diffuse large B-cell lymphoma. Blood. 2016;**127**(11):1410-1416

[100] Leonard JP, Gregory SA, Smith H, Horner TJ, Williams VC, Giampietro P, et al. CHOP chemotherapy followed by tositumomab and iodine-131 tositumomab for previously untreated diffuse large B-cell lymphoma. Clinical Lymphoma Myeloma and Leukemia. 2016;**16**(4):191-196

[101] Kraeber-Bodere F, Pallardy A, Maisonneuve H, Campion L, Moreau A, Soubeyran I, et al. Consolidation anti-CD22 fractionated radioimmunotherapy with 90 Y-epratuzumab tetraxetan following R-CHOP in elderly patients with diffuse large B-cell lymphoma: A prospective, single group, phase 2 trial. The Lancet Haematology. 2017;**4**(1):e35-e45

[102] Pro B, Advani R, Brice P, Bartlett NL, Rosenblatt JD, Illidge T, et al. Brentuximab vedotin (SGN-35) in patients with relapsed or refractory systemic anaplastic large-cell lymphoma: Results of a phase II study. Journal of Clinical Oncology. 2012;**30**(18):2190-2196

[103] Thieblemont C, Tilly H, Gomes da Silva M, Casasnovas R-O, Fruchart C, Morschhauser F, et al. Lenalidomide maintenance compared with placebo in responding elderly patients with diffuse large B-cell lymphoma treated with first-line rituximab plus cyclophosphamide, doxorubicin, vincristine, and prednisone. Journal of Clinical Oncology. 2017;**72**:6984

[104] Leonard JP, Kolibaba KS, Reeves JA, Tulpule A, Flinn IW, Kolevska T, et al. Randomized phase II study of R-CHOP with or without bortezomib in previously untreated patients with non–germinal center B-cell-like diffuse large B-cell lymphoma. Journal of Clinical Oncology. 2017;**73**:784

[105] Assouline SE, Nielsen TH, Yu S, Alcaide M, Chong L, MacDonald D, et al. Phase 2 study of panobinostat with or without rituximab in relapsed diffuse large B-cell lymphoma. Blood. 2016;**128**(2):185-194

[106] Ansell SM, Geyer SM, Hurvitz S, Fernando D, Habermann TM, Inwards DJ, et al. Phase I/II study of Ipilimumab (MDX-010), an anti-CTLA-4 monoclonal antibody, in patients with follicular non-hodgkin lymphoma. Blood. 2006;**108**(11):2729

[107] Zinzani PL, Ribrag V, Moskowitz CH, Michot J-M, Kuruvilla J, Balakumaran A, et al. Phase 1b study of pembrolizumab in patients with relapsed/refractory primary mediastinal large B-cell lymphoma: Results from the ongoing Keynote-013 trial. Blood. 2016:619-619

[108] Flinn IW, Bartlett NL, Blum KA, Ardeshna KM, LaCasce AS, Flowers CR, et al. A phase II trial to evaluate the efficacy of fostamatinib in patients with relapsed or refractory diffuse large B-cell lymphoma (DLBCL). European Journal of Cancer. 2016;**54**:11-17

[109] Crump M, Leppä S, Fayad L, Lee JJ, Di Rocco A, Ogura M, et al. Randomized, double-blind, phase III trial of enzastaurin versus placebo in patients achieving remission after first-line therapy for high-risk diffuse large B-cell lymphoma. Journal of Clinical Oncology. 2016;**34**(21):2484-2492

Chapter 4

Liquid Biopsy in Multiple Myeloma

Sridurga Mithraprabhu and Andrew Spencer

Additional information is available at the end of the chapter

http://dx.doi.org/10.5772/intechopen.72652

Abstract

Liquid biopsies represent an innovative methodology for cancer diagnostics and disease monitoring. The analysis of circulating cell-free nucleic acids (CFNA) and circulating tumour cells (CTC) are rapidly being adopted for quantitative and qualitative characterisation of the tumour genome and as a mode of non-invasive therapeutic monitoring. Circulating cell-free DNA (cfDNA) and CTC are representative of the underlying mutational profile of a cancer whereas the evaluation of extracellular RNA (exRNA) can be utilised as a prognostic biomarker thus providing critical biological information both at the time of diagnosis and during disease evolution. In this chapter, we will review the emerging utility of CFNA and CTC as biomarkers of prognosis and for both mutational characterisation and monitoring disease progression, and how these have the potential to provide additional information as an adjunct to bone marrow biopsies and conventional disease markers in multiple myeloma (MM). Emerging data suggest that liquid biopsies might offer a potentially simple, non-invasive, repeatable analysis that can aid in diagnosis, prognostication and therapeutic decision making in MM, with particular applicability in subsets of patients where conventional markers of disease burden may be less informative.

Keywords: cell-free nucleic acids, multiple myeloma, liquid biopsy, circulating tumour cells, non-invasive, diagnostics, disease burden

1. Introduction

1.1. Multiple myeloma

Multiple Myeloma (MM) is a multi-focal genetically heterogeneous clonal plasma cell (PC) malignancy that at diagnosis is present at multiple intra-medullary sites within the bone marrow (BM, **Figure 1**). It is the second most common haematological malignancy after lymphomas [1]. MM is preceded by a usually unrecognised asymptomatic clonal PC disorder exclusively confined to the BM called monoclonal gammopathy of undetermined significance (MGUS) [2, 3]. During disease progression the PCs evolve the capacity to grow independently of the BM milieu and thus proliferate outside of the BM, manifesting as extramedullary (EM) MM and/or plasma cell leukaemia (PCL), with published observations showing that PCL represents a more genetically abnormal sub-clone that evolves from the original intra-medullary PC population [4]. The incidence of EM soft-tissue plasmacytomas in newly diagnosed (ND) patients ranges from 7 to 18% with an incidence of almost 20% at the time of relapse [5, 6]. The diagnosis and monitoring of MM relies on sequential BM biopsies and the quantitation of biomarkers of disease burden in the blood and/or urine - clonal immunoglobulin (paraprotein, PP) and/or isotype restricted free-light chains (Serum Free light chains, SFLC or Bence Jones Proteinuria) and in 15–20% of patients the MM cells secrete only SFLC, so called light chain MM [7]. Notably, the routine biomarkers of tumour burden are not informative in subsets of patients with oligo-secretory (OS)-MM or non-secretory (NS)-MM, which are subsets of MM that have low or no measureable levels of PP (<10 g/L) and/or SFLC (<100 mg/L), respectively, and constitute about 10% of MM patients at diagnosis (Australian National Myeloma and Related Diseases Registry, [8]). Moreover, patients with secretory MM at the time of initial diagnosis can transform to NS-MM or OS-MM at the time of relapse and patients with advanced disease are significantly more likely to have OS-MM disease compared to ND patients [8]. These low or immeasurable levels of PP prevent a patient's disease from

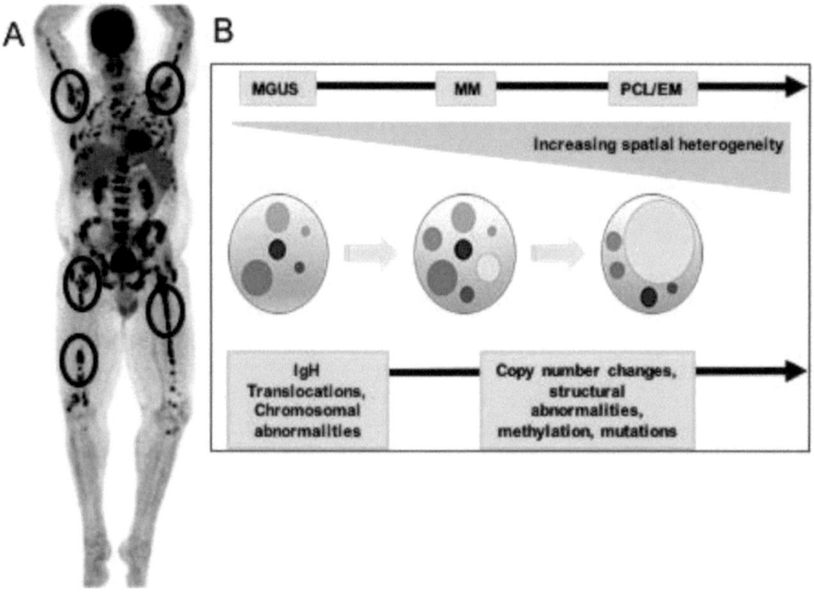

Figure 1. Multiple myeloma (MM) is a multi-focal malignancy manifesting at several sites black within the BM at diagnosis and in EM tissues in more advanced stages. (A) A PET image of a patient with MM is shown here, demonstrating disease foci at multiple sites (shown in the circles) with the potential that the tumour genome at these individual sites may demonstrate clonal heterogeneity. (B) Representation of the potential changes in clonal and sub-clonal fractions (represented in the different sized circles) are shown with the increasing spatial heterogeneity thought to be present during disease progression. Primary translocations of the IgH gene locus and chromosomal aneuploidies occur during MGUS and chromosomal abnormalities along with primary and secondary driver mutations emerge during MM progression.

being monitored using traditional blood and urine tests and as such OS-MM and NS-MM patients are typically ineligible to participate in clinical trials of newer anti-MM therapeutics. Conventionally, therefore, treatment response in these patients is determined via sequential BM biopsies, where available, and whole-body PET/CT or MRI represent the only accepted non-invasive modality for following response in NS-MM. Therefore, despite well-established diagnostic and monitoring modalities, there remains a critical need to address specific subsets of patients where these conventional markers are inadequate.

The treatment of MM has witnessed significant progress with the introduction of proteasome inhibitors (PI) and immunomodulatory agents (IMID), however, the disease remains incurable. MM cells acquire resistance to systemic therapies through the accumulation of mutations that are often not present during the initial stages of the disease [9] with this genetic evolution providing the more resistant clones with a growth and survival advantage (**Figure 1**, [10]). Mutational characterisation of MM utilising whole genome sequencing (WGS) or whole exome sequencing (WES) of single-site BM biopsies predominantly of ND patients have indicated that the MM mutational spectrum is both complex and heterogeneous with recurring mutations in KRAS, NRAS, TP53, BRAF, IRF4, MAX, ATM, ATR, CCND1, CYLD, DIS3, BRAF, FGFR3, RB1, HIST1H1E, EGR1, TRAG3, FAM46C and LTB [11–14]. The MM mutational landscape is dominated by RAS-MAPK pathway mutations (45–50%) and while these mutations can be targeted therapeutically, the biological implication of the presence of these mutations remains controversial. Chng WJ and co-authors observed that the presence of KRAS mutations, but not NRAS mutations, was associated with inferior overall survival (OS) and a more aggressive disease phenotype [15]. However, it has been recently demonstrated that NRAS mutations may confer reduced sensitivity to bortezomib but not dexamethasone, while the presence of KRAS mutations does not appear to correlate with drug sensitivity [16]. Conversely, more recent studies have concluded that harbouring RAS mutations has no significant impact on disease outcome [13, 14]. In contrast, available data suggests that the presence of mutations involving the DNA damage response genes (TP53, ATM and ATR) is associated with a negative impact on survival [14]. Recently, mutational analysis of PCs from 33 MGUS patients indicated that while the number of somatic mutations was significantly lower when compared to MM the spectrum of mutations mirrored that of MM with KRAS, NRAS, DIS3, HIST1H1E, EGR1 and LTB mutations being observed [17]. Importantly, mutations in the DNA damage response genes were not found, indicating that these are secondary drivers accounting for disease progression and drug resistance. Notably, one patient harboured both KRAS and NRAS mutations highlighting that diversification and heterogeneity in this pathway may exist before the development of symptomatic MM [17]. To date the mutational characterisation of MM has utilised single site BM biopsies, however, it is now increasingly recognised that such an approach may fail to capture the spatial and temporal genetic heterogeneity of this multi-focal disease, self-evidently with EM MM, but also, based on emerging data, in patients with 'typical MM' manifesting intra-clonal heterogeneity [11, 18–20]. Moreover, both spatial and temporal genetic heterogeneity are now recognised as adding to the genetic complexity of the disease as it evolves [21]. This is exemplified by recent observations from comparisons of BM and targeted biopsies of EM disease that sub-clones absent from the BM may be present at EM sites and critically, that these disease foci may respond differentially to treatment (**Figure 2**, [9, 22]). Therefore, despite the pivotal BM-based studies that currently inform our understanding of

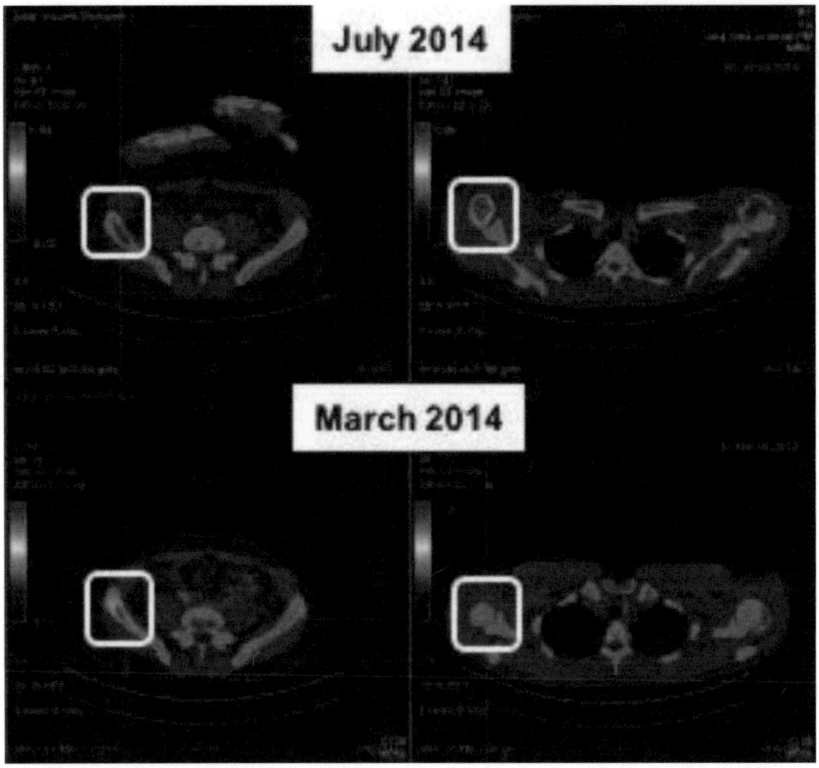

Figure 2. Different sites in a MM patient may respond differentially to treatment. PET image of a MM patient receiving thalidomide therapy taken 2 months apart showing regression of disease at one site (pelvis), while tumour growth is observed at another site (humerus).

the mutational spectrum in MM, the evident shortcomings of these approaches necessitates the adoption of newer and more novel strategies to enable the more comprehensive genomic characterisation of the disease.

1.2. Liquid biopsy

The utilisation of liquid biopsies continues to generate significant attention as it represents a platform that has the potential to provide rapidly evaluable and non-invasive, genomic characterisation of a patient's cancer. In simple terms, liquid biopsy refers to analyses that utilise blood or bodily fluids that contain circulating tumour cells (CTC) and/or fragments of nucleic acids or proteins that are derived from primary and/or secondary tumour sites. This material can then be interrogated to provide comprehensive information about the tumour genome and other biological characteristics of the disease. Moreover, liquid biopsies can be used to monitor the effects of therapy and may provide early evidence of recurrence or relapse of disease enabling early and informed changes in disease treatment. In this section, the two most widely studied types of liquid biopsy sources, CTC and cell-free nucleic acids (CFNA), will be discussed.

1.2.1. Circulating tumour cells (CTC)

CTC are intact tumour cells that disengage from tumour sites thus entering the circulation and are a recognised feature of metastatic cancers [23–25]. Historically, CTC were considered to be present only in a sub-set of ND, untreated or end-stage MM patients. Now with the advent of highly sensitive next-generation (NG) flow cytometry techniques the detection of CTC in pre-malignant MGUS and at different stages in MM has become feasible [26–28] and CTC can be detected in the peripheral blood of a substantial proportion of MM patients evaluated in this fashion [29, 30]. Importantly, the numbers of CTC in the peripheral blood in MM patients with active disease is known to be significantly higher than in patients with inactive disease, with higher numbers of CTC being a risk factor for progression to symptomatic MM for patients with either MGUS or smouldering MM (SMM) [29–33]. The number of CTC in ND and RR patients is also known to be an independent prognostic factor for survival [34–37]. Finally, the absolute numbers of CTC was found in one study to be a better predictor of disease activity than SFLC ratios [30].

1.2.2. Circulating cell-free nucleic acids (CFNA)

CFNA, refers to cfDNA and extracellular RNA (exRNA - includes mRNA and miRNA), and are being widely assessed in an ongoing fashion for their potential utility as blood biomarkers for cancer diagnostics. CFNA are derived predominantly through necrosis, spontaneous or chemotherapy induced apoptosis and active cellular release [38, 39]. Given that CFNA is also present at higher levels in certain physiological conditions and clinical scenarios (reviewed in [40]), it is critical to determine if the nucleic acids released are tumour-specific in cancer patients. In this section the different types of CFNA and their potential clinical utility will be discussed.

1.2.3. Cell-free DNA

The presence of CFNA in body fluids was first described by Mandel and Metais in 1948 [41]. One of the earliest observations in relation to cfDNA was that patients with malignant disease had higher levels of cfDNA in their serum than normal individuals, and that patients with persistently high levels of cfDNA demonstrated a lack of treatment response [42–44]. Mutated RAS fragments and microsatellite alterations in cfDNA were later observed in cancer patients and critically these alterations were not detected in paired tissue biopsies, highlighting the concept, very early-on, that isolated tissue biopsies may not represent the optimal material for defining the tumour genome [45, 46]. The development and utilisation of NGS technologies, WGS and/or WES of cfDNA containing tumour-derived DNA has identified mutations, tumour-derived chromosomal aberrations and gene rearrangements associated with acquired resistance to therapy without the need to perform sequential tumour biopsies [47–51]. Furthermore, it is evident that secondary mutations are more readily detectable in the plasma than via re-biopsy of primary tumours validating the utility of plasma-based analysis for the characterisation of potentially targetable oncogenes and the identification of resistance-associated mutations that are acquired during disease progression, thus informing therapeutic changes [48, 52, 53]. Available evidence would also suggest that cfDNA may be more representative of the entire tumour genome than the information derived from single BM or nodal/tumour biopsies, as emerging evidence supports the notion that a range of haematologic malignancies including MM are likely to harbour significant sub-clonal and spatial genetic heterogeneity. In MM, levels of cfDNA are significantly higher than in both normal volunteers and non-MM cancers [54, 55] and the potential utility of cfDNA in MM will be discussed below.

1.2.4. Extracellular RNA (mRNA and miRNA)

The presence of extracellular RNA (exRNA) in plasma/serum was also described some decades ago [41, 56, 57] with significantly higher levels in cancer patients compared to healthy individuals [58]. Additionally, tumour burden was shown to correlated with the level of circulating mRNA [59]. The exRNA released into the circulation is surprisingly stable owing to its protection from RNAse-mediated degradation through packaging into exosomes, which are shed into the blood stream [60–64]. Biomarker studies measuring cancer-specific circulating mRNA have identified higher level of mRNA and correlation with disease status in a number of malignancies including nasopharyngeal carcinoma [65], prostate [66, 67], gastrointestinal [68–72], breast [73–76], hepatocellular carcinoma [77], lung [78, 79], cervical [80], lymphoma [81] and thyroid [82]. These findings highlight the potential utility of exRNA in cancer diagnostics, and while promising, it will be critical to assess exRNA in larger and annotated sample sets to establish specific circulating mRNAs as reliable non-invasive biomarkers.

Similarly, extracellular miRNA are found in virtually all fluid compartments of the body including blood where they can circulate bound to proteins, high-density lipoproteins or apoptotic bodies, or within exosomes, thus providing stability against RNases (reviewed in [83]). The levels of circulating miRNA have been described in a number of cancers with one of the earliest reports being in diffuse large B-cell lymphoma (DLBCL) demonstrating a correlation between the level of specific miRNAs and prognosis [84]. Subsequently, several publications of circulating miRNA in malignancy have demonstrated increased miRNA in cancer patients when compared to healthy individuals and a decrease in levels following tumour debulking surgery (reviewed in [85–87]). Circulating miRNA expression profiles are also known to have signatures correlative to disease stage, diagnosis and relapse [88–91]. The origin of circulating RNA subtypes is, however, not as well understood as for cfDNA, as these can potentially be sourced from tumour cells, the supporting micro-environment or immune cells [92]. While mRNA has not been assessed in MM, there are a number of studies of miRNA and the prognostic utility of these will be discussed in the next section.

2. Biological and clinical implications of liquid biopsy analysis in MM

Liquid biopsy is gaining momentum in MM due to the inherent nature of the disease and the obvious limitations associated with BM biopsy. A summary of the potential utility of CTC and CFNA evaluation are presented in this section (**Figure 3**).

2.1. Determining the tumour genome composition

Given the clonal genomic heterogeneity that exists within MM, particularly with disease progression, it is theoretically necessary to perform repeated BM biopsies to track tumour

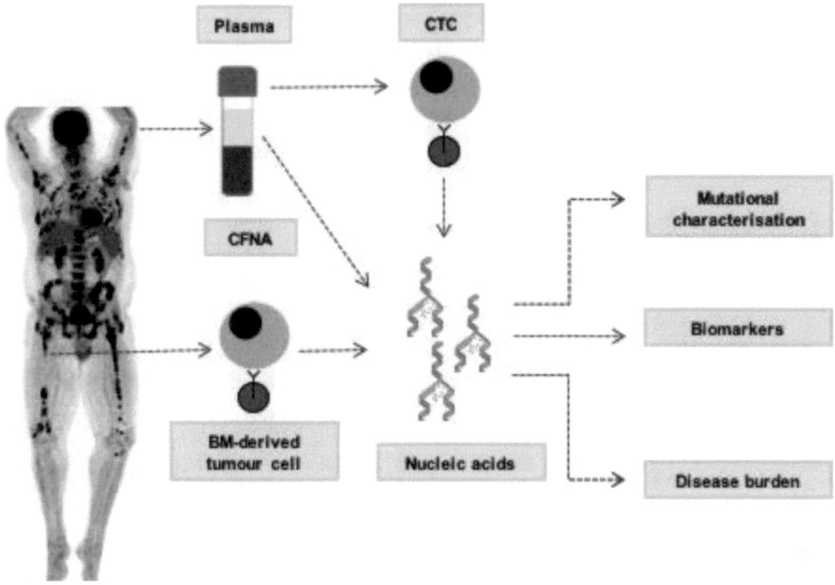

Figure 3. Currently in MM, BM-derived tumour cells are utilised for mutational characterisation, biomarker identification and to define disease burden. Peripheral blood can be utilised to obtain both CTC and CFNA. DNA and RNA can be derived from both sources and as both CTC and CFNA are derived from multiple tumour sites they theoretically will provide a more comprehensive profile of the disease in comparison to a single-site BM biopsy.

genomic evolution within any particular patient. Such an approach, however, remains an unattractive proposition as BM biopsies are invasive, not without complications, subject to sampling error and cannot capture the increasing spatial heterogeneity present with disease evolution. Therefore, the capacity to perform sequential mutational characterisation using a more 'holistic' and non-invasive approach would be a highly desirable alternative option. Both CTC and CFNA have been explored for this purpose in MM, however, the field is relatively unestablished with only a small number of publications addressing this concept. One of the earliest reports by Zandecki et al. evaluated CTC and matched BM-MM cells and demonstrated that chromosomal abnormalities were consistent between these two compartments [93]. The recent development of both NG flow cytometry and contemporary sequencing technologies has enabled the analysis of CTC at the single-cell level [27] but to date only small numbers of patients have been evaluated using this approach. Analysis of 9 patients with single cell WGS revealed that all BM-defined mutations were similarly present in CTC [27]. Further analysis was done on CTC in two patients with low disease burden (one with treated MM and one with MGUS). The CTC of the MM patient harboured readily detectable somatic mutations in BRAF, TP53 and IRF4, with reappearance of the mutations when the patient relapsed, indicating that the treatment had not eradicated these particular sub-clones. CTC analysis of the patient with MGUS revealed the presence of a NRAS mutation, also present in the BM. The concordance with BM genetic composition was also confirmed by Mishima et al. utilising NGS when analysing 8 paired CTC and BM aspirates [28]. Clonal, defined as a > 0.90 mutant allele fraction (MAF), mutations were present in >99% of CTC and BM, while subclonal shared mutations (defined as >0.05 MAF) were concordant in >80%, with 16% of subclones (<0.05 MAF) discordant between the two compartments consistent with spatial heterogeneity [28]. Similarly, copy number alternations (CNA) were assessed and found to be 92% concordant. Likewise, RNA-seq at the single cell level also accurately predicted the recognised non-random chromosomal translocations that manifest in MM responsible for overexpression of key MM-associated oncogenes [27]. Overall, for both somatic mutations and CNA, CTC appear to harbour more variances indicating that they are likely sourced from multiple tumour sites and the manifestations of spatial heterogeneity may thus be more accurately captured by this type of analysis.

The evaluation of cfDNA for mutational characterisation and monitoring of disease burden in MM has also recently been described [54, 55, 94, 95]. Importantly, and for the first time, spatial and clonal heterogeneity on a large scale in MM was confirmed by our study evaluating paired BM-derived CD138 selected MM cells and cfDNA utilising a highly sensitive targeted sequencing platform consisting of a panel of 96 cancer-associated mutations including mutations of KRAS, NRAS, BRAF and TP53. This demonstrated that 21% of MM patients had mutations detectable only in the plasma and that the prevalence of spatial heterogeneity increased with disease evolution [55]. Numerous signalling pathways are known to be mutated in MM [13, 14], with previous BM WES studies demonstrating that activating mutations of the RAS-MAPK pathway were present in approximately 50% of patients. In contrast, our study demonstrated RAS-MAPK activating mutations in 69% of cases and the co-existence of multiple mutated sub-clones in a significant proportion, with >3 activating mutations in 23% of patients (range, 3–17 mutations per patient) representing a hitherto unrecognised mutational convergence on the RAS-MAPK pathway. This had remained largely undiscovered in single-site BM WES studies owing presumably to the relative insensitivity of the methodologies used and the presence of clonal heterogeneity at sites distant to the BM biopsy site. While it is likely, with high-sensitivity approaches, that there will be a MAF threshold for minor BM sub-clones that enables them to be reproducibly detected in the plasma, this will not be relevant with less sensitive strategies like WES and targeted amplicon sequencing that cannot detect smaller sub-clonal mutations, thus explaining, and consistent with, the 96% concordance between BM and PL demonstrated using NGS technologies [54]. Interestingly, mutations in PIK3CA, which have only rarely been described in MM, were found in a recent study to be present, but only in the plasma, indicating that these could be a feature of EM disease [54]. However, confirmatory studies with larger cohorts of patients and more comprehensive and targeted panels of MM-associated mutations are required to validate these observations. Theoretically, therefore, plasma cfDNA analysis of MM patients, particularly in the case of EM-MM, would not only provide information on the underlying biology of this disease, but could also furnish information on response to therapy through quantitative sequential tracking of plasma-only mutations. Moreover, RNA-seq of plasma cfRNA derived from MM patients is also theoretically possible to provide information on single nucleotide polymorphisms (SNP), although this has not yet been described in the published literature. So, while in the short-term it is unlikely that plasma cfDNA evaluation will replace BM biopsy, as the latter remains necessary in MM for diagnostic purposes, we believe cfDNA analysis as an adjunct to BM biopsy for comprehensive mutational characterisation is likely to become a reality in the near future.

To date, the analysis of CTC or cfDNA with paired BM has largely been performed only at single time-points and has not been comprehensively utilised for longitudinal assessment using sequential specimens that would be critical to identify the evolution of the clonal architecture of the disease during therapy. The prognostic significance of mutational profiling in MM also remains largely unknown, with only a few genes thought to have prognostic significance. Furthermore, it should be recognised that the prognostic impact of certain mutations has been based on studies profiling material sourced from BM aspirates and therefore may not have been representative of the entire tumour genome. This shortfall could be potentially overcome using CTC and/or ctDNA as an adjunct to BM biopsy for mutational analysis and consequently, for prognostic profiling.

2.2. Biomarkers

The establishment of single-cell RNA-seq methodology in CTC from MM patients [27] presents an important opportunity for the identification of biomarkers that may define differing sub-sets and stages of the disease. Theoretically, this may represent a technically feasible and hence more reliable strategy than evaluation of exRNA as the RNA would be derived from tumour cells that should overcome some of the stability issues that may be associated with exRNA. Furthermore, CTC-derived RNA should address the issue of spatial heterogeneity and hence provide a more inclusive RNA-signature during disease evolution, as compared to present data based on single-site BM biopsies. To date, the potential of exRNA for differentiating the continuum of plasma cell dyscrasias ranging from MGUS to intra-medullary, EM MM and PCL has been explored in MM, but mainly through the analysis of miRNA and not mRNA (reviewed in [83]). Available evidence would suggest that MM cells contain differing populations of miRNA species at defined disease stages [96–100], therefore an approach identifying miRNA biomarkers non-invasively utilising exRNA would represent a readily accessible and novel approach. However, while circulating miRNA biomarker studies, including patients from different disease stages, have defined relative differences in both the expression of specific miRNAs and the absolute levels of circulating miRNAs as potential biomarkers [101–109] there is widespread discordance between the published studies with respect to the specific miRNAs identified [83]. For example, Yoshizawa et al. found significant downregulation of miR-92a in patients with symptomatic MM when compared to normal subjects, conversely, Besse et al. when comparing serum miRNA profiles between healthy, ND and EM patients, demonstrated that miR-130a expression was significantly decreased in the EM patients, hence a potential biomarker for EM disease, but no correlation with patient outcome was evident [101]. Jones et al., identified that a combination of miR-1246 and miR-1308 could distinguish MGUS from MM patients [106], whereas miR-25 was shown to correlate with conventional serum markers of MM at both diagnosis and at complete response (CR) post autologous stem-cell transplantation (ASCT) [103]. Some of the studies also identified a prognostic correlation with the actual levels of circulating miRNA. Rocci et al. demonstrated that miR-16 and 25 were significantly associated with OS in ND MM [102]. Qu et al. identified miR-483-5p as a potential predictor of MM survival [110]. Hao et al. showed that lower expression of miR-19a predicted poor OS [107], while Kubiczkova et al. concluded that a combination of miR-34a and let-7e can distinguish MM patients from normal individuals, and that patients with lower levels of miR-744 and let-7e had shorter OS [105]. In parallel with these studies, an evaluation of exosome-derived miRNA demonstrated that both let-7b and miR-18a were significantly associated with progression-free survival (PFS) and OS [111]. Unlike CTC, one of the significant shortcoming of assessing circulating miRNA levels is that expression levels might be impacted upon by both the biological characteristics of the disease and the tumour burden, thereby presenting significant challenges when it comes to identifying correlations with prognosis. Moreover, the discrepancy between these studies highlights the lack of concordance between the analytical methodologies, study populations and treatment regimens employed. A recent publication that provided a systematic review and meta-analysis of 7 circulating miRNA studies in MM established that utilising a combination of miRNAs rather than single miRNAs would be more effective in the diagnosis and prognostic classification of MM [112].

2.3. Therapeutic monitoring

Longitudinal and dynamic monitoring of CTC and CFNA could provide an avenue for detecting loss of response in patients before the emergence of clinical relapse. This could be particularly useful in patients with minimal residual disease (MRD) or when conventional markers are inadequate. MM treatment has witnessed significant progress with the utilisation of novel therapies including PI and IMID with approximately 75% of patients achieving a near-complete response (CR) or CR with front-line therapy. In this context the attribution of MRD negativity has emerged as a paradigm that may be critical in informing treatment decisions. While MM invariably relapses, MRD-negative patients consistently demonstrate more prolonged PFS and may represent a group where therapeutic de-escalation or modification can be safely considered [113, 114]. Consequently, the necessity for highly sensitive assays to detect MRD is critical and this has led to the development and increasing adoption of NGS MRD approaches [115–119]. Currently, MRD status is determined via single site BM biopsy, which clearly has its limitations. Given that the numbers of CTC in the peripheral blood in MM patients with active disease is known to be significantly higher than in patients with inactive disease and the developments in the detection of CTC in MM, the possibility of assessing the overall numbers/presence of CTC in patients during therapy for MRD assessment is imminent [29–33]. Recently, CTCs were monitored to predict response to in MM patients treated within an open-label, randomised, multicenter phase III clinical trial MM5 of newly diagnosed MM patients with the authors concluding that CTC detection in conjunction with BM for MRD detection [120]. Likewise, cfDNA has been used for dynamic monitoring following surgery/radiotherapy for the detection of residual disease in a number of solid cancers, with persistently high or increasing levels of cfDNA detectable mutations post-surgery/radiotherapy associated with a lack of treatment response and a much greater risk of relapse [42], while patients with undetectable levels of somatic mutations in cfDNA have demonstrated fewer or no recurrences [121]. The monitoring of MRD using cfDNA in diffuse large-cell B Lymphoma has also demonstrated that the persistence of cfDNA mutations identifies patients at risk of recurrence before the emergence of clinical relapse [122]. However, any correlation between the presence or re-emergence of cfDNA detectable mutations and disease progression has not yet been assessed in MM.

Currently, only three studies in MM have utilised liquid biopsy in comparison with conventional markers of disease burden in sequential plasma samples, of which only one study has compared CTC and ctDNA for therapeutic monitoring. All three studies utilised different approaches. Oberle and colleagues assessed clonotypic V(D)J rearrangement in CTC and cfDNA in a cohort of 27 MM patients. Overall, an association between both the presence of cfDNA and CTC V(D)J detectable rearrangements with response was demonstrated [94].

Notably, the study detected V(D)J rearrangement in cfDNA in all patients assessed while rearrangements in CTC were only detectable in 70% of patients, indicating that cfDNA, derived from CTC, BM and EM tissue, may represent a better medium for disease evaluation than CTC alone. Long-term monitoring of recurrently occurring mutations in sequential serum samples from 11 patients over a period of 7 years has also been performed in MM [95]. While the majority of patients assessed demonstrated a correlation between PP and the quantifiable levels of specific mutations in sequential plasma samples, there were clearly some patients where analysis of cfDNA was able to identify impending relapse prior to the emergence of clinical relapse, showing the potentially higher sensitivity of cfDNA analysis for disease monitoring. However, a major limitation of sequentially monitoring an initially identified mutant clone is the possibility a sub-clonal mutations not detectable at diagnosis evolving during relapse or being present at an undetectable level initially and subsequently predominating due to selection pressure. Indeed, this appeared to be evident in one of the patients studied, where the initial detection of a BRAF V600E mutation was not maintained despite the continued serologically persisting disease [95]. The evolution of the tumour genome during therapy was also clearly demonstrated in our study, in which 7 patients were monitored sequentially [55]. One patient in particular demonstrated the potential complexities presented by genomic disease evolution. Initially the patient manifested both TP53 R273H and NRAS G13R mutated clones that were responsive to therapy with lenalidomide and dexamethasone (Rd). Subsequently a rapid increase in SFLC consistent with light-chain escape was coincident with the emergence of two new KRAS clones, KRAS G12A and KRAS G12 V. The clonal fraction of both KRAS clones reduced with a switch to Ixazomib-cyclophosphamide-dexamethasone (ICd) therapy coinciding with a serological response. However, the NRAS G13R clone that was responsive to Rd. progressed on ICd in contrast to the TP53 R273H clone that continued to respond,

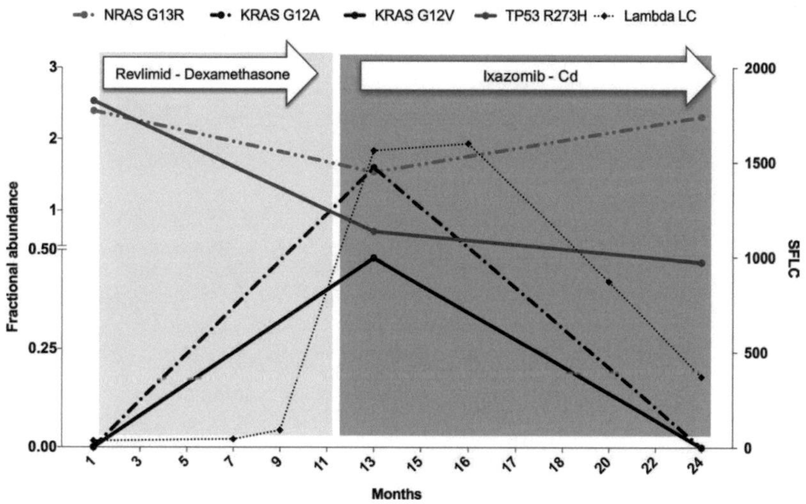

Figure 4. Line graph represents the clonal fraction of 4 mutant clones (left Y-axis) and lambda LC (right Y-axis) in sequential PL of relapsed patients collected at months 1, 13 and 24 during therapy. Patient relapsed on revlimid and dexamethasone with increase in levels of two mutant clones KRAS G12 V and KRAS G12A at month 13 coinciding with lambda LC, however, TP53 R273H and NRAS G13R were found to decrease. A switch to Ixazomib, cyclophosphamide and dexamethasone (cd) at month 13 decreased levels of KRAS G12A and KRAS G12 V with increasing levels of NRAS G13R suggesting differential response of mutant clones to treatment. Image reproduced from [55].

highlighting the differential responses of the 4 mutant clones to two different lines of therapy (**Figure 4**). These observations signify that comprehensive mutational analysis in sequential plasma is critical to define therapeutic response in a timely manner. Plasma ctDNA analysis may also represent a novel and informative strategy for disease monitoring in OS-MM and NS-MM patients as demonstrated in our recent publication [55]. Sequential plasma ctDNA analysis in a ND NS-MM patient over a period of 19 months showed that relapsed disease was associated with the reappearance of mutant KRAS G12 V and KRAS G12D clones that had been present at diagnosis in the BM and the emergence of two new clones, NRAS G13D and NRAS Q61K, with the former showing refractoriness to both Thalidomide – dexamethasone, cyclophosphamide, etoposide and cisplatin (T-DCEP) and re-treatment with bortezomib (velcade) – cyclophosphamide – dexamethasone (VCD) and persisting until the patient died shortly thereafter from progressive disease (**Figure 5**). Interestingly the BM biopsy at month 19 showed apparent reduction in disease burden coincident with reintroduction of VCD but droplet digital PCR (ddPCR) of plasma ctDNA showed an increasing clonal fraction of the NRAS G13D clone consistent with VCD-refractory disease distant to the site of BM biopsy. This first-time observation indicates that ctDNA represents a readily accessible non-invasive biomarker of disease burden that may be superior to BM biopsy for monitoring treatment response in NS-MM. Overall, all three studies demonstrated the potential for ctDNA to be used in monitoring MM patients. Clearly, there were limitations due to small sample sizes, lack of homogenous patient treatment and the critical need to be more comprehensive in mutational identification to address tumour genome evolution. Future studies should therefore incorporate sequential cfDNA assessment adopting NGS-based approaches,

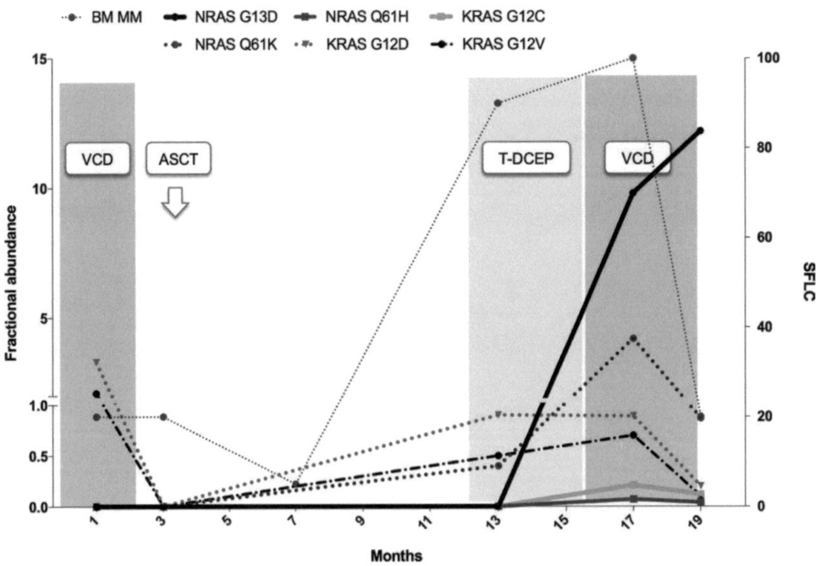

Figure 5. Line graph represents the clonal fraction of mutant clones by ddPCR in a non-secretory patient, patient #2. PL was collected at 1, 3, 13, 17 and 19 months post- diagnosis. The proportion of BM MM cells is shown with an increasing clonal fraction of 4 clones coinciding with BM relapse at month 13, only 9 months post-autologous stem cell transplantations (ASCT). At month 19 a BM response to VCD was evident but with an increasing abundance of the NRAS G13D clone. The patient succumbed to refractory progressive disease shortly afterwards. Image reproduced from [55].

at diagnosis and subsequent relapses, to quantify previously detected and emergent clones, in larger annotated sample sets, thus enabling the comprehensive tracking of mutations and assessment of disease burden with correlation to conventional serum biomarkers.

3. Methodologies and challenges

An increasing number of publications have proven the utility of liquid biopsy for cancer screening, diagnosis and disease monitoring. However, for this paradigm to be more widely incorporated into the clinical setting a standardised approach for both the pre-analytical processing and the analytical platforms utilised is necessary. Identification and isolation of MM CTC has been established through the utilisation of ultra-sensitive NGS multicolour flow cytometry techniques [26–28]. Lohr et al. devised a combination methodology that allowed for isolation of CTC using the standard markers (CD138+ CD38+ CD56 variable, CD45 low) and serial dilutions to single cells through fluorescence microscopy to improve the detection of CTC [27]. Currently, these are the only described methodologies for isolation of CTC and more studies are required to standardise the methodologies described.

CFNA analysis relies on the standardisation of collection, processing and optimal storage of cfDNA and exRNA, which can now be streamlined with commercially available specialised collection tubes that can stabilise blood at room temperature and preserve the white blood cells to avoid rupture and therefore contamination with cellular DNA in the plasma (Streck, PAXgene, Roche, NORGEN BIOTEK, etc.). Isolation of genomic DNA or RNA from both CTC and CFNA, to a large extent, has also been simplified through the use of commercially available specific isolation kits, although the performance of each of these kits in comparison to other conventional methods is controversial [123]. The choice of the NGS methodologies to address specific questions is however, more complicated and is confounded by the type of nucleic acid being analysed, assay sensitivity and specificity and the heterogeneous content of tumour-derived nucleic acids. A substantial technical challenge to overcome in optimising cfDNA analysis is the level of sensitivity of the various NGS methodologies, as cfDNA may contain low-frequency mutant alleles that might not be readily detectable in WES and targeted amplicon sequencing, which have a sensitivity between 1 and 5%. This is being addressed with the utilisation of unique molecular indices that provide further resolution [48, 124] and such approaches are currently offered by a number of commercial companies (Rubicon genomics, QIAGEN, Agilent).

Analysis of exRNA is more complicated as a technology-of-choice needs to be determined for large-scale identification of potential biomarkers. Additionally, the validation and diagnostic implication of circulating RNA sub-types currently relies on 'internal controls' which are often not suited for this type of analysis. This could be addressed using absolute quantification methods, a plausible approach utilising ddPCR, which provides a more robust approach by quantitating targets per unit in serum or plasma, as done in cfDNA studies.

For CFNA and CTC, unfortunately, to date, few of the described methodologies are as yet validated or standardised, complicating generalisability and inter-study comparisons. Overall, the field would benefit from establishment of certain guidelines for each aspect of sample analysis to allow for comparison of studies of similar kind. These limitations not withstanding, the analysis of ctDNA has gained significant momentum is the past couple of years, with numerous commercial companies offering 'liquid biopsy' testing. Such analysis is now frequently integrated into clinical trials and plasma DNA EGFR mutation testing for non-small cell lung cancer has recently been approved by the FDA [125–127]. Further commercialisation of these 'liquid biopsies' as diagnostics is rapidly evolving, but currently is largely limited to informing treatment choices in late stage cancers.

4. Conclusions

Liquid biopsy analysis can provide a dynamic and comprehensive picture of the genomic landscape in MM. Specifically, serial analysis can provide a non-invasive approach to monitor tumour burden and genomic evolution that also incorporates characterisation of the spatial and temporal genomic heterogeneity, which predominates over time, in this multi-focal disease. Accumulating published evidence and imminent developments in the field indicate that this type of analysis will provide critical information for precision medicine and likely transform the management of more problematic sub-groups of MM including NS, OS patients and those with EM disease. In the future, instead of utilising extensive imaging and invasive and potentially misrepresentative BM biopsies, liquid biopsies could be used to inform real-time clinical decision thus further improving the outcome for MM patients.

Author details

Sridurga Mithraprabhu[1,2*] and Andrew Spencer[1,2,3]

*Address all correspondence to: durga.mithraprabhu@monash.edu

1 Myeloma Research Group, Australian Centre for Blood Diseases, Alfred Hospital – Monash University, Melbourne, Victoria, Australia

2 Malignant Haematology and Stem Cell Transplantation, Alfred Hospital, Melbourne, Victoria, Australia

3 Department of Clinical Haematology, Monash University, Melbourne, Victoria, Australia

References

[1] Siegel RL, Miller KD, Jemal A. Cancer statistics, 2016. CA: a Cancer Journal for Clinicians. 2016;**66**(1):7-30

[2] Landgren O et al. Monoclonal gammopathy of undetermined significance (MGUS) consistently precedes multiple myeloma: A prospective study. Blood. 2009;**113**(22):5412-5417

[3] Weiss BM et al. A monoclonal gammopathy precedes multiple myeloma in most patients. Blood. 2009;**113**(22):5418-5422

[4] Kalff A et al. A rare case of IGH/MYC and IGH/BCL2 double hit primary plasma cell leukemia. Haematologica. 2015;**100**(2):E60-E62

[5] Blade J et al. Soft-tissue plasmacytomas in multiple myeloma: Incidence, mechanisms of extramedullary spread, and treatment approach. Journal of Clinical Oncology. 2011;**29**(28):3805-3812

[6] Varettoni M et al. Incidence, presenting features and outcome of extramedullary disease in multiple myeloma: A longitudinal study on 1003 consecutive patients. Annals of Oncology. 2010;**21**(2):325-330

[7] Kyle RA et al. Review of 1027 patients with newly diagnosed multiple myeloma. Mayo Clinic Proceedings. 2003;**78**(1):21-33

[8] Larson D, Kyle RA, Rajkumar SV. Prevalence and monitoring of Oligosecretory myeloma. New England Journal of Medicine. 2012;**367**(6):580-581

[9] Egan JB et al. Extramedullary myeloma whole genome sequencing reveals novel mutations in Cereblon, proteasome subunit G2 and the glucocorticoid receptor in multi drug resistant disease. British Journal of Haematology. 2013;**161**(5):748-751

[10] Egan JB et al. Whole-genome sequencing of multiple myeloma from diagnosis to plasma cell leukemia reveals genomic initiating events, evolution, and clonal tides. Blood. 2012;**120**(5):1060-1066

[11] Bolli N et al. Heterogeneity of genomic evolution and mutational profiles in multiple myeloma. Nature Communications. 2014;**5**

[12] Chapman MA et al. Initial genome sequencing and analysis of multiple myeloma. Nature. 2011;**471**(7339):467-472

[13] Lohr JG et al. Widespread genetic heterogeneity in multiple myeloma: Implications for targeted therapy. Cancer Cell. 2014;**25**(1):91-101

[14] Walker BA et al. Mutational Spectrum, copy number changes, and outcome: Results of a sequencing study of patients with newly diagnosed myeloma. Journal of Clinical Oncology. 2015;**33**(33):3911-3920

[15] Chng WJ et al. Clinical and biological significance of RAS mutations in multiple myeloma. Leukemia. 2008;**22**(12):2280-2284

[16] Mulligan G et al. Mutation of NRAS but not KRAS significantly reduces myeloma sensitivity to single-agent bortezomib therapy. Blood. 2014;**123**(5):632-639

[17] Mikulasova A et al. Somatic mutation spectrum in monoclonal gammopathy of undetermined significance indicates a less complex genomic landscape compared to multiple myeloma. Haematologica. 2017;**102**(9):1617-1625

[18] de Haart SJ et al. Comparison of intramedullary myeloma and corresponding extramedullary soft tissue plasmacytomas using genetic mutational panel analyses. Blood Cancer Journal. 2016;**20**(6):e426

[19] Melchor L et al. Spatiotemporal analysis of Intraclonal heterogeneity in multiple myeloma: Unravelling the impact of treatment and the propagating capacity of subclones using whole exome sequencing. Blood. 2015;**126**:371

[20] Weinhold N et al. Extensive regional intra-clonal heterogeneity in multiple myeloma - implications for diagnostics, risk stratification and targeted treatment. Blood. 2016;**128**:3278

[21] Rasche L et al. Spatial genomic heterogeneity in multiple myeloma revealed by multi-region sequencing. Nature Communications. 2017;**8**(1):268

[22] Kumar AK et al. Extramedullary progression of multiple myeloma despite concomitant medullary response to multiple combination therapies and autologous transplant: A case report. Journal of Medical Case Reports. 2014;**8**:299

[23] Masuda T et al. Clinical and biological significance of circulating tumor cells in cancer. Molecular Oncology. 2016;**10**(3):408-417

[24] Allard WJ et al. Tumor cells circulate in the peripheral blood of all major carcinomas but not in healthy subjects or patients with nonmalignant diseases. Clinical Cancer Research. 2004;**10**(20):6897-6904

[25] Cristofanilli M et al. Circulating tumor cells, disease progression, and survival in metastatic breast cancer. The New England Journal of Medicine. 2004;**351**(8):781-791

[26] Paiva B et al. Detailed characterization of multiple myeloma circulating tumor cells shows unique phenotypic, cytogenetic, functional, and circadian distribution profile. Blood. 2013;**122**(22):3591-3598

[27] Lohr JG et al. Genetic interrogation of circulating multiple myeloma cells at single-cell resolution. Science Translational Medicine. 2016;**8**(363):363ra147

[28] Mishima Y et al. The mutational landscape of circulating tumor cells in multiple myeloma. Cell Reports. 2017;**19**(1):218-224

[29] Rawstron AC et al. Circulating plasma cells in multiple myeloma: Characterization and correlation with disease stage. British Journal of Haematology. 1997;**97**(1):46-55

[30] Witzig TE et al. Quantitation of circulating peripheral blood plasma cells and their relationship to disease activity in patients with multiple myeloma. Cancer. 1993;**72**(1):108-113

[31] Bianchi G et al. High levels of peripheral blood circulating plasma cells as a specific risk factor for progression of smoldering multiple myeloma. Leukemia. 2013;**27**(3):680-685

[32] Kumar S et al. Prognostic value of circulating plasma cells in monoclonal gammopathy of undetermined significance. Journal of Clinical Oncology. 2005;**23**(24):5668-5674

[33] Gonsalves WI et al. Quantification of circulating clonal plasma cells via multiparametric flow cytometry identifies patients with smoldering multiple myeloma at high risk of progression. Leukemia. 2017;**31**(1):130-135

[34] Witzig TE et al. Peripheral blood monoclonal plasma cells as a predictor of survival in patients with multiple myeloma. Blood. 1996;**88**(5):1780-1787

[35] Nowakowski GS et al. Circulating plasma cells detected by flow cytometry as a predictor of survival in 302 patients with newly diagnosed multiple myeloma. Blood. 2005;**106**(7):2276-2279

[36] Gonsalves WI et al. Quantification of clonal circulating plasma cells in relapsed multiple myeloma. British Journal of Haematology. 2014;**167**(4):500-505

[37] Gonsalves WI et al. Quantification of clonal circulating plasma cells in newly diagnosed multiple myeloma: Implications for redefining high-risk myeloma. Leukemia. 2014;**28**(10):2060-2065

[38] Jahr S et al. DNA fragments in the blood plasma of cancer patients: Quantitations and evidence for their origin from apoptotic and necrotic cells. Cancer Research. 2001;**61**(4):1659-1665

[39] Stroun M et al. The origin and mechanism of circulating DNA. Annals of the New York Academy of Sciences. 2000;**906**:161-168

[40] Wan JC et al. Liquid biopsies come of age: Towards implementation of circulating tumour DNA. Nature Reviews. Cancer. 2017;**17**(4):223-238

[41] Mandel P, Metais P. Les acides nucléiques du plasma sanguin chez l'homme. Comptes Rendus des Seances de la Societe de Biologie et de Ses Filiales. 1948;**142**(3-4):241-243

[42] Leon SA et al. Free DNA in the serum of cancer patients and the effect of therapy. Cancer Research. 1977;**37**(3):646-650

[43] Shapiro B et al. Determination of circulating DNA levels in patients with benign or malignant gastrointestinal disease. Cancer. 1983;**51**(11):2116-2120

[44] Stroun M et al. Isolation and characterization of DNA from the plasma of cancer patients. European Journal of Cancer & Clinical Oncology. 1987;**23**(6):707-712

[45] Chen XQ et al. Microsatellite alterations in plasma DNA of small cell lung cancer patients. Nature Medicine. 1996;**2**(9):1033-1035

[46] Vasioukhin V et al. Point mutations of the N-ras gene in the blood plasma DNA of patients with myelodysplastic syndrome or acute myelogenous leukaemia. British Journal of Haematology. 1994;**86**(4):774-779

[47] Chan KC et al. Cancer genome scanning in plasma: Detection of tumor-associated copy number aberrations, single-nucleotide variants, and tumoral heterogeneity by massively parallel sequencing. Clinical Chemistry. 2013;**59**(1):211-224

[48] Forshew T et al. Noninvasive identification and monitoring of cancer mutations by targeted deep sequencing of plasma DNA. Science Translational Medicine. 2012;**4**(136):136ra68

[49] Heitzer E et al. Tumor-associated copy number changes in the circulation of patients with prostate cancer identified through whole-genome sequencing. Genome Medicine. 2013;**5**(4):30

[50] Leary RJ et al. Detection of chromosomal alterations in the circulation of cancer patients with whole-genome sequencing. Science Translational Medicine. 2012;**4**(162):162ra154

[51] Murtaza M et al. Non-invasive analysis of acquired resistance to cancer therapy by sequencing of plasma DNA. Nature. 2013;**497**(7447):108-112

[52] Demetri GD et al. Mutational analysis of plasma DNA from patients (pts) in the phase III GRID study of regorafenib (REC) versus placebo (PL) in tyrosine kinase inhibitor (TKI)-refractory GIST: Correlating genotype with clinical outcomes. Journal of Clinical Oncology. 2013;**31**(15):10503

[53] Demetri GD et al. Detection of oncogenic kinase mutations in circulating plasma DNA and correlation with clinical benefit in the phase III GRID study of regorafenib vs placebo in TKI-refractory metastatic GIST. Cancer Research. 2013;**73**(8):LB-295

[54] Kis O et al. Circulating tumour DNA sequence analysis as an alternative to multiple myeloma bone marrow aspirates. Nature Communications. 2017;**8**:15086

[55] Mithraprabhu S et al. Circulating tumour DNA analysis demonstrates spatial mutational heterogeneity that coincides with disease relapse in myeloma. Leukemia. 2017;**31**(8):1695-1705

[56] Kamm RC, Smith AG. Nucleic acid concentrations in normal human plasma. Clinical Chemistry. 1972;**18**(6):519-522

[57] Shutack JG, Baxt J, Wasniewski JJ Jr. A study of the RNA levels of normal blood serum. The Journal of the American Osteopathic Association. 1968;**67**(9):1051-1053

[58] Wieczorek AJ, Rhyner C, Block LH. Isolation and characterization of an RNA-proteolipid complex associated with the malignant state in humans. Proceedings of the National Academy of Sciences of the United States of America. 1985;**82**(10):3455-3459

[59] Wieczorek AJ et al. Diagnostic and prognostic value of RNA-proteolipid in sera of patients with malignant disorders following therapy: First clinical evaluation of a novel tumor marker. Cancer Research. 1987;**47**(23):6407-6412

[60] Cocucci E, Racchetti G, Meldolesi J. Shedding microvesicles: Artefacts no more. Trends in Cell Biology. 2009;**19**(2):43-51

[61] Orozco AF, Lewis DE. Flow cytometric analysis of circulating microparticles in plasma. Cytometry. Part A. 2010;**77**(6):502-514

[62] Tsui NB, Ng EK, Lo YM. Stability of endogenous and added RNA in blood specimens, serum, and plasma. Clinical Chemistry. 2002;**48**(10):1647-1653

[63] El-Hefnawy T et al. Characterization of amplifiable, circulating RNA in plasma and its potential as a tool for cancer diagnostics. Clinical Chemistry. 2004;**50**(3):564-573

[64] Garcia JM et al. Extracellular plasma RNA from colon cancer patients is confined in a vesicle-like structure and is mRNA-enriched. RNA. 2008;**14**(7):1424-1432

[65] Lo KW et al. Analysis of cell-free Epstein-Barr virus associated RNA in the plasma of patients with nasopharyngeal carcinoma. Clinical Chemistry. 1999;**45**(8 Pt 1):1292-1294

[66] Deligezer U et al. Post-treatment circulating plasma BMP6 mRNA and H3K27 methylation levels discriminate metastatic prostate cancer from localized disease. Clinica Chimica Acta. 2010;**411**(19-20):1452-1456

[67] March-Villalba JA et al. Cell-free circulating plasma hTERT mRNA is a useful marker for prostate cancer diagnosis and is associated with poor prognosis tumor characteristics. PLoS One. 2012;**7**(8):e43470

[68] Xu W et al. Combination of circulating CXCR4 and Bmi-1 mRNA in plasma: A potential novel tumor marker for gastric cancer. Molecular Medicine Reports. 2009;**2**(5):765-771

[69] Garcia JM et al. Prognostic value of LISCH7 mRNA in plasma and tumor of colon cancer patients. Clinical Cancer Research. 2007;**13**(21):6351-6358

[70] Kang Y et al. Circulating cell-free human telomerase reverse transcriptase mRNA in plasma and its potential diagnostic and prognostic value for gastric cancer. International Journal of Clinical Oncology. 2013;**18**(3):478-486

[71] Wong SC et al. Quantification of plasma beta-catenin mRNA in colorectal cancer and adenoma patients. Clinical Cancer Research. 2004;**10**(5):1613-1617

[72] Silva JM et al. Detection of epithelial tumour RNA in the plasma of colon cancer patients is associated with advanced stages and circulating tumour cells. Gut. 2002;**50**(4):530-534

[73] Silva JM et al. Detection of epithelial messenger RNA in the plasma of breast cancer patients is associated with poor prognosis tumor characteristics. Clinical Cancer Research. 2001;**7**(9):2821-2825

[74] Chen XQ et al. Telomerase RNA as a detection marker in the serum of breast cancer patients. Clinical Cancer Research. 2000;**6**(10):3823-3826

[75] Joosse SA et al. Circulating cell-free cancer-testis MAGE-A RNA, BORIS RNA, let-7b and miR-202 in the blood of patients with breast cancer and benign breast diseases. British Journal of Cancer. 2014;**111**(5):909-917

[76] Garcia V et al. Free circulating mRNA in plasma from breast cancer patients and clinical outcome. Cancer Letters. 2008;**263**(2):312-320

[77] Miura N et al. Serum human telomerase reverse transcriptase messenger RNA as a novel tumor marker for hepatocellular carcinoma. Clinical Cancer Research. 2005;**11**(9):3205-3209

[78] Sueoka E et al. Detection of plasma hnRNP B1 mRNA, a new cancer biomarker, in lung cancer patients by quantitative real-time polymerase chain reaction. Lung Cancer. 2005;**48**(1):77-83

[79] Zhou D et al. Clinical verification of plasma messenger RNA as novel noninvasive biomarker identified through bioinformatics analysis for lung cancer. Oncotarget. 2017;**8**(27):43978-43989

[80] Zhang X et al. Detection of circulating Bmi-1 mRNA in plasma and its potential diagnostic and prognostic value for uterine cervical cancer. International Journal of Cancer. 2012;**131**(1).165-172

[81] Garcia V et al. Extracellular tumor-related mRNA in plasma of lymphoma patients and survival implications. PLoS One. 2009;**4**(12):e8173

[82] Barzon L et al. Evaluation of circulating thyroid-specific transcripts as markers of thyroid cancer relapse. International Journal of Cancer. 2004;**110**(6):914-920

[83] Hocking J et al. Liquid biopsies for liquid tumors: Emerging potential of circulating free nucleic acid evaluation for the management of hematologic malignancies. Cancer Biology & Medicine. 2016;**13**(2):215-225

[84] Lawrie CH et al. Detection of elevated levels of tumour-associated microRNAs in serum of patients with diffuse large B-cell lymphoma. British Journal of Haematology. 2008;**141**(5):672-675

[85] Kosaka N, Iguchi H, Ochiya T. Circulating microRNA in body fluid: A new potential biomarker for cancer diagnosis and prognosis. Cancer Science. 2010;**101**(10):2087-2092

[86] Larrea E et al. New concepts in cancer biomarkers: Circulating miRNAs in liquid biopsies. International Journal of Molecular Sciences. 2016;**17**(5)

[87] Singh R et al. Circulating microRNAs in cancer: Hope or hype? Cancer Letters. 2016;**381**(1):113-121

[88] Mitchell PS et al. Circulating microRNAs as stable blood-based markers for cancer detection. Proceedings of the National Academy of Sciences of the United States of America. 2008;**105**(30):10513-10518

[89] Ng EK et al. Differential expression of microRNAs in plasma of patients with colorectal cancer: A potential marker for colorectal cancer screening. Gut. 2009;**58**(10):1375-1381

[90] Roth C et al. Circulating microRNAs as blood-based markers for patients with primary and metastatic breast cancer. Breast Cancer Research. 2010;**12**(6):R90

[91] Verma AM et al. Circulating plasma microRNAs as a screening method for detection of colorectal adenomas. Lancet. 2015;**385**(Suppl 1):S100

[92] Turchinovich A, Weiz L, Burwinkel B. Extracellular miRNAs: The mystery of their origin and function. Trends in Biochemical Sciences. 2012;**37**(11):460-465

[93] Zandecki M et al. Involvement of peripheral blood cells in multiple myeloma: Chromosome changes are the rule within circulating plasma cells but not within B lymphocytes. Leukemia. 1997;**11**(7):1034-1039

[94] Oberle A et al. Monitoring multiple myeloma by next-generation sequencing of V(D)J rearrangements from circulating myeloma cells and cell-free myeloma DNA. Haematologica. 2017;**102**(6):1105-1111

[95] Rustad EH et al. Monitoring multiple myeloma by quantification of recurrent mutations in serum. Haematologica. 2017;**102**(7):1266-1272

[96] Pichiorri F et al. MicroRNAs regulate critical genes associated with multiple myeloma pathogenesis. Proceedings of the National Academy of Sciences of the United States of America. 2008;**105**(35):12885-12890

[97] Chen L et al. miR-17-92 cluster microRNAs confers tumorigenicity in multiple myeloma. Cancer Letters. 2011;**309**(1):62-70

[98] Corthals SL et al. MicroRNA signatures characterize multiple myeloma patients. Leukemia. 2011;**25**(11):1784-1789

[99] Gutierrez NC et al. Deregulation of microRNA expression in the different genetic subtypes of multiple myeloma and correlation with gene expression profiling. Leukemia. 2010;**24**(3):629-637

[100] Lionetti M et al. Identification of microRNA expression patterns and definition of a microRNA/mRNA regulatory network in distinct molecular groups of multiple myeloma. Blood. 2009;**114**(25):e20-e26

[101] Besse L et al. Circulating serum MicroRNA-130a as a novel putative marker of extramedullary myeloma. PLoS One. 2015;**10**(9):e0137294

[102] Rocci A et al. Circulating miRNA markers show promise as new prognosticators for multiple myeloma. Leukemia. 2014;**28**(9):1922-1926

[103] Navarro A et al. A serum microRNA signature associated with complete remission and progression after autologous stem-cell transplantation in patients with multiple myeloma. Oncotarget. 2015;**6**(3):1874-1883

[104] Huang JJ et al. Circulating microRNA expression is associated with genetic subtype and survival of multiple myeloma. Medical Oncology. 2012;**29**(4):2402-2408

[105] Kubiczkova L et al. Circulating serum microRNAs as novel diagnostic and prognostic biomarkers for multiple myeloma and monoclonal gammopathy of undetermined significance. Haematologica. 2014;**99**(3):511-518

[106] Jones CI et al. Identification of circulating microRNAs as diagnostic biomarkers for use in multiple myeloma. British Journal of Cancer. 2012;**107**(12):1987-1996

[107] Hao M et al. Low serum miR-19a expression as a novel poor prognostic indicator in multiple myeloma. International Journal of Cancer. 2015;**136**(8):1835-1844

[108] Yoshizawa S et al. Downregulated plasma miR-92a levels have clinical impact on multiple myeloma and related disorders. Blood Cancer Journal. 2012;**2**(1):e53

[109] Jung SH et al. Circulating microRNA expressions can predict the outcome of lenalidomide plus low-dose dexamethasone treatment in patients with refractory/relapsed multiple myeloma. Haematologica. 2017;**102**(11):e456-e459

[110] Qu X et al. Circulating microRNA 483-5p as a novel biomarker for diagnosis survival prediction in multiple myeloma. Medical Oncology. 2014;**31**(10):219

[111] Manier S et al. Prognostic role of circulating exosomal miRNAs in multiple myeloma. Blood. 2017;**129**(17):2429-2436

[112] Zhang L et al. A panel of circulating miRNAs as diagnostic biomarkers for screening multiple myeloma: A systematic review and meta-analysis. International Journal of Laboratory Hematology. 2016;**38**(6):589-599

[113] Rawstron AC et al. Minimal residual disease assessed by multiparameter flow cytometry in multiple myeloma: Impact on outcome in the Medical Research Council myeloma IX study. Journal of Clinical Oncology. 2013;**31**(20):2540-2547

[114] Rawstron AC et al. Minimal residual disease in myeloma by flow cytometry: Independent prediction of survival benefit per log reduction. Blood. 2015;**125**(12):1932-1935

[115] Martinez-Lopez J et al. Prognostic value of deep sequencing method for minimal residual disease detection in multiple myeloma. Blood. 2014;**123**(20):3073-3079

[116] Martinez-Lopez J et al. Analytical and clinical validation of a novel in-house deep-sequencing method for minimal residual disease monitoring in a phase II trial for multiple myeloma. Leukemia. 2017;**31**(6):1446-1449

[117] Paiva B et al. Phenotypic and genomic analysis of multiple myeloma minimal residual disease tumor cells: A new model to understand chemoresistance. Blood. 2016;**127**(15):1896-1906

[118] Paiva B et al. Is this the time to introduce minimal residual disease in multiple myeloma clinical practice? Clinical Cancer Research. 2015;**21**(9):2001-2008

[119] Paiva B, van Dongen JJ, Orfao A. New criteria for response assessment: Role of minimal residual disease in multiple myeloma. Blood. 2015;**125**(20):3059-3068

[120] Huhn S et al. Circulating tumor cells as a biomarker for response to therapy in multiple myeloma patients treated within the GMMG-MM5 trial. Bone Marrow Transplantation. 2017;**52**(8):1194-1198

[121] Garcia-Murillas I et al. Mutation tracking in circulating tumor DNA predicts relapse in early breast cancer. Science Translational Medicine. 2015;**7**(302):302ra133

[122] Roschewski M et al. Circulating tumour DNA and CT monitoring in patients with untreated diffuse large B-cell lymphoma: A correlative biomarker study. The Lancet Oncology. 2015;**16**(5):541-549

[123] Fong SL et al. Comparison of 7 methods for extracting cell-free DNA from serum samples of colorectal cancer patients. Clinical Chemistry. 2009;**55**(3):587-589

[124] Newman AM et al. An ultrasensitive method for quantitating circulating tumor DNA with broad patient coverage. Nature Medicine. 2014;**20**(5):548-554

[125] Schwarzenbach H, Hoon DS, Pantel K. Cell-free nucleic acids as biomarkers in cancer patients. Nature Reviews. Cancer. 2011;**11**(6):426-437

[126] cobas EGFR Mutation Test v2. 2016. http://www.fda.gov/Drugs/InformationOnDrugs/ApprovedDrugs/ucm504540.htm

[127] Siravegna G et al. Integrating liquid biopsies into the management of cancer. Nature Reviews. Clinical Oncology. 2017;**14**(9):531-548

Chapter 5

Quantitative-Morphological and Cytological Analyses in Leukemia

Cecília Lantos, Steven M. Kornblau and
Amina A. Qutub

Additional information is available at the end of the chapter

http://dx.doi.org/10.5772/intechopen.73675

Abstract

Leukemia, a blood cancer originating in the bone marrow, presents as a heterogeneous disease with highly variable survival rates. Leukemia is classified into major types based on the rate of cancerous cell growth and cell lineage: chronic or acute and myeloid or lymphoid leukemia. Histological and cytological analysis of the peripheral blood and the bone marrow can classify these major leukemia categories. However, histological analyses of patient biopsies and cytological microscopic assessment of blood and bone marrow smears are insufficient to diagnose leukemia subtypes and to direct therapy. Hence, more expensive and time-consuming diagnostic tools routinely complement histological-cytological analysis during a patient's diagnosis. To extract more accurate and detailed information from patient tissue samples, digital pathology is emerging as a powerful tool to enhance biopsy- and smear-based decisions. Furthermore, digital pathology methods integrated with advances in machine learning enable new diagnostic features from leukemia patients' histological and cytological slides and optimize patient classification, thus providing a cheaper, more robust, and faster diagnostic tool than current standards. This review summarizes emerging approaches to automatically diagnose leukemia from morphological and cytological-histological analyses.

Keywords: blood cancer, acute leukemia, machine learning, digital pathology, classification, supervised learning

1. Introduction

Leukemia is a very heterogeneous cancer that arises from the combination of many genetic and epigenetic mutation events, all of which alter hematopoiesis [1–3]. Hematopoiesis is the proliferation of blood cells in the bone marrow (BM). Blood cells differentiate in the BM and, then, when mature, spread out to the peripheral blood (PB) system. In normal circumstances, the multipotent progenitor hematopoietic stem cells in the bone marrow reproduce and commit to differentiate into common myeloid or lymphoid progenitor cells. Myeloid and lymphoid progenitor cells differentiate into two main cell lineages containing unipotential precursor cells. Each precursor matures through multiple stages to become a red blood cell (RBC), a platelet, or a white blood cell (WBC) type. Myeloid cells consist of RBCs, platelets, segmented neutrophils, monocytes, eosinophils, basophils, and mast cells; lymphoid cells are T and B lymphocytes, dendritic cells, or natural killer (NK) cells (**Figure 1**) [1, 4].

Malignant proliferation in the myeloid or lymphoid cell linage causes myeloid or lymphoid leukemia. The diseased cells stop maturing, halt differentiation, and then accumulate, hence blocking the development of healthy progenitor cells. Cell maturation in chronic leukemia is blocked at a later stage, and it has a longer course of development compared to acute leukemia, where lineage proliferation is arrested at an early stage of differentiation leading to a very aggressive, fast-growing disease [4, 5].

Based on these two major differences, myeloid or lymphoid and chronic or acute, four major leukemia types are distinguished: acute myeloid leukemia (AML), acute lymphoid leukemia (ALL), chronic myeloid leukemia (CML), and chronic lymphoid leukemia (CLL). Each type has a distinguishable morphology, and diagnosis is based on histological analysis of each patient's bone marrow biopsy and cytological microscopic assessment of bone marrow smear or peripheral blood smear [5, 6].

However, full classification requires more refined categories than the four major leukemia types, and modern classification also includes mutation analysis, cytogenetics, and flow cytometry data. Therefore, older morphological-based classification systems (French-American-British (FAB)) cannot be fully matched with the World Health Organization (WHO) scheme, which utilizes all of these features. The FAB classification system is predominantly used for the 30–40% of AML cases that are not otherwise specified, while in special cases, a morphological

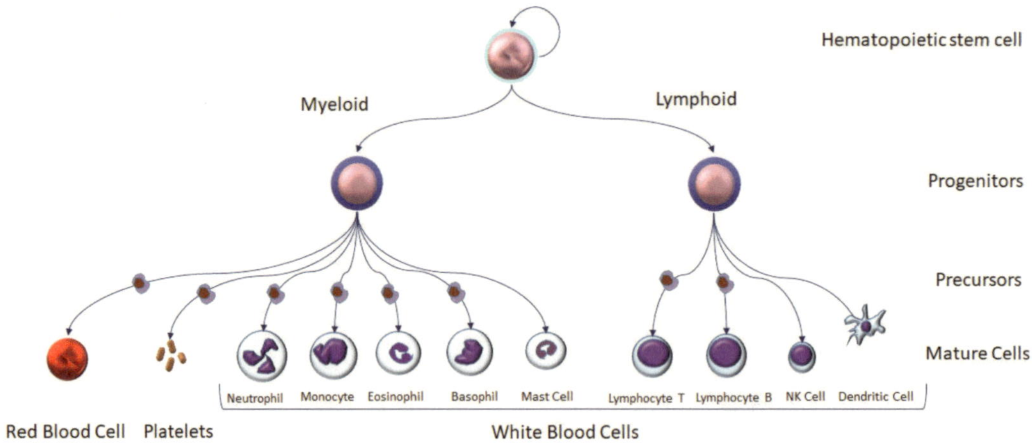

Figure 1. Schematic chart of hematopoiesis.

pattern can be matched to an individual gene mutation or clinical criteria (e.g., AML t(8;21)(q22; q22.1)/RUNX1-RUNX1T1 or AML with myelodysplasia-related changes) [7]. To enable more personalized therapy, diagnosis and therapy selection require the analysis of histology and cytology in combination with all clinical and genetic data of the patient including cytogenetics, gene mutation analysis, and gene expression data obtained from flow cytometry [5, 6, 8, 9].

The ancillary diagnostic tests are costly and time-consuming, currently often requiring a week or more, compared to the histological-cytological analysis, which can typically be performed in a day. The delay in diagnosis can lead to delays in treatment, seriously impacting patients suffering from acute leukemia. A faster, less time-consuming, and more precise automated histology- and cytology-based diagnostic tool would facilitate diagnosis and personalized, rapid treatment [10].

Due to the development of whole slide imaging (WSI), which yields large digital images of an entire tissue sample, patients' histological-cytological data are stored in an image bank format to allow easy access to study their pathology. A digital tissue bank fosters the computational, automated analysis of the histological-cytological images [11–14]. This review describes possible solutions to integrate morphometrics obtained from images of biopsy and smear samples with standard clinical covariates to optimize diagnosis and direct therapy for leukemia.

2. Morphological diagnosis in leukemia

The current major standard diagnostic test in leukemia is histological-cytological analysis. This includes basic light microscopy of routinely stained bone marrow biopsy, bone marrow smear, and peripheral blood smear.

Diagnosis from the smear is established based on the complete blood count and differential count (the proportion of specific cell types in the specimen). A biopsy can confirm the percentage of the specific cell types in the smear. Normal PB smear contains mature cells and up to 1–2% immature cells. The presence of immature cells at a significantly higher percentage leads to the diagnosis of leukemia. Leukemia in the BM smear is detected based on the irregular proportion of specific immature cells and their morphological alterations [1].

Based on abnormally high proportions of specific blood cells and morphological dysplasia in the biopsy and smear specimen, the French-American-British (FAB) system describes a morphologically based classification for acute leukemia. AML subtypes are divided into eight different groups (M0–M7) and ALL subtypes into three different groups (L1–L3). Such classification system for chronic leukemia is less precise, where the subtypes are overlapping [5, 9].

Although the FAB classification system is based on cellular appearance, some immature cells do not have distinguishable morphological characteristics. Immunophenotyping confirms the diagnosis, especially in ALL T- and B-cell lineage and AML minimally differentiated (M0) and AML megakaryoblastic (M7) subtypes [5].

As a result, histology and cytology are major diagnostic tools: however, their current prognostic potential is limited, as the majority of genetic events do not have known, defining morphological characteristics [5, 10]. Thanks to emerging computer technologies, a pathologist's qualitative decision can be supported by an automated quantitative decision tool. Morphometrics of the pathological slides can both provide new diagnostic information not visible to the naked eye and improve the prognostic ability of histological-cytological analyses [15, 16].

3. Digital cytology analysis

Statistical analysis of cells and cellular features can guide a pathologist's diagnosis of leukemia. The number of RBCs, WBCs, and platelets, the proportion of specific immature and mature cells, and more detailed morphological features recognized by automated WSI can all help direct a diagnosis. Digital image analysis of BM biopsy has been applied to study relapse in AML [17, 18]. The focus of most prior studies has been recognition of the acute leukemia FAB subtypes or differentiation of acute and chronic leukemia from the PB and BM smears. While PB and BM smears can differ in the type and maturation of their cells, the quantitative process to recognize the cell types and extract morphometric information is similar. We describe it below:

Following steps a pathologist would take, computer-based digital pathology aims to detect, localize, and recognize the specific cell type under study (**Figure 2**). An acquired image is preprocessed through image enhancement steps; then, cells are detected, and cell boundaries are traced out using segmentation algorithms for morphometric analysis.

Processing steps to automate the analysis of leukemia smear images are shown in **Figure 2**. A whole slide image (WSI) of a Wright-Giemsa-stained bone marrow smear is shown in **Figure 2a**. This is a typical smear image annotated by a pathologist. The Wright-Giemsa-stained image reveals RBCs as smaller pink cells without nuclei (either distributed as single cells or clustered) and a few WBCs of different sizes with dark purple nuclei. Notably, image acquisition techniques, staining methods, and digitization protocols can differ in each laboratory. Furthermore, environmental effects can introduce artifacts and degrade the quality of the image. Image preprocessing steps can improve the image quality and correct for differences in protocols and in illumination. Methods of image correction techniques include illumination

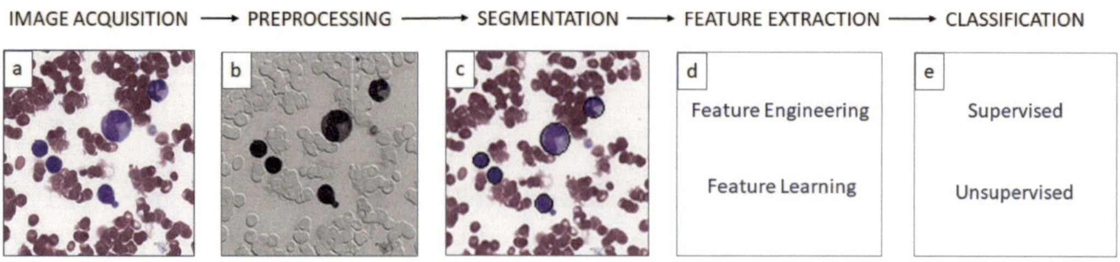

Figure 2. Image processing pipeline (a–e: Image from Carlos Bueso-Ramos, MD, PhD, MD Anderson Cancer Center).

normalization, color or stain correction for image enhancement, contrast enhancement and smoothing, contrast stretching, and histogram equalization [19–21].

Leukemia is detected based on the number, type, and proportion of various cell types in the blood. Segmentation algorithms enable identification of individual cells from smear images (**Figure 2b**); these algorithms can distinguish overlapping cells from individual cells in order to extract cell-based features and can also divide each WBC into its components: cell membrane, nucleus, and cytoplasm (**Figure 2c**) [19, 21–37]. Following segmentation, metrics can be extracted from the WBCs and their subcellular components (cell size, nuclear size, etc.).

4. Quantification of cytology using machine learning

To computationally classify tissue types from smear images, identified cells and tissues in the images have to be transformed into a vector of features. Conventional machine learning algorithms typically utilize a domain-specific approach to classify cell and tissue types based on a series of handcrafted features. These algorithms extract metrics from images based on a human engineering process that requires domain knowledge [38, 39].

Features of the smear sample can be extracted from an individual cell in the image or across the entire slide. Once a WBC is segmented within the image, features are extracted either from the whole WBC or separately from the nucleus and cytoplasm. The major discriminating cellular characteristics to classify WBCs are (a) geometric features such as shape (e.g., roundness) and size (e.g., nucleus-cytoplasm size ratio); (b) color features; (c) texture features such as density, granularity, and Fourier descriptors for texture quantification calculated by the two-dimensional Fourier transform; and (d) irregularity or boundary roughness measured by fractal dimension [10, 23, 33, 35, 40–49]. Although the analysis at the single cell level provides useful information, it is not sufficient for the diagnosis of a very heterogeneous disorder such as leukemia. In addition to single cell data, characteristics of multicellular groups need to be studied [1]. New studies have extended cell-based morphometric analysis to distinguish major leukemia types and subtypes (**Table 1**).

The common characteristics in these studies are general steps of the image processing pipeline: preprocessing, segmentation, feature engineering, and supervised classification (**Table 1**). They discriminate cancerous vs. healthy tissue, AML vs. ALL, CL vs. AL, or AML and ALL subtypes. The main differences across the various studies are the choice of the specific engineered features and the choice of the classification method as illustrated below.

Most of the digital pathology studies of leukemia analyze PB. A healthy blood smear is distinguished from a leukemic smear if one or more immature cells are present. This can be determined from the nucleus structure or from whole cell characteristics. Discriminating features that classify healthy tissue, AML and ALL in the PB are extracted from the cell nucleus. BM is more heterogeneous than PB, and features of BM images are extracted from the whole cells or separately from the nuclei and the cytoplasm. Commonly used features include texture-based metrics and morphology. Texture is based on the spatial variation of the gray-level pixel intensities which can be characterized by their homogeneity, energy, and correlation, among other metrics represented in the gray-level co-occurrence matrix (GLCM). Shape is based on geometrical parameters such as area, perimeter, compactness, minor axis,

Reference	Leukemia type	Extracted features	Classification
Reta et al. 2015 [58]	**BM (Bone marrow):** AML vs ALL, M2 vs M3 vs M5 vs vs L1 vs L2	**Cell + nucleus + cytoplasm:** Shape: area, perimeter, circularity, width, Length, elongation, major axis, minor axis, eccentricity, extent, equivalent diameter, Euler number, Convex area Size Ratio: Nucleus/Cytoplasm area, Nucleus/Cell area and perimeter Color/Pixel Intensity Statistics: Mode, Mean, Standard deviation, Variance, Sum Texture: Homogeneity, Contrast, Correlation, Energy, Entropy 10 Eigenvalues (PCA) of R, G, B channel of RGB image and of gray image	k-nearest neighbor (kNN), Random Forest (RF), Simple Logistic (SL), Support Vector Machines (SMV), Random Committee (RC)
Kazemi et al. 2016 [57]	**PB (Peripheral blood):** AML vs Healthy, M2 vs M3 vs M4 vs vs M5 vs (M1+M6+M7)	**Nucleus:** Shape: Area, Permieter, Elongation, Major and Minor axis, Solidity, Eccentricity, Form Factor, Compactness, Size Ratio: Nuclues/Cytoplasm Color: Mean, Standard deviation, Variance Texture: Energy, Entropy, Contrast, Correlation, Homogeneity Fractal: Hausdorff dimension (HD) Nucleus boundary Irregularity	Support vector machine (SVM)
Madhukar et al. 2012 [54]	**PB:** AML vs Healthy	**Nucleus:** Texture: Gray-Level Co-occurrence Matrix: Contrast, Homogeneity, Energy, Entropy, Correlation **Image Slide:** Fractal: HD dimension	Support vector machine (SVM)
Agaian et al. 2014 [53]	**PB:** AML vs Healthy	**Nucleus:** Shape: Area, Parameter, Compactness, Minor and Major Axis, Eccentricity, FormFactor, Elongation, Solidity Color: Standard deviation, Mean, Energy Texture: GLCM: Homogeneity, Contrast, Correlation Fractal: HD dimension **Image Slide:** Fractal: HD dimension	Support Vector Machine (SVM)

Reference	Leukemia type	Extracted features	Classification
Vaghela et al. 2016 [62]	**PB:** CLL vs CML	**Nucleus:** Roundness + Count	Not applied
Jacob et al. 2016 [50]	**PB:** AML vs ALL vs Healthy	**Nucleus:** Shape: Area, Parameter, Compactness, Minor and Major Axis, Eccentricity, FormFactor, Elongation, Solidity Texture: GLCM: Homogeneity, Energy, Contrast, Correlation Fractal: HD dimension	Support Vector Machine (SVM)
Supardi et al. 2012 [55]	**PB:** ALL vs AML	**Cell:** Shape: Size: Area, Radius, Perimeter Second order central moment Color: std and mean variance of Red, Green, Blue and intensities of RGB color	k-Nearest-Neighbor (kNN)
Gumble et al. 2017 [51]	**PB:** ALL vs Healthy	**Nucleus & cytoplasm (Binary gray):** Shape/Texture: Area, Total White Cells, Total Black Pixels, Perimeter, Eccentricity, Solidity, Form Factor, Bounding Box	k-Nearest-Neighbor (kNN)
Harun et al. 2011 [56]	**PB:** AML vs ALL	**Cell & cytoplasm & nucleus:** Shape: Area, Nucleus/ Cytoplasm Size Ratio **Cell & Nucleus:** Shape: Perimeter	Hybrid Multilayer Perceptron Neural Network (HMLP NN)
Escalante et al. 2012 [59]	**BM:** ALL vs AML, L1 vs L2, M2 vs (M3+M5), M3 vs (M2+M5), M5 vs (M2+M3), M1 vs M3 vs M5, L1 vs L2 vs M1 vs vs M3 vs M6	**Cell & nucleus:** Shape: Area, Perimeter, Circularity, Width, Height, Elongation, Major and Minor Axis, Eccentricity, Extension, Diameter, Euler number, Convex number, Solidity Pixel intensity Statistics: Mode, Mean, Standard deviation, Variance, IOD, avg. IOD Texture: Entropy, Contrast, Correlation, Energy, Homogeneity Eigenvalues (PCA) - R,G,B, grayscale **Cytoplasm:** Shape: Area Pixel Intensity Statistics: Mode, Mean, Standard deviation, Variance Eigenvalues (PCA) - R,G,B, grayscale	Ensemble Particle Swarm Model Selection (ESPMS)
Mohapatra et al. 2014 [52]	**PB:** ALL vs Healthy	**Nucleus & cytoplasm& cell:** Shape: Area **Nucleus & Cytoplasm:** Color: mean intensity of R,G,B and Hue, Saturation, Lightness components Texture: Wavelet	Ensemble of Classifiers (EOC), Naive Bayesian (NB), K-nearest neighbor (KNN), Multilayer Perceptron (MLP NN), Radial Basis Functional Network

Reference	Leukemia type	Extracted features	Classification
		coefficients and GLCM statistics: Contrast, Correlation, Energy, Homogeneity, Entropy **Nucleus:** Shape: Form Factor, Roundness, Compactness, Elongation, Perimeter Color: mean intensity of R,G,B and Hue, Saturation, Lightness components Texture: Fourier transform: Mean, variance, skewness, kurtosis of the frequency components Boundary roughness: Fractal HD dimension Contour signature: Variance, skewness, kurtosis (center-contour)	(RBFN), Support Vector Machine (SVM)
Mohapatra thesis 2013 [61]	**PB:**L1 vs L2 vs L3	**Nucleus & Cytoplasm & Cell:** Shape: Area **Nucleus & Cell:** Shape: Size ratio: Nucleus / Cell **Nucleus & Cytoplasm:** Color: RGB and HSV components **Cytoplasm:** Vacuole count **Nucleus:** Shape: Form Factor, Roundness, Compactness, Elongation, Perimeter Nucleus Indentation, Nucleoli count, Texture: Frourier descriptor, Wavelet and Haralick coefficients (GLCM statistics): Contrast, Correlation, Energy, Homogeneity, Entropy	Ensemble of classifiers (EOC), Naive Bayesian (NB), K-nearest neighbor (KNN), Multilayer Perceptron (MLP NN), Radial Basis Functional Network (RBFN), Support Vector Machine (SVM)
Mohapatra thesis 2013 [61]	**PB:** ALL vs AML	**Nucleus & cytoplasm & cell** Shape: Size **Cytoplasm:** Color: RGB and HSV components Texture: Coarseness Intensity and shape: Auer Rodes as Cytoplasmic Holes **Nucleus:** Nucleoli count Texture: Frourier descriptor, Wavelet and Haralick coefficients (GLCM statistics): Contrast, Correlation, Energy, Homogeneity, Entropy	Ensemble of Classifiers (EOC), Naive Bayesian (NB), K-nearest neighbor (KNN), Multilayer Perceptron (MLP NN), Radial Basis Functional Network (RBFN), Support Vector Machine (SVM)

Table 1. Leukemia subtype classification.

major axis, eccentricity, form factor, elongation, and solidity. Fractal or Hausdorff dimension (HD) represents the nucleus boundary roughness (Jacob and Mundackal) [50].

4.1. Examples of digital pathology for leukemia

To provide examples of digital pathology's impact in leukemia classification, we summarize here a few of the recent studies. In one study, ALL cells were distinguished from healthy PB cells from shape and texture features extracted from the nucleus and cytoplasm (Gumble and Rode). These features included area, total white blood cells, total black pixels, perimeter, eccentricity, solidity, form factor, and bounding box parameters [51]. In another study, Mohapatra et al. added color and the Fourier descriptor as a cell-based nuclear feature to the shape, fractal, and texture parameters to distinguish ALL from healthy lymphoblasts/lymphocytes [52].

What literally do these features mean? In the Mohapatra et al. study, color features of a cell were calculated from the mean intensity of the nucleus color components in RGB or HSV color space and from a grayscale intensity map. In the case of RGB images, the mean intensity of the red, green, and blue channels and, in the case of HSV images, the mean intensity of the hue, saturation, and lightness components were computed. The same color features were calculated for the cytoplasm. The Fourier descriptors were the mean, variance, skewness, and kurtosis of the texture in the frequency domain. The fractal/HD of the nucleus boundary roughness was considered, as was the variance, skewness, and kurtosis computed between the cell's center and each contour point. Texture features from the cytoplasm included wavelet coefficients and metrics derived from the GLCM including contrast, correlation, energy, homogeneity, and entropy values. The area was calculated for the nucleus, cytoplasm, and the whole cell [52].

In addition to determining leukemia from cell-based features, AML can be distinguished from healthy tissue by extracting whole tissue−/slide-based features as illustrated in two other studies (Madhukar et al., Agaian et al.) [53, 54].

Furthermore, AML can also be distinguished from ALL through comparing cellular features in patient smears, as shown by Jacob and Mundackal [50], Supardi et al. [55], and Harun et al. [56]. Jacob et al. and Supardi et al. used cellular metrics based on texture, shape, and Hausdorff dimension, while Harun et al. classified the two leukemias by cell and nuclear perimeters, areas of the cytoplasm and whole cells, and nucleus-cytoplasm ratio [56].

More specifically, AML and ALL subtypes have been discriminated based on cell-based features in three different studies. To classify AML subtypes, Kazemi et al. predicted five AML groups (M2, M3, M4, M5, and all the remaining subtypes (M0, M1, M6, M7) considered as one group) based on handcrafted morphological features from blood microscopic images. The features used were extracted from cells' nuclei: irregularity, Hausdorff dimension, shape, color, and texture features complemented by the nucleus-cytoplasm ratio. The same set of features allowed more accurate discrimination of healthy tissue vs. AML tissue than AML tissue vs. ALL tissue [57]. Reta et al. performed a similar analysis which discriminated L1, L2, M3, M3, and M5 subtypes in ALL and AML based on cellular features, with nucleus features proving to be the most discriminative [58]. An earlier study (Escalante et al.) was also able to discriminate multiple leukemia tissue types from the BM: ALL vs. AML, L1 vs. L2, M2 vs. M3 + M5, M3 vs. M2 + M5, M5 vs. M2 + M3, M1 vs. M3 vs. M5, and L1 vs. L2 vs. M1 vs. M3 vs. M5 [59]. However, in the latter study, there was no significant difference in model performance using features extracted from the nucleus and cytoplasm vs. the whole cell.

This contradicts other studies that suggest classification based on subcellular morphometry improves AML [60] and ALL [61] subtype recognition. In particular, these groups found that color and shape information in the cytoplasmic holes, which indicate vacuoles, and color and shape information on the nucleus, which indicate nucleoli, can reveal the presence of Auer rods discriminating AML from ALL where Auer rods are absent [61].

In addition to the large number of publications characterizing acute forms of leukemia, studies (Vaghela et al.) have suggested measurements of WBC roundness and counts can discriminate chronic myeloid vs. chronic lymphoid leukemia [62].

4.2. Classification methods

4.2.1. Traditional machine learning methods

Support vector machine (SVM) is a common classification method in leukemia (Jacob et al. [50]; Agaian et al. [53]; Kazemi et al. [57]; Madhukar et al. [54]). However, other methods (Supardi et al., Gumble and Rode) have been applied with success to classify AML and ALL histology and cytology images including k-nearest neighbor classifiers [51, 55], a hybrid multilayer neural network (HMLNN) (Harun et al.) [56], and an ensemble particle swarm model selection method (EPSMS) (Escalante et al.) [59]. Alternatively, Kumar et al. suggested using a shallow neural network (NN) classifier after the AML slide is processed using wavelet transformation [37]. Other groups (Mohapatra et al.; Reta et al.; Escalante et al.) have compared multiple classifiers on leukemia image datasets and found that depending on the target, different classification methods appear to be the optimal solution [52, 58, 59].

When a small amount of data is available, conventional feature engineering-based machine learning algorithms provide fairly accurate predictions [39]. The accuracy of feature engineering proposed models depends on the distinct leukemia databases studied, the number and quality of the images, and the image acquisition mode; these require different data preprocessing steps. These methods are mainly based on supervised classification of leukemia subtypes. When the set of quantitative morphological features of the leukemia subtype is trained on a labeled dataset, then classifiers have been able to predict the four major leukemia types or the FAB classes applied to a test set. In case of insufficient number of training samples, Kasmin et al. proposed reinforcement learning to classify ALL, AML, CLL, and CML from PB cellular nucleus' geometrical, texture, color, and statistical parameters [63].

Although these previous studies found new morphological features from the digitalized leukemia patient histology slides, and were successfully able to identify the major leukemia types and M0–M7 and L1–L3 subtypes, morphological features from the leukemia cells were not correlated with non-morphological information such as genetic mutations and clinical data. The morphological classification methods currently are not sufficient to recognize the majority of the underlying molecular abnormalities and cannot be used to direct therapy. In addition, the subtype groups' underlying genetic patterns are not unique per subtype. Should morphological classification match genetic backgrounds, this could help speed up the diagnosis process. One study attempted to correlate morphological quantitative features in order to classify ALL lymphoblasts into the WHO subtypes and compare the results with flow cytometry analysis. To this aim, an unsupervised feature selection method was applied, and an optimal subset of the features was extracted to match the WHO classification [61]. This study and others that follow are helping pave the way for increasingly sophisticated means of classifying leukemia by images that enable incorporation of genetic and epigenetic details. Advances in computational methods are too, as the next section describes.

4.2.2. Deep learning methods

Although engineered feature-based conventional machine learning algorithms provide fairly accurate predictions, they do not reach the capability of human perception. The feature engineering process requires defining a carefully chosen set of features. This is a laborious process, and the feature parameters are very sensitive to the specific training set from where they were extracted. Due to this rigidity, a conventional machine learning algorithm likely could not be applied to a second dataset without parameter tweaking. To overcome these limitations, deep learning algorithms trained on large amounts of data can extract generalized features to perform human-level pattern recognition [64, 65].

When a large amount of data is available, for identifying morphological features in leukemia, a deep learning approach can be applied. Deep learning can self-discover new, hierarchical features in images (feature learning) allowing better pattern recognition for classification. These features are identified without human knowledge, and the learning approach is called "domain-agonistic," where the computational system alone is able to distinguish distinct tissue types in any type of cancer. Today, with the increasing computing capacity of modern computers and the availability of big data storage, huge amounts of data can now be extracted and analyzed to identify key features for classification. This has enabled deep learning methods to outperform previous conventional machine learning approaches and to achieve higher accuracy [39, 66].

Deep learning is the extension of conventional, artificial neural networks where, instead of a single-layered network, a multilayered connected network processes input data and generates output. The network design is dependent on the input dataset and classification target. For pattern classification problems, convolutional neural networks (CNNs) are the ideally suited network design. The network learns from the example images fed to it and extracts hierarchical features automatically layer by layer (e.g., from low-level features like edges to higher-level features such as the cell, tissue, and then organ) without expert human intervention while retaining highly expressive power (**Figure 3**) [65–67].

The input of the CNN is a series of images, cropped from the whole slide image, and the images are processed in batch. For WBC classification, one cropped image contains one whole cell. Contrary to the cell-based analysis, for tissue classification, the images are slide-based, so the features are learned directly from the spatial pattern. The image size and the number of images fed to the network should be chosen carefully, and the variety of images should represent the

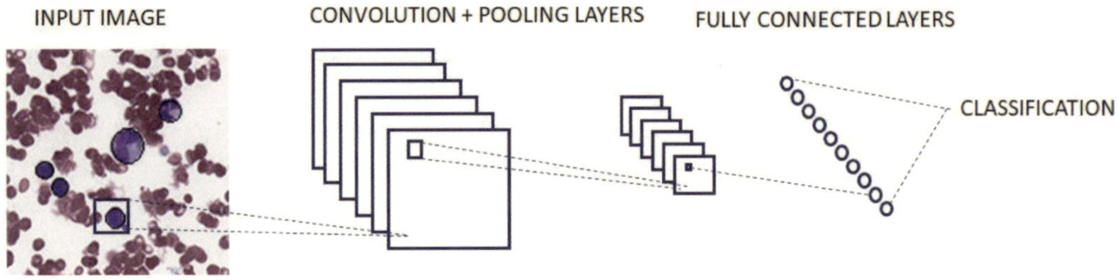

Figure 3. Feature learning for classification.

variability of the tissue type. Grayscale images are two-dimensional: width and height. Color images have a third dimension, depth, representing the RGB color channels [38, 65, 67, 68].

Once the set of images is defined and labeled, feature maps are created by sliding a series of filters representing shapes, textures, or colors over the input image (convolution), thus identifying local dependencies. The filters representing the features are learned during the training process through backpropagation and a gradient descent algorithm. After convolution, an activation process introduces nonlinear properties to the linear convolution to improve the model accuracy and to avoid overfitting. The convolutional layer then is down-sampled (pooling). This is successively repeated as many times as necessary according to the hierarchical complexity of the image. The last feature map is then flattened into a one-dimensional vector to feed a fully connected layer for neural network (NN) classification. The NN classification process can be replaced by a different classification scheme such as an SVM or random forest [38, 65, 67, 68].

Convolutional neural networks are ideally suited for pattern recognition and medical image analysis. In fact, CNNs have been successfully applied to feature learning to detect and diagnose a number of different cancers, including leukemia cells. Deep learning methods have been used for white blood cell detection and classification [68], lymphocyte detection [38], and lymphoma subtype classification [38] by identifying three subtypes of lymphoma: chronic lymphocytic leukemia (CLL), follicular lymphoma (FL), and mantle cell lymphoma (MCL). It also has been applied to the analysis of ALL cellular images to classify ALL subtype histopathology [67, 69].

Although the current research in pattern recognition is dominated by the supervised deep learning approach, the unsupervised approach is expected to provide breakthrough results in the near future, and extensive research is currently ongoing to optimize these algorithms [65, 66].

5. Conclusions and future outlook

Standard leukemia diagnosis and therapy are currently based on morphological classification of patients' bone marrow smears and biopsies, peripheral blood smears, and molecular and cytogenetic analyses to identify genetic abnormalities. However, morphological and genetic classification analysis is insufficient to fully predict appropriate response to therapy, while emerging nonstandard methods to improve and personalize leukemia classification can be expensive and time-consuming. Digital pathology is emerging as a powerful, inexpensive tool to enhance biopsy- and smear-based decisions.

This review discussed how computational cytology can help improve leukemia diagnosis by enhancing pathologist smear-based decisions and improve leukemia diagnosis with automated, biologically meaningful pattern recognition. Techniques summarized in this review extract quantitative imaging features from stained bone marrow and peripheral blood smear samples to detect and classify leukemia. To identify morphological features, conventional machine learning approaches have been broadly applied to classify leukemia types and subtypes based on feature engineering. However, to acquire a new set of morphological features in leukemia, a deep learning approach would provide higher accuracy.

For most of the cases reviewed in this chapter, the image processing pipeline implements a supervised classification scheme, where the morphometric features are extracted from a set of labeled data (ALL vs. AML, FAB, M1, etc.) and then are validated on a test dataset. In future studies, supervised morphological analysis can be complemented with unsupervised classification schemes such as unbiased clustering. This approach could reveal whether entirely new classification schemes should be implemented for ALL or AML, independent from known acute or chronic leukemia subtype morphological classification. It also could potentially reveal common underlying genetic or proteomic patterns.

Emerging omics analysis methods are determining protein expression signatures for leukemia patients; however, these new processes can be time and labor intensive. To determine genetic information and protein signature membership rapidly and without the time delay required for proteomic-based signature assignment, advances in digital pathology offer potentially exciting, inexpensive, rapid alternatives. If morphological surrogates that reliably correlate with clinical, genetic, or proteomic features, either individually or in combinatorial patterns, can be identified directly from histology images, then this could significantly speed up leukemia diagnosis, reduce the cost of the diagnostic workup, optimize the assignment of patients to a particular therapy, and potentially uncover new pathways for drug targeting.

Cell metrics can be predefined manually, and often metrics are those known to be pertinent to leukemia cells. These algorithms, which together are employed as part of a "feature engineering process," extract metrics from images based on features of cells (e.g., size or nucleus shape). Using a supervised classification approach, the metrics are extracted from predefined leukemia subtypes. As an example, a set of quantitative morphological features defining a leukemia subtype are trained on a labeled dataset according to the FAB morphological classes, and the resulting developed classifier is then used to predict the leukemia subtypes on a test set.

In the unsupervised classification approach, new clusters of leukemia subtypes are created from the engineered features. Contrary to the feature engineering process, learning algorithms self-discover features representative of leukemia cell types (feature learning) where features are learned from annotated (supervised) or unannotated (unsupervised) data (**Figure 2**).

Acknowledgements

This work is supported by Gulf Coast Consortia, Computational Cancer Biology Fellowship, and funded by CPRIT (Cancer Prevention and Research Institute of Texas) Grant Number RP170593.

Author details

Cecília Lantos[1]*, Steven M. Kornblau[2] and Amina A. Qutub[1]

*Address all correspondence to: cecilia.lantos@rice.edu

1 Department of Bioengineering, Rice University, Houston, TX, USA

2 Department of Leukemia and Department of Stem Cell Transplantation, The University of Texas, Houston, TX, USA

References

[1] Rodak BF, Carr JH. Clinical Hematology Atlas. St. Louis, Missouri, USA: Elsevier Saunders; 2013

[2] Li S, Mason C, Melnick A. Genetic and epigenetic heterogeneity in acute myeloid leukemia. Current Opinion in Genetics & Development. 2016;**36**:100-106

[3] Guièze R, Wu CJ. Genomic and epigenomic heterogeneity in chronic lymphocytic leukemia. Blood. 2015;**126**(4):445-453

[4] Shafat MS, Gnaneswaran B, Bowles KM, Rushworth SA. Review. The bone marrow microenvironment – Home of the leukemic blasts. Blood Reviews. 2017;**31**:277-286

[5] Szczepanski T, Velden VHJ v d, Dongen JJ v. Classification systems for acute and chronic leukaemias. Best Practice & Research Clinical Haematology. 2003;**16**(4):561-582

[6] Cotelingam JD, Article R. Bone marrow biopsy: Interpretive guidelines for the surgical pathologist. Advances in Anatomic Pathology. 2003;**10**(1):8-26

[7] Swerdlow SH, Campo E, Harris NL, Jaffe ES, Pileri S, Stein H, Thiele J. WHO Classification of Tumours of Haematopoietic and Lymphoid Tissues. WHO Classification of Tumours: WHO Press, The International Agency for Research on Cancer; 2017

[8] Rose D, Haferlach T, Schnittger S, Perglerová K, Kern W, Haferlach C. Subtype-specific patterns of molecular mutations in acute myeloid leukemia. Leukemia. 2017;**31**:11-17

[9] Pui C-H. Current Clinical Oncology: Treatment of Acute Leukemias: New Directions for Clinical Research. Totowa, NJ, USA: Humana Press Inc.; 2003

[10] Tuzel O, Yang L, Meer P, Foran DJ. Classification of hematologic malignancies using texton signatures. Pattern Analysis and Applications. 2007;**10**(4):277-290

[11] Isse K, Lesniak A, Grama K, Roysam B, Minervini MI, Demetris AJ. Digital transplantation pathology: Combining whole slide imaging, multiplex staining, and automated image analysis. American Journal of Transplantation. 2012;**12**(1):27-37

[12] Gurcan MN, Boucheron L, Can A, Madabhushi A, Rajpoot N, Yener B. Histopathological image analysis: A review. IEEE Reviews in Biomedical Engineering. 2009;**2**:147-171

[13] Pantanowitz L. Digital images and the future of digital pathology. Journal of Pathology Informatics. 2010;**1**:15

[14] Wilbur DC. Digital cytology: Current state of the art and prospects for the future. Acta Cytologica. 2011;**55**:227-238

[15] Beck AH, Sangoi AR, Leung S, Marinelli RJ, Nielsen TO. Systematic analysis of breast cancer morphology uncovers stromal features associated with survival. Science Translational Medicine. 2011;**3**(108):1-11

[16] J. Yao, S. Wang, X. Zhu and J. Huang, Imaging Biomarker Discovery For Lung Cancer Survival Prediction. Athens, Greece: MICCAI; 2016

[17] Huang H-Q, Fang X-Z, Shi J, Hu J. Abnormal localization of immature precursors (ALIP) detection for early prediction of acute myelocytic leukemia (AML) relapse. Medical & Biological Engineering & Computing. 2014;**52**:121-129

[18] Cao G, Li L, Chen W, Yu Y, Shi J, Zhang G, Liu X. Effective identification and localization of immature precursors in bone marrow biopsy. Medical & Biological Engineering & Computing. 2015;**53**:215-226

[19] Mahaja S, Golait SS, Meshram A, Jichlkan N. Review: Detection of types of acute leukemia. International Journal of Computer Science and Mobile Computing. 2014;**3**(3):104-111

[20] Liu Z, Liu J, Xiao X, Yuan H, Li X, Chang J, Zheng C. Segmentation of white blood cells through nucleus mark watershed operations and mean shift clustering. Sensors. 2015;**15**: 22561-22586

[21] N. Brieu, O. Pauly, J. Zimmermann, G. Binnig and G. Schmidt, Slide-Specific Models for Segmentation of Differently Stained Digital Histopathology Whole Slide Images. San Diego, California, USA: Medical Imaging 2016: Image Processing; 2016

[22] Bergen T, Steckhan D, Wittenberg T, Zerfaß T. Segmentation of leukocytes and erythrocytes in blood smear images, in 30th annual international IEEE EMBS conference, Vancouver, British Columbia, Canada. August. 2008;**20-24**:2008

[23] Shivhare S, Shrivastava R. Automatic bone marrow white blood cell classification using morphological granulometric feature of nucleus. International Journal of Scientific & Technology Research. 2012;**1**(4):125-131

[24] Mohapatra S, Patra D, Kumar K. Unsupervised Leukocyte Image Segmentation Using Rough Fuzzy Clustering. ISRN Artificial Intelligence. 2012;**2012**:923946

[25] Nee LH, Mashor MY, Hassan R. White blood cell segmentation for acute leukemia bone marrow images. In: International Conference on Biomedical Engineering (ICoBE); Penang, Malaysia. 2012

[26] Rajivegandhi C, Mrinal A, Sanjana N, Shekhar S. Acute mylogenous leukemia detection using blood microscopic images. International Journal for Research in Applied Science & Engineering. 2015;**3**(4):610-616

[27] Mao-jun S, Zhao-bin W, Hong-juan Z, Yi-de M. A new method for blood cell image segmentation and counting based on PCNN and autowave. 3rd International Symposium on Communications, Control and Signal Processing (ISCCSP); Malta. 2008

[28] Sobhy NM, Salem NM, Dosoky ME. A comparative study of white blood cells segmentation using Otsu threshold and watershed transformation. Journal of Biomedical Engineering and Medical Imaging. 2016;**3**(3):15-24

[29] Saritha M, Prakash BB, Sukesh K, Shrinivas B. Detection of blood cancer in microscopic images of human blood samples: A review. International Conference on Electrical, Electronics, and Optimization Techniques (ICEEOT); Chennai, India. 2016

[30] Bajcsy P, Cardone A, Chalfoun J, Halter M, Juba D, Kociolek M. Survey statistics of automated segmentations applied to optical imaging of mammalian cells. BMC Bioinformatics. 2015;**16**:330

[31] Raje C, Rangole J. Detection of Leukemia in Microscopic Images Using Image Processing. In: International Conference on Communication and Signal Processing, April 3-5, 2014; Chennai, India. 2014

[32] Belekar JS, Chougule SR. WBC segmentation using morphological operation and SMMT operator—A review. International Journal of Innovative Research in Computer and Communication Engineering. 2015;**3**(1):434-440

[33] Prinyakupt J, Pluempitiwiriyawej C. Segmentation of white blood cells and comparison of cell morphology by linear and naïve Bayes classifiers. Biomedical Engineering Online. 2015;**14**:63

[34] Vaghela HP, Modi H, Pandya M, Potdar M. Leukemia Detection Using Digital Image Processing Techniques. In: International Journal of Applied Information Systems (IJAIS); New York, USA. 2015

[35] Piuri V, Scotti F. Morphological Classification of Blood Leucocytes by Microscope Images. In: IEEE lntemational Conference on Computational Intelligence far Memrement Systems and Applications (CIMSA); Boston, MA, USA. 2004

[36] Amin MM, Kermani S, Talebi A, Oghli MG. Recognition of acute lymphoblastic leukemia cells in microscopic images using K-means classifier. Journal of Medical Signals and Sensors. 2015;**5**(1):49-58

[37] Kumar IR, Kumar DH. Classification of acute Myelogenous leukemia using multilevel wavelet transform and neural network for bio-medical applications. International Journal of Innovative Technologies. 2015;**3**(8):1498-1505

[38] Janowczyk A, Madabhushi A. Deep learning for digital pathology image analysis: A comprehensive tutorial with selected use cases. Journal of Pathology Informatics. 2016;**7**:29

[39] Shen D, Wu G, Suk H-I. Deep learning in medical image analysis. Annual Review of Biomedical Engineering. 2017;**19**:221-248

[40] Deshmukh P, Jadhav C. Survey on detection of leukemia using white blood cell. International Journal of Modern Trends in Engineering and Research. 2015;**2**(12):294-298

[41] Rajendran S. Image Retrieval Techniques, Analysis and Interpretation for Leukemia Data Sets. In: 12th ACIS International Conference on Software Engineering, Artificial Intelligence, Networking and Parallel/Distributed Computing; Sydney, NSW, Australia. 2011

[42] Alférez S, Merino A, Bigorra L, Rodellar J. Characterization and automatic screening of reactive and abnormal neoplastic B lymphoid cells from peripheral blood. International Journal of Laboratory Hematology. 2016;**38**:209-219

[43] Mathur A, Tripathi AS, Kuse M. Scalable system for classification of white blood cells from Leishman stained blood stain images. Journal of Pathology Informatics. 2013;**4**:15

[44] Theera-Umpon N, Dhompongsa S. Morphological Granulometric features of nucleus in automatic bone marrow white blood cell classification. IEEE Transactions on Information Technology in Biomedicine. 2007;**11**(2):353-359

[45] Neoh SC, Srisukkham W, Zhang L, Todryk S, Greystoke B, Lim CP, Hossain MA, Aslam N. An intelligent decision support system for Leukaemia diagnosis using microscopic blood images. Scientific Reports. 2015;**5**:14938

[46] Scotti F. Automatic Morphological Analysis for Acute Leukemia Identification in Peripheral Blood Microscope Images. In: CIMSA 2005 – IEEE International Conference on Computational Intelligence for Measurement Systems and Applications; Giardini-Naxos, Italy. 2005

[47] Khashman A, Abbas HH. ALL identification using blood smear images and a neural classifier. In: Advances in Computational Intelligence. Berlin Heidelberg: Springer-Verlag; 2013. pp. 80-87

[48] Alférez S, Merino A, Bigorra L, Mujica L, Ruiz M, Rodellar J. Automatic recognition of atypical lymphoid cells from peripheral blood by digital image analysis. American Journal of Clinical Pathology. 2015;**143**:168-176

[49] Bigorra L, Merino A, Alférez S, Rodellar J. Feature analysis and automatic identification of leukemic lineage blast cells and reactive lymphoid cells from peripheral blood cell images. Journal of Clinical Laboratory Analysis. 2017;**31**, p. e22024

[50] Jacob A, Mundackal FA. Automated screening system for acute leukemia detection and type classification. International Journal of Advanced Research in Electrical, Electronics and Instrumentation Engineering. 2016;**5**(4):2426-2432

[51] Gumble PM, Rode S. Analysis & Classification of acute lymphoblastic leukemia using KNN algorithm. International Journal on Recent and Innovation Trends in Computing and Communication. 2017;**5**(2):94-98

[52] Mohapatra S, Patra D, Satpathy S. An ensemble classifier system for early diagnosis of acute lymphoblastic leukemia in blood microscopic images. Neural Computing and Applications. 2014;**24**:1887-1904

[53] Agaian S, Madhukar M, Chronopoulos AT. Automated screening system for acute myelogenous leukemia detection in blood microscopic images. IEEE Systems Journal. 2014;**8**(3):995-1004

[54] Madhukar M, Agaian S, Chronopoulos AT. Deterministic Model for Acute Myelogenous Leukemia Classification. In: IEEE International Conference on Systems, Man, and Cybernetics; Seoul, Korea. 2012

[55] Supardi NZ, Mashor MY, Harun NH, Hassan FAR. Classification of Blasts in Acute Leukemia Blood Samples Using K-Nearest Neighbour. In: IEEE 8th International Colloquium on Signal Processing and its Applications; Malacca, Malaysia. 2012

[56] Harun N, Mashor M, Nasir AA, Rosline H. Automated Classification of Blasts in Acute Leukemia Blood Samples Using HMLP Network. In: 3rd International Conference on Computing and Informatics, ICOCI; Bandung, Indonesia. 2011

[57] Kazemi F, Naiafabadi TA, Araabi BN. Automatic recognition of acute Myelogenous leukemia in blood microscopic images using K-means clustering and support vector machine. Journal of Medical Signals and Sensors. 2016;**6**(3):183-193

[58] Reta C, Altamirano L, Gonzalez JA, Diaz-Hernandez R, Peregrina H, Olmos I, Alonso JE, Lobato R. Segmentation and classification of bone marrow cells images using contextual information for medical diagnosis of acute Leukemias. PLoS One. 2015;**10**(6, p. e0130805)

[59] Escalante HJ, Montes-y-Gómez M, González JA, Gómez-Gil P, Altamirano L, Reyes CA, Reta C, Rosales A. Acute leukemia classification by ensemble particle swarm model selection. Artificial Intelligence in Medicine. 2012;**55**:163-175

[60] Sandhu RK, Maini R. Automated detection of leukemia. International Journal of Advanced Research in Computer Science. 2017;**8**(5):210-212

[61] Mohapatra S. Hematological Image Analysis for Acute Lymphoblastic Leukemia Detection and Classification [Thesis]. Rourkela, India: National Institute of Technology Rourkela; 2013

[62] Vaghela H, Modi H, Pandya M, Potdar MB. A novel approach to detect chronic leukemia using shape based feature extraction and identification with digital image processing. International Journal of Applied Information Systems (IJAIS). 2016;**11**(5):9-16

[63] Kasmin F, Prabuwono AS, Azizi A. Detection of leukemia in human blood sample based on microscopic images: A study. Journal of Theoretical and Applied Information Technology. 2012;**46**(2):579-586

[64] Patel AB, Nguyen T, Baraniuk RG. A Probabilistic Theory of Deep Learning, arXiv: 1504.00641v1 [stat.ML], 2015

[65] Goodfellow I, Yoshua B, Courville A. Deep Learning. Cambridge, MA, USA: MIT Press; 2016

[66] LeCun Y, Bengio Y, Hinton G. Deep learning. Nature. 2015;**521**:436-444

[67] Litjens G, Kooi T, Bejnord BE, Setio AAA, Ciompi F, Ghafoorian M, Laak JAvd, Ginneken Bv, Sánchez CI. A Survey on Deep Learning in Medical Image Analysis, arXiv:1702.05747v2, p. https://arxiv.org/abs/1702.05747v2, 2017

[68] Zhao J, Zhang M, Zhou Z, Chu J, Cao F. Automatic detection and classification of leukocytes using convolutional neural networks. Medical & Biological Engineering & Computing. 2017;**55**(8):1287-1301

[69] Sipes RK. Using Convolutional Neural Networks for Fine Grained Image Classification of Acute Lymphoblastic Leukemia [Master Thesis]. Cheney, WA, USA: Eastern Washington University; 2016

Chapter 6

Myeloid Sarcoma: The Other Side of Acute Leukemia

Bhaskar Kahali

Additional information is available at the end of the chapter

http://dx.doi.org/10.5772/intechopen.74931

Abstract

Myeloid sarcomas are extramedullary myeloid masses with associated tissue damage. Myeloid sarcomas usually arise before, during or after diagnosis of acute leukemia, most often AML. Majority of the patients with myeloid sarcoma respond to upfront systemic chemotherapy and sometimes bone marrow transplant, but it is unclear which patients will benefit from which treatments. This is primarily due to the paucity of knowledge on myeloid sarcoma. At present, there are no prognostic biomarkers for myeloid sarcoma, which can help in risk stratification in patients with myeloid sarcoma. Several studies have suggested that myeloid sarcoma is more likely to occur with certain translocations such as CBF and MLL rearrangements. In addition, sequencing analysis has identified several mutations in genes such as FLT3, NPM1, EZH2, and KIT. Nevertheless, there is still lack of knowledge to understand why particular leukemia migrates to the skin and soft tissues and becomes refractory to systemic therapy.

Keywords: extramedullary infiltration, myeloid sarcoma, acute leukemia

1. Introduction

Myeloid Sarcoma (MS) constitutes a rare pathological condition of extramedullary manifestation of leukemic cells of primarily myeloid origins that destroy the normal tissue architecture at the site of origin. Presence of the enzyme myeloperoxidase (MPO), gives the tumors its characteristic green hue, leading to the term, 'chloroma' (Greek, Chloros, meaning green) coined by a British physician, A. Burns in 1811 [1, 2]. Alternatively, MS is also referred as, Granulocytic sarcoma or Myeloblastoma. In the majority of the cases, MS is associated with acute myeloid leukemia (AML), however, it may also manifest in non-leukemic individuals. In addition, MS has also been reported in cases of myeloproliferative neoplasms (MPN), or myelodysplastic disorders (MPD) [3, 4]. At present, MS represents a major subgroup of myeloid neoplasms and acute leukemia in WHO classification [5].

2. Epidemiology

MS can manifest under different clinical scenarios including, (1) MS with concurrent AML, (2) as an isolated tumor and may precede the blood and bone marrow involvement or without any history of myeloid neoplasia and, (3) extramedullary relapse of AML [1, 3, 6–9]. However, with a limited number of prospective studies, the exact frequency and the extent of MS are not well described. Based on the retrospective and the autopsy studies, the occurrence of MS in AML patients is reported to be ~10% across genders and all age groups [3, 10, 11]. In depth analysis however revealed that MS primarily affects pediatric patients (>50% of all MS patients) with slight male biasness [7, 12, 13]. In 15–35% of cases, MS can appear concomitantly with AML, whereas, in 50% of cases MS appears following the diagnosis of AML. In rare instances (<1%), MS has also been diagnosed after allogenic stem cell transplantation (allo-SCT), which manifests as an isolated tumor with or without accompanying blood and bone marrow relapse [14, 15].

3. Mechanisms

The precise mechanism underlying the development of MS is unclear. However, extramedullary infiltration by acute leukemia strongly implicates the presence of an alternative homing signal that enables the blast cells to re-localize to these secondary sites. In this context, strong evidence was provided by the studies demonstrating the presence of different chemokine receptors on blast cells in MS and concurrent AML involving blood and bone marrow [16]. Taken together, these observations led to the proposal that unusual manifestations of adhesion molecules dictate the migration of AML subclones to surrounding tissues. Stefanidakis et al. provided further insights into the migratory capacity of blast cells. In their study, the authors reported that a major factor for the migration of AML cells into non-myeloid regions is the interactions between matrix metalloproteinase (MMP) – 9 and leukocyte β2 integrin along with some unidentified proteins [2]. Stefanidakis et al. termed the complex, 'invadosome' [2]. The observations that highly invasive AML cell lines express high level of MMP-2 and tissue inhibitor of metalloproteinase 2 (TIMP2) further support the conclusion of Stefanidakis and colleagues [17]. In a recent study, Zhu et al. has reported a correlation between high expression of enhancer of Zeste 2 (EZH2), the catalytic subunit of polycomb repressor complex 2 (PRC2), and extramedullary infiltration of AML [18]. The authors have indicated that increased expression of EZH2 attenuates the expression of TIMPs, which result in the upregulation of MMPs. The uninhibited MMPs ultimately degrades the extracellular matrix (ECM) and thus aid in the escape of the blast cells in the extramedullary space [18].

4. Sites of involvement and symptoms

MS can manifest in different anatomical sites. However, there is a lack of study to establish a correlation between AML and predilection for sites by MS. The most commonly involved sites of MS are skin, bone and lymph nodes [3, 10, 11]. In addition, other sites associated with MS include central nervous system (CNS), oral and nasal mucosa, breasts, genitourinary tract, chest wall, testis etc. Skin is the primary sites for the development of MS in pediatric patients (~54%), followed by ocular region [3, 10, 11].

In majority of instances, MS is asymptomatic. Even so, depending on the size and location of the tumor, the most common signs and symptoms associated with MS are compression accompanied by pains, bleeding, fever and fatigues [1].

5. Diagnosis and disease pathology

At present, there is no specific diagnosis for MS. Given the fact that MS in majority of cases is asymptomatic and does not elicit any specific symptoms, it often poses serious diagnostic challenge for a clinician. Consequently, MS is often misdiagnosed as large cell lymphoma, malignant melanoma, extramedullary hematopoiesis or inflammation. However, diagnosis of MS in association with existing leukemia is comparatively easier than isolated MS. Detection and identification of MS requires the coordinated intervention of different medical procedure. Computed tomography (CT) and magnetic resonance imagery (MRI) are generally used for the detection of the tumors [19]. Following the detection of tumors biopsies are conducted to confirm the malignancy of the mass.

However, accurate diagnosis of MS requires histological examination and immunophenotypic analysis. Histological analysis of MS generally elicits myeloid cells at different stages of maturation. The infiltrating leukemic cells generally elicit irregular large nuclei and large cytoplasm-to-nuclear ratio. Depending on the predominant cell types in the tumors, MS are classified into granulocytic, monoblastic and myelomonocytic. In addition, depending on the maturity of the cells, MS are further subdivided into immature, mature and blastic types [11]. In addition to morphology, cytochemical stainings on imprints may allow for confirming the myeloid affiliation and differentiating granulocytic-lineage and monoblastic forms. According to the WHO 2016 classification, cytochemical stains may include myeloperoxidase and naphthol AS-D chloroacetate esterase (positive in granulocytic MS), as well as non-specific esterase (positive in monoblastic MS) [5]. The diagnosis is further validated by immunophenotyping. Flow cytometric analysis on cell suspensions can be performed; however, immunohistochemistry on paraffin-embedded tissue sections is more commonly used for the detection of lineage affiliation and evaluation of maturation. MS are usually positive for myeloid and monocytic markers, i.e. CD33, CD68, lysozyme, the more immature markers such as CD117 and CD34, CD61, glycophorin, CD4, etc. CD99 and TdT may also be positive. CD56 can be detected in

Immunophenotypic profiles	Most common markers
Myeloid	Myeloperoxidase (MPO), CD33, CD68 (detected by KP1 monoclonal antibody but not by PG-M1), CD34, CD117
Promyelocytic	Myeloperoxidase (MPO), CD15, CD117, lacking CD34 and TdT
Myelomonocytic	Homogeneous expression of CD68 (KP1), while CD68 (PG-M1) and MPO in distinct subpopulations
Monoblastic	CD68 (PG-M1), CD14, lacking MPO, CD163, CD11c
Megakaryoblastic	CD61, von Willebrand factor
Erythroid	CD71, glycophorin A, glycophorin C

Table 1. Common immunophenotypes.

around 20% of MS cases [1, 12]. NPM1 cytoplasmic and nuclear staining indicates *NPM1* gene mutations. To exclude the possibility of lymphoma the tumors should be interrogated for different T and B lineage markers such as, CD3, CD20, and CD79a. Aberrant expression of B/T-cell markers is possible, however, if criteria for a mixed-lineage leukemia are fulfilled the case is not classified as MS according to WHO 2016. Particular antigenic constellations may more precisely define subtypes shown in **Table 1**.

MS is also associated with several cytogenetic and chromosomal abnormalities (please see next section for detailed report). Consequently, fluorescence in situ hybridization (FISH) should be employed as a part diagnostic work up for patient stratification [20].

6. Cytogenetics and molecular genetics of myeloid sarcoma

Cytogenetic analysis conducted with bone marrow and peripheral blood blasts in MS patients has demonstrated cytogenetic abnormalities in more than 50% of instances [21]. Nonetheless, the rates of specific cytogenetic abnormalities associated with MS are rather diverse. Studies have elicited the frequent association of between MS and core binding factor (CBF) leukemia and AML with *MLL* rearrangements [22]. The most common chromosomal abnormality, t(8;21), is associated with pediatric MS or in patients with ocular involvement [21, 23, 24]. The second predominant chromosomal aberration associated with pediatric MS is inv16 [3, 25]. However, studies by Pileri et al. showed the relative rarity of t(8,21) in adult MS patients [21]. Instead, trisomy 8, monosomy 7 and *MLL* rearrangements constitute the majority of the cases [21]. The prevalence of inv16 was also not well documented in adult patients. In addition, other chromosomal aberrations including monosomy 5, 7 or 8 were reported in isolated cases. *Nucleophosmin (NPM)-1* mutations have been reported to be in 15% of MS patients. This particular variant of MS elicits clinical attributes similar to *NPM-1* positive AML and manifest primarily in M4 and M5 French American British (FAB) subclasses of AML [26]. *NPM-1* mutant positive MS is also associated with the loss of CD34 expression and normal karyotype. Studies conducted by Ansari-Lari et al. have reported the presence of *FLT3-ITD* mutation in ~33% (three of nine) of MS patients with concurrent AML [27]. However, the implications of *NPM-1* and *FLT3-ITD* mutations on prognosis of MS are still not clear and data are too scarce for definite conclusions. In their retrospective study, Vega-Ruiz et al. showed that 3% of patients with acute promyelocytic leukemia (APL) manifest MS, predominantly in CNS [28]. Studies conducted by several groups have also attributed the development of MS to the use of all-trans retinoic acid (ATRA) or with conventional chemotherapy [29].

7. Imaging as a diagnostic tool

Timely identification of MS has a significant impact on the treatment outcomes and achieving remission in case of AML. As often, these extramedullary tumors serve as sanctuary sites for future relapse. However, detection and simultaneous identification of MS is challenging. The standard AML diagnosis does not include MS, nor there are any specific diagnostic regimens for MS. Consequently, in majority of cases diagnosis of MS is either significantly delayed or remain undetected. In this context, multimodal imaging procedure can be beneficial for early detection of tumors [30]. This generally involves employment of traditional imaging techniques such as, positron emission tomography (PET), CT and MRI [25]. Particularly, in the last decades, PET/CT is becoming an essential tool for disease detection [25]. In this context, 18F-fluorodeoxygenase (18F-FDG)PET/CT has been recognized as a very potent instrument for the identification of not only leukemia but also extramedullary invasion of blast cells [8, 31, 32]. In a prospective study, Stölzel et al. have successfully employed whole-body 18F-FDG PET/CT in 94 AML patients, consisting of both newly diagnosed and relapsed cases of AML for detection of MS [33]. In a different study, Aschoff et al. have demonstrated the sensitivity of 18F-FDG PET/CT by reducing the number of false-positive associated with traditional PET imaging [34]. In addition, 18F-FDG PET/CT has also been able identify new sites of MS, which is not identified by traditional imaging techniques [8].

Although, encouraging, 18F-FDG PET/CT does have some restrictions. Several reports have shown that 18F-FDG PET/CT is not sensitive enough to pick up extramedullary infiltration in the soft tissues such as skin meninges and mucus membranes. In addition, 18F-FDG is not a tumor specific marker but rather depends on the glucose uptake by the cells [8]. As such, there is an increase chance of false-positive signals associated with 18F-FDG PET/CT specifically, in brain and kidney that have high basal glucose metabolism [9]. As an alternative, various groups have used 18F-fluorodeoxythymidine (FLT), a thymidine analogue and proliferating marker, as a tracer for PET/CT in place of 18F-FDG [8]. Unlike 18F-FDG, 18F-FLT has generally low uptake in different organs, such as brain and kidney and therefore elicits comparatively less background [35]. Although, as of now there has been no prospective/retrospective study with 18F-FLT PET/CT for MS detection, but the sensitivity and accuracy of 18F-FLT PET/CT has been demonstrated in different cancers including, non-small cell lung cancer (NSCLC) and NPM-ALK-Positive lymphoma [8, 36].

8. Treatment

Given the scarcity of positively diagnosed MS and randomized prospective trials, there is at present no consensus MS specific therapeutic regimen. The current routine includes conventional AML-type chemotherapy and radiotherapy for both isolated and MS or MS with concomitant AML. Studies led by different groups have shown that standard AML therapy exhibits better overall survival in case of isolated MS incidents [10]. Nevertheless, there is a lack of data addressing a particular chemotherapeutic regimen for MS. Existing data indicates cytarabine to be an essential drug in this regard [37].

The use of radiotherapy is also not well studied as a prospective means of treatment of MS. Although, in some instances, radiation is used in combination with chemotherapy to treat MS. However, no added advantage was observed in those cases [11, 38]. In addition, hematopoietic stem cell transplantation is also used, albeit retrospectively, in MS patients [1]. Reported data does suggest an advantage of auto- or allo-HSCT in MS patients with or without concomitant AML irrespective of age, gender, anatomic location, clinical presentation or cytogenic status [1, 3, 11]. In addition, retrospective chemotherapy trials conducted by the Children's Cancer Group demonstrated a better event-free survival for children with isolated MS than patients with concurrent AML [38].

Taken together, however, no studies ever compared the different prognostic factors in MS patients with or without AML and consequently, their effects on the treatment regimens. The published data, nevertheless, do suggest a difference in prognosis between patients with isolated MS and with concurrent or relapsed AML. Traditionally, the simultaneous expression of MS at diagnosis of AML is considered as poor prognosis. However, there is evidence contrary to this observation.

As stated above, till now there is no specific treatment for MS. Consequently, to a large extent the treatment of MS depends on the site, volume as well as the timing of diagnosis of the extramedullary tumor. Based on these factors, the clinicians determine the treatment plan by employing singly chemotherapy, radiation therapy or bone marrow transplantation or in combination. A detailed discussion of these different therapeutic regimens is discussed below.

9. Chemotherapy

Systemic chemotherapy is the primary choice of treatment for both isolated MS and MS with simultaneous bone marrow involvement. This is largely due to the fact that even if there is no primary bone marrow involvement, isolated or primary MS ultimately gives rise to AML in majority of the cases [3, 39]. Consequently, the chemotherapy regimens for MS generally follow the same protocol as AML. All these regimens mainly include cytarabine with fludarabine, idarubicin, or both. In some instances, granulocyte colony-stimulating factor (G-CSF), daunorubicin and cyclophosphamide are also used [32, 37, 40]. In particular, combination therapy with cytarabine and daunorubicin has been demonstrated to achieve complete remission in ~65% of MS patients. In addition, chemotherapy has also shown to be effective in attenuating AML development in isolated MS cases (~71%) in both adult and pediatric population [37, 41]. However, at present there is not enough data to identify a specific chemotherapy plan that is beneficial for MS.

10. Radiotherapy

In some instance, radiation is also used as a part of the treatment plan for MS. However, existing data does suggest that radiation alone may not be sufficient enough to completely eradicate MS. Study conducted by Bakst et al. has demonstrated that patients with isolated MS generally respond better to systemic chemotherapy compared to radiotherapy [39]. In addition, there is also no conclusive data demonstrating that radiotherapy in MS alone can prevent the development of systemic leukemia involving bone marrow (~40%). Consequently, in most cases radiation is used in combination with chemotherapy in treating MS [42].

11. Bone marrow transplantation

Allo-SCT has also been demonstrated to be beneficial in treating isolated MS. Consequently, many investigators/clinicians considered allo-SCT as a primary line treatment following remission in MS patients [21, 43]. However, in a retrospective study, Chevallier et al. have showed that there is no difference in 5-year survival rate in patients with isolated or MS with leukemia when treated with allo-SCT [43]. In both the cases, the average survival was ~48% for 5-year survival. In a different study, Pileri et al. showed that MS patients receiving transplantation demonstrated a better overall survival rate (~70%), than patients who did not receive transplantation (0%) as a part of the treatment plan [21]. In subgroup analysis, transplantation did not display any biasness depending on age, tumor site, timing of diagnosis etc. [21].

Taken together, these reports do suggest that transplantation should be considered as a part of the consolidation therapy following remission in both isolated and leukemic MS in adult and pediatric patients. However, one should be cautious as there are reports of manifestation of MS postallo-SCT, most likely due to reduced graft-versus-leukemia (GVL) state at extramedullary sites [25].

At present, there is not enough data in the field to make an informed choice for the best course of treatment for different variants of MS. Based on the existing data, it is reasonable to consider systemic chemotherapy as the best course of action, in association with radiotherapy and allo-SCT depending on the bone marrow involvement. Given the fact that most of the reports are isolated, single center analysis with small patient pool, it is not possible to develop a consensus therapeutic regimen. To achieve such MS specific therapy, large multicenter collaboration and development of prospective clinical trials is imperative.

12. Targeted therapy: a possibility for the future?

Next-generation sequencing (NGS) and mutational analysis have uncovered significant insights into the pathogenicity of leukemia. Consequently, the chances to develop targeted therapies for leukemia have become a distinct possibility. However, due to misdiagnosis and paucity of clinical samples, such comprehensive analysis for MS is still lacking. Nonetheless, studies conducted with small cohorts of patients did report mutations in genes such as *FLT3* and *NPM1*. Li et al. performed an NGS analysis with six patients with a custom panel targeting 21 common genes associated with AML and myelodysplastic syndrome (MDS) [44]. In addition to *FLT3* and *NPM1*, the authors were also able to identify mutations in several genes such as *KIT, TET2, EZH2, SF3B1* and *ASXL1* akin to AML [44]. This report does provide substantial evidence of an underlying similarity in the pathogenicity between MS and AML. The importance of targeted therapy is further accentuated by Piccaluga and colleagues [45]. In this study, the authors used an anti-CD33 monoclonal antibody to treat MS patients with concurrent CD33-positive AML. Two out five patients in the study elicited a complete remission of both MS and AML, while two patients showed reductions of extramedullary disease only [45]. In a different study, treatment of MS patients with BCR-ABL1, FLT3-ITD and FIP1L1-PDGFRA mutations by tyrosine kinase inhibitors (TKIs) also showed encouraging outcome [46].

Taken together these observations does suggest that akin to AML a similar sequencing (whole genome, whole exome, and RNA seq.) base analysis should be employed in case of MS. However, the success of such an endeavor depends on the obtainability of large cohorts of samples, which unfortunately is a rarity in case of MS. Large multicenter collaboration is essential to circumvent this problem.

13. Conclusion

Myeloid sarcoma is acknowledged as a separate disease entity for a significant period. It is an extremely rare hematological malignancy and is often associated with poor prognosis. Due to the scarcity of samples, there is no risk assessment study for MS. There are several unanswered questions for MS. Specifically, is there a bias for certain AML (such as CBF leukemia) to induce extramedullary infiltration. If yes, what is the primary mechanism(s) that drives the processes? Does MS represent alternate molecular landscapes, clonal evolution, from the original bone marrow disease? It can be argued that MS reflects a state of reduced immune surveillance in a patient at diagnosis or following hematopoietic stem cell transplantation. Consequently, this raises the possibility that MS may serve as a sanctuary site for leukemic relapse. The observation supports this implication that isolated MS ultimately gives rise to leukemia involving bone marrow.

MS is often challenging to identify and even more challenging to diagnose. Owing to its similarity with solid tumors, MS is often misdiagnosed, particularly as non-Hodgkin lymphoma. Accurate diagnosis of MS required an orchestrated approach involving whole body imaging (PET/CT, MRI), broad panels of immunohistochemical staining, and FISH assay for cytogenetic and chromosomal abnormalities. Also, bone marrow biopsy should be that part of the diagnosis. In fact, all isolated MS cases should be prophylactically treated for AML even if there is no detectable leukemia. Caution should be exercised when analyzing immunohistochemistry for MS. For example, CD43 and CD68, although, a reliable indicator of AML, should be correlated with CD33, myeloperoxidase staining for accurate MS diagnosis. Treatment should involve systemic chemotherapy as the first line of treatment with radiotherapy and allo-HCT as part of the consolidation therapy. Surgery should be employed for tumor resection, if possible.

We need more prospective studies with larger patient cohorts to understand the mechanism(s) of MS development. In addition, future studies should be directed to whole genome sequencing of MS samples to understand the different genetic abnormalities associated with MS and how they differ from the corresponding bone marrow disease. Genetic information will also help in better patient stratification. As evident from the whole-body PET/CT imaging, the incidence of MS is more prevalent than expected indicating that we most likely have underestimated the impact and implications of MS.

Author details

Bhaskar Kahali

Address all correspondence to: bhaskar.kahali@stjude.org

Bone Marrow Trans and Cell Therapy, St Jude Children's Research Hospital, Memphis, United States

References

[1] Avni B, Koren-Michowitz M. Myeloid sarcoma: Current approach and therapeutic options. Therapeutic Advances in Hematology. 2011;**2**(5):309-316

[2] Stefanidakis M, Karjalainen K, Jaalouk DE, Gahmberg CG, O'Brien S, Pasqualini R, Arap W, Koivunen E. Role of leukemia cell invadosome in extramedullary infiltration. Blood. 2009;**114**(14):3008-3017

[3] Bakst RLTM, Douer D, Yahalom J. How I treat extramedullary acute myeloid leukemia. Blood. 2011;**118**:3785-3793

[4] Ravandi-Kashani F, Cortes J, Giles FJ. Myelodysplasia presenting as granulocytic sarcoma of mediastinum causing superior vena cava syndrome. Leukemia & Lymphoma. 2000;**36**(5–6): 631-637

[5] Arber DA, Orazi A, Hasserjian R, Thiele J, Borowitz MJ, Le Beau MM, Bloomfield CD, Cazzola M, Vardiman JW. The 2016 revision to the World Health Organization classification of myeloid neoplasms and acute leukemia. Blood. 2016;**127**(20):2391-2405

[6] Fleckenstein K, Geinitz H, Grosu A, Goetze K, Werner M, Molls M. Irradiation for conjunctival granulocytic sarcoma. Strahlentherapie und Onkologie. 2003;**179**(3):187-190

[7] Neiman RS, Barcos M, Berard C, Bonner H, Mann R, Rydell RE, Bennett JM. Granulocytic sarcoma: A clinicopathologic study of 61 biopsied cases. Cancer. 1981;**48**(6):1426-1437

[8] Stolzel F, Rollig C, Radke J, Mohr B, Platzbecker U, Bornhauser M, Paulus T, Ehninger G, Zophel K, Schaich M. (1)(8)F-FDG-PET/CT for detection of extramedullary acute myeloid leukemia. Haematologica. 2011;**96**(10):1552-1556

[9] van Veen S, Kluin PM, de Keizer RJ, Kluin-Nelemans HC. Granulocytic sarcoma (chloroma). Presentation of an unusual case. American Journal of Clinical Pathology. 1991;**95**(4):567-571

[10] Avni B, Rund D, Levin M, Grisariu S, Ben-Yehuda D, Bar-Cohen S, Paltiel O. Clinical implications of acute myeloid leukemia presenting as myeloid sarcoma. Hematological Oncology. 2012;**30**(1):34-40

[11] Lan TY, Lin DT, Tien HF, Yang RS, Chen CY, Wu K. Prognostic factors of treatment outcomes in patients with granulocytic sarcoma. Acta Haematologica. 2009;**122**(4):238-246

[12] Campidelli C, Agostinelli C, Stitson R, Pileri SA. Myeloid sarcoma: Extramedullary manifestation of myeloid disorders. American Journal of Clinical Pathology. 2009;**132**(3):426-437

[13] Kawamoto K, Miyoshi H, Yoshida N, Takizawa J, Sone H, Ohshima K. Clinicopathological, cytogenetic, and prognostic analysis of 131 myeloid sarcoma patients. The American Journal of Surgical Pathology. 2016;**40**(11):1473-1483

[14] Bain EE, Rothman I, Lin L. De novo myeloid sarcoma in a 4-month-old infant: A case report and review of the literature. Journal of Cutaneous Pathology. 2013;**40**(3):321-325

[15] Yoo SW, Chung EJ, Kim SY, Ko JH, Baek HS, Lee HJ, Oh SH, Jeon SC, Lee WS, Park CK, et al. Multiple extramedullary relapses without bone marrow involvement after second allogeneic hematopoietic stem cell transplantation for acute myeloid leukemia. Pediatric Transplantation. 2012;**16**(4):E125-E129

[16] Faaij CM, Willemze AJ, Revesz T, Balzarolo M, Tensen CP, Hoogeboom M, Vermeer MH, van Wering E, Zwaan CM, Kaspers GJ, et al. Chemokine/chemokine receptor interactions in extramedullary leukaemia of the skin in childhood AML: Differential roles for CCR2, CCR5, CXCR4 and CXCR7. Pediatric Blood & Cancer. 2010;**55**(2):344-348

[17] Wang C, Chen Z, Li Z. The essential roles of matrix metalloproteinase-2, membrane type 1 metalloproteinase and tissue inhibitor of metalloproteinase-2 in the invasive capacity of acute monocytic leukemia SHI-1 cells. Leukemia Research. 2010;**34**:1083-1090

[18] Zhu Q, Zhang L, Li X, Chen F, Jiang L, Yu G, Wang Z, Yin C, Jiang X, Zhong Q, et al. Higher EZH2 expression is associated with extramedullary infiltration in acute myeloid leukemia. Tumour Biology. 2016;**37**(8):11409-11420

[19] Pui MH, Fletcher BD, Langston JW. Granulocytic sarcoma in childhood leukemia: Imaging features. Radiology. 1994;**190**(3):698-702

[20] Wilson CS, Medeiros LJ. Extramedullary manifestations of myeloid neoplasms. American Journal of Clinical Pathology. 2015;**144**(2):219-239

[21] Pileri SA, Ascani S, Cox MC, Campidelli C, Bacci F, Piccioli M, Piccaluga PP, Agostinelli C, Asioli S, Novero D, et al. Myeloid sarcoma: Clinico-pathologic, phenotypic and cytogenetic analysis of 92 adult patients. Leukemia. 2007;**21**(2):340-350

[22] Park KU, Lee DS, Lee HS, Kim CJ, Cho HI. Granulocytic sarcoma in MLL-positive infant acute myelogenous leukemia: Fluorescence in situ hybridization study of childhood acute myelogenous leukemia for detecting MLL rearrangement. The American Journal of Pathology. 2001;**159**(6):2011-2016

[23] Klco JM, Welch JS, Nguyen TT, Hurley MY, Kreisel FH, Hassan A, Lind AC, Frater JL. State of the art in myeloid sarcoma. International Journal of Laboratory Hematology. 2011;**33**(6):555-565

[24] Schwyzer R, Sherman GG, Cohn RJ, Poole JE, Willem P. Granulocytic sarcoma in children with acute myeloblastic leukemia and t(8;21). Medical and Pediatric Oncology. 1998;**31**(3): 144-149

[25] Ohanian MFS, Ravandi F, Pemmaraju N, Garcia-Manero G, Cortes J, Estrov Z. Is acute myeloid leukemia a liquid tumor. International Journal of Cancer. 2013;**133**:534-544

[26] Falini B, Mecucci C, Tiacci E, Alcalay M, Rosati R, Pasqualucci L, La Starza R, Diverio D, Colombo E, Santucci A, et al. Cytoplasmic nucleophosmin in acute myelogenous leukemia with a normal karyotype. The New England Journal of Medicine. 2005;**352**(3):254-266

[27] Ansari-Lari MA, Yang CF, Tinawi-Aljundi R, Cooper L, Long P, Allan RH, Borowitz MJ, Berg KD, Murphy KM. FLT3 mutations in myeloid sarcoma. British Journal of Haematology. 2004;**126**(6):785-791

[28] Vega-Ruiz A, Faderl S, Estrov Z, Pierce S, Cortes J, Kantarjian H, Ravandi F. Incidence of extramedullary disease in patients with acute promyelocytic leukemia: A single-institution experience. International Journal of Hematology. 2009;**89**(4):489-496

[29] Specchia G, Lo Coco F, Vignetti M, Avvisati G, Fazi P, Albano F, Di Raimondo F, Martino B, Ferrara F, Selleri C, et al. Extramedullary involvement at relapse in acute promyelocytic leukemia patients treated or not with all-trans retinoic acid: A report by the Gruppo Italiano Malattie Ematologiche dell'Adulto. Journal of Clinical Oncology. 2001;**19**(20): 4023-4028

[30] Cunningham I. A basis for updating our approach to resistant acute leukemia. American Journal of Hematology. 2012;**87**(3):251-257

[31] Kuenzle K, Taverna C, Steinert HC. Detection of extramedullary infiltrates in acute myelogenous leukemia with whole-body positron emission tomography and 2-deoxy-2-[18F]-fluoro-D-glucose. Molecular Imaging and Biology. 2002;**4**(2):179-183

[32] Rao S, Langston A, Galt JR, Halkar RK. Extramedullary acute myeloid leukemia and the use of FDG-PET/CT. Clinical Nuclear Medicine. 2009;**34**(6):365-366

[33] Friedrich Stölzel TL, Parmentier SB, Paulus T, Kuithan F, Kramer M, Alakel N, Sockel K, Taube F, Kotzerke J, Röllig C, Bornhäuser M, Ehninger G, Zoephel K, Schaich M. The prevalence of extramedullary AML detected by 18-FDG/PET-CT: Results from the prospective PET-AML trial. Blood. 2014;**124**(21):2270

[34] Aschoff P, Hantschel M, Oksuz M, Werner MK, Lichy M, Vogel W, Pfannenberg C. Integrated FDG-PET/CT for detection, therapy monitoring and follow-up of granulocytic sarcoma. Initial results. Nuklearmedizin. 2009;**48**(5):185-191

[35] Chandrasekaran S, Hollander A, Xu X, Benci JL, Davis JJ, Dorsey JF, Kao G. 18F-fluorothymidine-pet imaging of glioblastoma multiforme: Effects of radiation therapy on radiotracer uptake and molecular biomarker patterns. Scientific World Journal. 2013;**2013**: 796029

[36] Li Z, Graf N, Herrmann K, Junger A, Aichler M, Feuchtinger A, Baumgart A, Walch A, Peschel C, Schwaiger M, et al. FLT-PET is superior to FDG-PET for very early response prediction in NPM-ALK-positive lymphoma treated with targeted therapy. Cancer Research. 2012;**72**(19):5014-5024

[37] Yamauchi K, Yasuda M. Comparison in treatments of nonleukemic granulocytic sarcoma: Report of two cases and a review of 72 cases in the literature. Cancer. 2002;**94**(6):1739-1746

[38] Dusenbery KE, Howells WB, Arthur DC, Alonzo T, Lee JW, Kobrinsky N, Barnard DR, Wells RJ, Buckley JD, Lange BJ, et al. Extramedullary leukemia in children with newly diagnosed acute myeloid leukemia: A report from the Children's cancer group. Journal of Pediatric Hematology/Oncology. 2003;**25**(10):760-768

[39] Bakst R, Wolden S, Yahalom J. Radiation therapy for chloroma (granulocytic sarcoma). International Journal of Radiation Oncology, Biology, Physics. 2012;**82**(5):1816-1822

[40] Bleul CC, Fuhlbrigge RC, Casasnovas JM, Aiuti A, Springer TA. A highly efficacious lymphocyte chemoattractant, stromal cell-derived factor 1 (SDF-1). The Journal of Experimental Medicine. 1996;**184**(3):1101-1109

[41] Crazzolara R, Kreczy A, Mann G, Heitger A, Eibl G, Fink FM, Mohle R, Meister B. High expression of the chemokine receptor CXCR4 predicts extramedullary organ infiltration in childhood acute lymphoblastic leukaemia. British Journal of Haematology. 2001;**115**(3): 545-553

[42] Aiuti A, Webb IJ, Bleul C, Springer T, Gutierrez-Ramos JC. The chemokine SDF-1 is a chemoattractant for human CD34+ hematopoietic progenitor cells and provides a new mechanism to explain the mobilization of CD34+ progenitors to peripheral blood. The Journal of Experimental Medicine. 1997;**185**(1):111-120

[43] Chevallier PMM, Lioure B, Michel G, Contentin N, Deconinck E, Bordigoni P, Vernant JP, Hunault M, Vigouroux S, Blaise D, Tabrizi R, Buzyn A, Socie G, Michallet M, Volteau C, Harousseau JL. Allogeneic hematopoietic stem-cell transplantation for myeloid sarcoma: A retrospective study from the SFGM-TC. Journal of Clinical Oncology. 2008;**26**: 4940-4943

[44] Li Z, Stolzel F, Onel K, Sukhanova M, Mirza MK, Yap KL, Borinets O, Larson RA, Stock W, Sasaki MM, et al. Next-generation sequencing reveals clinically actionable molecular markers in myeloid sarcoma. Leukemia. 2015;**29**(10):2113-2116

[45] Piccaluga PP, Martinelli G, Rondoni M, Malagola M, Gaitani S, Isidori A, Bonini A, Gugliotta L, Luppi M, Morselli M, et al. Gemtuzumab ozogamicin for relapsed and refractory acute myeloid leukemia and myeloid sarcomas. Leukemia & Lymphoma. 2004;**45**(9):1791-1795

[46] Vedy D, Muehlematter D, Rausch T, Stalder M, Jotterand M, Spertini O. Acute myeloid leukemia with myeloid sarcoma and eosinophilia: Prolonged remission and molecular response to imatinib. Journal of Clinical Oncology. 2010;**28**(3):e33-e35

Section 3

Benign Hematological Diseases

Chapter 7

Understanding the Clotting Cascade, Regulators, and Clinical Modulators of Coagulation

Vijaya S. Pilli

Additional information is available at the end of the chapter

http://dx.doi.org/10.5772/intechopen.75141

Abstract

The circulatory system plays a vital role in the survival of an organism by supplying it with essential nutrients, signaling molecules and eliminating the waste or toxic products from the body. This flow is tightly regulated by various factors, procoagulants support the formation of hemostatic plugs to prevent the leakage or blood loss and anticoagulants prevent the formation of unwanted clots. Disruption or dysregulation of procoagulants and anticoagulants lead to clinical complexities. In this chapter defects in the coagulation system, hereditary, acquired coagulation disorders, their diagnosis and recent clinical modulators of the coagulation system are discussed.

Keywords: coagulation, hemophilia, thrombosis, pro-coagulants and anticoagulants

1. Introduction

Blood carries a set of zymogen serine proteases called procoagulants these serine proteases are activated upon injury and promote the formation of a clot [1]. The clot formation initiates by two mechanisms [1–4]. One of the mechanisms is termed as tissue factor pathway or extrinsic pathway, and the other pathway is called as contact pathway or intrinsic pathway [2]. Extrinsic pathway or tissue factor pathway is initiated by the tissue factor (TF) released form the damaged cell [1–4]. TF proteolytically cleaves a zymogen factor VII (FVII) and activates it [1–4]. Activated factor VII (FVIIa) forms a complex with TF, forming a potent protease complex which activates the downstream cascade by limited proteolysis. TF-FVIIa complex converts the inactive factor IX (FIX) and factor X to activated factor IX (FIXa) and activated factor X (FXa). The activated FIXa binds to activated Factor VIIIa(FVIIIa) to form X-ase complex on the phosphatidylserine-rich membrane surface, this complex converts FX to FXa. Intrinsic/ contact pathway is initiated by artificial surfaces in the plasma. Artificial surfaces induce conformational change in factor XII (FXII) and results in activation of small amount of FXII. Activated factor XII (FXIIa) activates high molecular weight kininogen (HK) and plasma prekallikrein (PK) and this acts as a positive feedback loop for FXII activation [1–4]. Further, FXIIa activates Factor XI (FXI) to FXIa, which intern activates FIX. Both extrinsic and intrinsic pathways collaborate with a common pathway that involves activated FXa. FXa binds to activated factor V (FVa), forming prothrombinase complex and Prothrombinase complex cleaves prothrombin to generate activated thrombin. Thrombin cleaves fibrinogen to fibrin, these fibrin monomers polymerizes to form insoluble fibrin polymer (**Figure 1A**).

Along with the clotting factors, platelets play a vital role in regulating the hemostasis by forming a cellular plug at the site of injury. The circulating platelets get immobilized at the sub endothelial surface of the site of injury by binding to the von Willebrand factor (VWF) [3]. Platelet receptor GPIb-IXV is essential for this process. Similarly, receptor GPVI helps to anchor the platelets at the site of injury with the help of collagen. Further these platelets get activated and expose phosphatidylserine, which provides a lipid surface for the clotting factors [3]. Among the clotting factors, fibrin helps in activating the platelets by cleaving the protease activated receptors (PARs) that include PAR1 and PAR4 (**Figure 1B**).

Hemostasis is tightly monitored by feedback mechanisms, where anticoagulants inhibit the protease function of coagulation favors by directly inhibiting them or their cofactors [1–4]. The natural anticoagulants include tissue factor pathway inhibitor (TFPI), Activated protein C (APC), Protein S (PS) and Protein Z (PZ). These anticoagulants help in regulating blood clot

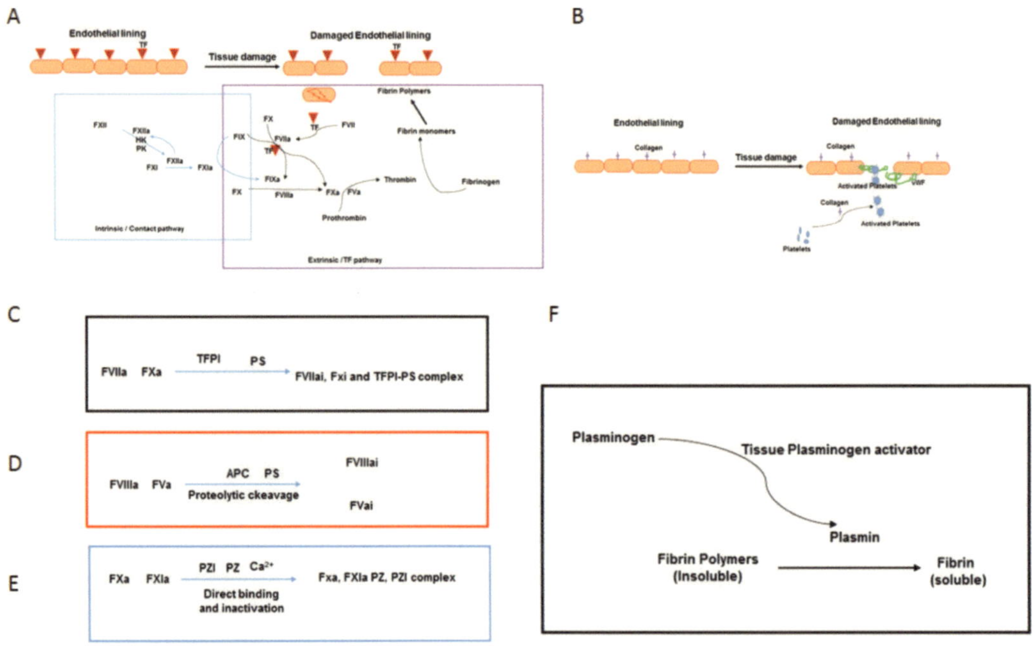

Figure 1. (A) Schematic representation of coagulation cascade. (B) Schematic representation of platelet plug formation. (C) TFPI pathway. (D) APC function. (E) PZI pathway. (F) Clot lysis.

formation [5–7]. TFPI directly binds to FVIIa and Xa complex and inhibits their function and the TFPI function is accelerated in presence of PS. APC proteolytically cleaves FVIIIa and FVa [7]. PS was discovered as a cofactor for TFPI, APC and recent reports demonstrated that PS can directly bind and inhibit the functions of FVa, FIXa and FXa [5–7]. Protein Z-dependent protease inhibitor inhibits FXa and FXIa, in the presence of PZ and calcium [8] (**Figure 1C-E**).

Blood clots from the healthy system are removed by fibrinolytic system [9]. In the fibrinolysis process tissue specific plasminogen activators (tPA) or urokinase plasminogen activator activates plasminogen by proteolytically cleaving it into activated plasmin. Plasmin cleaves the insoluble fibrin polymers into soluble peptides [9] (**Figure 1F**).

2. Defects in hemostasis

Quantitative or qualitative defects in the coagulation factors lead to hemostatic defects such as hemophilia or thrombosis [10, 11]. Hemophilia is characterized by defects in clotting factors and it is characterized by spontaneous or periodic bleedings [11]. Whereas, thrombosis is caused by the high amount of procoagulants in the plasma, hyper activation of procoagulants or defects in anticoagulants [10]. Thrombosis is characterized by systemic clots which impair the normal hemostasis. Bleeding disorders are also classified hereditary and acquired disorders. Hereditary disorders are associated with gene mutations and inherited to the offspring [11]. The major hereditary disorders are hemophilia, rare bleeding disorders and thrombosis. Acquired disorders are caused by several factors such as infections, habits and environmental effects [12].

3. Hemophilia

Hemophilia is an inherited bleeding disorder, caused by the deficiency of procoagulants. Deficiency of FVIII is known as hemophilia A, deficiency of FIX is known as hemophilia B and deficiency of FXI is known as hemophilia C [13–17]. The hemophilia A and B are X chromosome linked disorders and they are mainly observed in the male population [14, 15, 17]. Hemophilia A cases are observed in 1 in 5000 males whereas, hemophilia B cases are observed in 1 in 20,000 males (https://www.hemophilia.org/About-Us/Fast-Facts). Hemophilia is classified based on the functional antigen levels. Patients with <1% activity with spontaneous bleeding are termed as severe hemophilia, patients with 1–5% activity are called moderate hemophilia and individuals with >5%, <40% are termed as mild hemophilia [17].

3.1. Hemophilia a and factor VIII

Hemophilia A is majorly caused by deficiency in FVIII antigen levels or mutations in FVIII gene that effect FVIII functions [18, 19]. FVIII is encoded by the gene that localized on the long arm of X chromosome and the gene consists of 26 exons [18, 19]. A total of 2537 mutations are identified on FVIII gene [20]. FVIII is highly expressed in the liver [21, 22]. The mature FVIII protein consists of 2332 amino acids with 6 domains. These domains include A1, A2, B, A3, C1 and C2 [23, 24]. In the blood FVIII is activated by thrombin or FXa [25, 26]. Thrombin cleaves FVIII at R372, R740 and R1689 and removes B domain [26]. Similarly, FXa cleaves FVIII at

K36, R336, R562, R740, R1689 and R1721 [27]. FXa mediated cleavage of FVIII at K36 and R336 leads to inactivation of FVIIIa [27]. APC inactivates FVIII by proteolytically cleaving FVIIIa at R336 and R562 which leads to destabilization of A1 and A2 domain interaction [28, 29] (**Figure 2**). In 1960s, major treatment for hemophilia A is whole blood or plasma transfusion [30, 31]. This treatment has a drawback of viral transfusion along with the coagulation factors. Treatments of mild hemophilia A include vasopressin analogs to enhance the synthesis of FVIII, 1-Desamino-8d-arginine vasopressin (DDAVP) is a vasopressin analog clinically used to enhance the plasma levels of FVIII [32, 33]. Recombinant FVIIa and FVIII are also used to prevent bleeding events in the hemophilia patients [34].These clotting factors are also supplemented with FVIIa or factor FVII inhibitor bypassing agent (FEIBA) to enhance the function of FVIIa and FVIII, whereas FEIBA enhanced the risk of thrombosis [35, 36]. Recent studies elucidated that stabilized recombinant FVIII can be used as a therapeutic for hemophilia A, this includes more stable isoforms of FVIII such as B domain deleted FVIII (BDD FVIII) [37] (**Table 1**). The ongoing research is focusing on using BDD FVIII as a gene therapy by incorporating it into the viral vectors and delivering it into the patient [38].

3.2. Hemophilia B and its treatment

Hemophilia B is another bleeding disorder considered to be indistinguishable from hemophilia A whereas, recent evidences elucidated that hemophilia B patients have less severe bleeding phenotype lower bleeding frequency and better long term outcomes compared to hemophilia A [42]. Hemophilia B is caused due to FIX deficiency [43]. FIX is encoded by a gene present on X chromosome, FIX is a major component of intrinsic pathway of coagulation cascade and it is activated into FIXa by FXIa or FVIIa [44–46]. Activated FIX forms a X-ase complex with FVIIIa and phosphatidylserine [47]. Tenase complex converts X to Xa [47]. The bleeding tendency depends on FIX activity in the plasma [48]. FIX deficiencies are classified based on the plasma FIX activity and they are severe (<1% FIX activity), moderate (1–5%) and

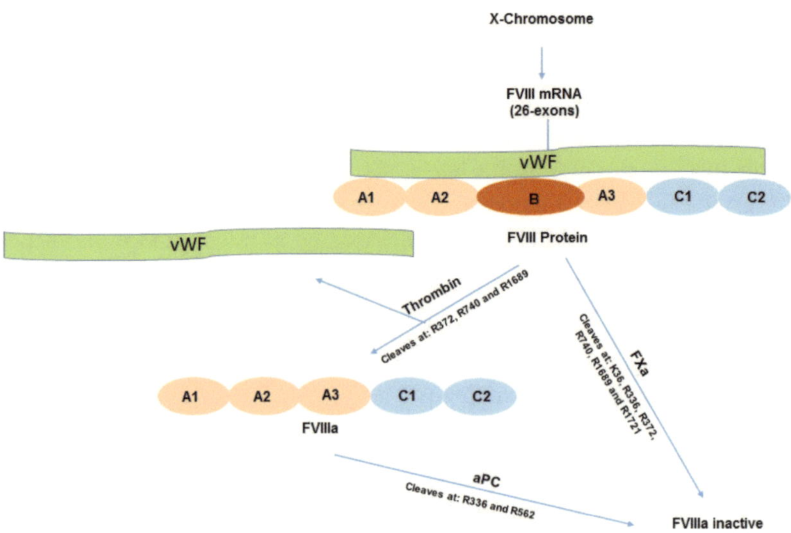

Figure 2. Schematic representation for FVIII biosynthesis and inactivation.

http://dx.doi.org/10.5772/intechopen.75141

FVIII-product	Half-life in hours
Full length Plasma derived [31]	14.8–17.5
Plasma derived FVIII-vWF complex [39]	12.2–17.9
Recombinant Full length FVII [34]	14.6 ± 4.9
B-Domain Deleted FVIII [34]	14.5 ± 5.3
BDD-PEGylated [40]	14.69 ± 3.79
BDD-rFVIII-Fc [41]	19.7 ± 2.3
BDD-rFVIII EHL single chain [30]	14.2

Table 1. Development of FVIII therapy for hemophilia.

mild (5–40%) [48]. Current therapies for hemophilia B include plasma derived FIX, recombinant FIX, recombinant FIX fused with polyethylene glycol (PEG), recombinant FIX fused with Fc portion of immunoglobulin G, FIX fused with albumin mutant FIX [48]. The disadvantages of plasma derived FIX is that it has a very short half-life in the patient plasma and plasma derived FIX has chances of viral contamination. Recombinant FIX is produced in Chinese hamster ovary cells [48]. rFIX has an increased half-life compared to plasma derived FIX, it over came the problem of viral contamination, however rFIX showed 30% less activity compared to plasma derived FIX, due to variations in the glycosylation. Conjugation of FIX with PEG is known as PEGylation. PEG serves as a shield for PEGylated FIX and protects it from proteolytic cleavage. PEGylated FIX's half-life is five times in mice compared to the half-life of rFIX [48]. FC fused FIX has a half-life of 48 h. The other FIX fusion protein in clinical trial is FIX fused with albumin. Single amino acid mutation in the catalytic domain of FIX (R338L) increased its Tenase activity by 2 fold and thrombin generation activity by 6 fold, therefore by FIX R338L usage in gene therapy is under investigation [49].

3.3. Hemophilia C

Hemophilia C is caused by FXI deficiency where factor XI activity of 15–20 U/dL or lower. Surprisingly FXI deficiency does not show a severe bleeding phenotype [16].

4. Platelets in hemophilia

Platelets are key components of primary coagulation system [50]. TF released from the damaged endothelial cells activates the platelets [51].Activated platelets get adhere to the site of damage with help of vWF [52]. Upon activation platelets expose phosphatidylserine which gives the lipid surface to the coagulation cascade [51]. Recent studies elucidate that platelets can play a major role in hemophilia, as hemophilia patients with same FIX or FVIII antigen levels has different clotting time due to variations in the platelet mediated coagulation activity [53–55]. Platelets store FVIII in the alpha granules therefore, platelets are being used as therapeutic components for hemophilia treatment, majorly in gene therapy. In a recent study, hemophilic dogs were transfused with genetically modified platelets (which can over express FVIII gene). Bleeding events were stopped in the hemophilic dogs after transfusing them with genetically altered platelets [53].

5. Rare bleeding disorders

Rare inherited bleeding disorders (RBDs) include deficiencies of coagulation factors such as fibrinogen, factor II (FII), FV, combined deficiency of FV and FVII, FVIII, FX, FXI, FXIII and vitamin K dependent factors. RBDs are mostly autosomal recessive disorders varying from 1 in 500,000 to 1 in 2–3 million [56]. These disorders are diagnosed by clotting assays such as thrombin time, prothrombin time and activated partial thromboplastin time followed by molecular diagnosis [56].

5.1. Fibrinogen deficiency

Fibrinogen is a 340 kDa hexamer assembled by the combination of 3 homologous polypeptide chains (Aα, Bβ and γ) [57]. Fibrinogen plays an important role in clot formation where thrombin converts fibrinogen into soluble fibrin which further forms an insoluble polymer mesh, fibrin also plays an active role in platelet aggregation by binding to glycoprotein IIb/IIIa on the activated platelets [57]. The genes encoding for Bβ (FGB), Aα (FGA) and γ (FGG) are located on chromosome 4 from centromere to telomere [58]. Fibrinogen is primarily synthesized in liver [59]. Fibrin deficiency is identified as two phenotypes termed as afibrinogenemia/hypofibrinogenemia and it is characterized by low plasma and platelet fibrinogen antigens whereas, dys/hypodysfibrinogenemia is characterized by the deficiency of functional fibrinogen levels [60, 61]. Afibrinogenemia is detected by prolonged prothrombin time, thrombin time, activated partial thromboplastin time, impaired platelet adhesion and impaired platelet aggregation induced by ADP [60, 62]. Clinical manifestations of fibrinogen include umbilical stump bleeding, possible gastrointestinal bleeding, recurrent episodes of intracranial hemorrhage [60, 63]. Treatment for fibrinogen deficiency include replacement therapy by cryoprecipitate [63].

5.2. Prothrombin deficiency

Prothrombin is a vitamin K dependent glycoprotein synthesized in the liver [64]. Prothrombin is encoded by 21 kb gene present on chromosome 11 [65, 66]. Prothrombin deficiency is observed in 1 in 2 million [65]. Prothrombin deficiency is classified into two types, hypoprothrombinemia caused by low prothrombin production and dysprothrombinemia is caused by deficiency of functional prothrombin [65]. Hypoprothrombinemia with less than 5% prothrombin antigen is characterized by severe bleeding whereas dysprothrombinemia causes variable bleeding tendencies [65]. Treatments for prothrombin deficiency include prothrombin complex concentrate and fresh frozen plasma [67].

5.3. Factor V deficiency

FV is a single polypeptide encoded by chromosome 1 and primarily synthesized in the liver and some evidences show that FV is also produced by megakaryocytes [68–70]. The activated FV acts as a cofactor for FXa, to form a prothrombinase complex and it also serves as a target for APC-PS complex in inhibiting the coagulation cascade [71]. Patients with FV deficiency surprisingly do not show bleeding phenotype. Recent evidences elucidated that platelets endocytose FV from plasma, modify them intracellularly and release it at the site of injury. This platelet released FV is resistant for inhibition. If symptomatic patients usually have umbilical stump bleeding, skin and mucosal tract hemorrhage [72].

5.4. FVII deficiency

FVII is a 50 Kda single chain polypeptide encoded by F7 gene located on chromosome 13 and FVII levels are influenced by age, sex and health condition such as blood cholesterol and triglyceride levels [73, 74]. FVII deficiency is observed in 1 in 500,000, with variable phenotypes [74]. Some patients do not show bleeding phenotype despite very low FVII levels, whereas others with similar FVII antigen levels show severe bleeding phenotype [74]. The bleeding phenotypes of FVII deficiency include central nervous system hemorrhage, epistatic and menorrhagia [74]. Frozen fresh plasma, prothrombin complex concentrates, plasma derived FVII concentrate, recombinant FVIIa are typically used to treat FVII deficiency [75, 76].

5.5. FX deficiency

Factor X is a single chain polypeptide with a molecular weight of 58,900 kDa and circulates in plasma with a concentration of 10 μg/ml [77]. FX is encoded by FX gene present on chromosome 13 [78]. FX deficiency is characterized by central nervous system and gastro intestinal bleeding [79, 80]. FX deficiency is one of the very rare disorders observed in 1 in 500,000–1000,000 [79, 80]. Treatments of FX deficiency include highly purified plasma FX, recombinant FX, fresh frozen plasma and prothrombin complex concentrates [79, 80].

5.6. FXI deficiency

FXI is a 80 kDa protein with a plasma concentration of 30 nM, encoded by a 23 kb gene present on chromosome 4 [81–83]. Mutations in the coding region are the major causes for FXI deficiency and the prevalence of FXI deficiency is 1 in 1000,000 [83, 84]. The common symptoms of FXI deficiency are oral and post-operative bleeding. FXI deficient women are prone to menorrhagia. Fresh frozen plasma, FXI concentrate and antifibrinolytic agents are used to treat FXI deficiency [84].

5.7. FXIII deficiency

The functional FXIII consist 2 catalytic A subunits (FXIII-A) and 2 carrier subunits (FXIIIB) [85]. FXIII-B is encoded by chromosome 6 and synthesized by the cells derived from bone marrow, whereas FXIIIA is encoded by chromosome 1 and secreted from liver [85, 86]. FXIII crosslinks α and γ subunits of fibrin thereby increases the strength of fibrin clot and increases fibrinolytic resistance [86]. Prevalence of FXIII deficiency is 1 in 2 million, patients with FXIII-A have high tendency of bleeding [87]. 2–5% plasma FXIII is sufficient to prevent bleeding, FXIII concentrates are usually used to treat FXIII deficiency and frozen fresh plasma and cryoprecipitate are also recommended [87].

5.8. Vitamin K dependent coagulation factors deficiency (VKCFD)

Procoagulants such as FII, FVII, FIX and FX, as well as anticoagulants Protein C, S and Z contain a Glutamic acid rich domain [88, 89]. The Glutamate residues require γ-carboxylation to enable these proteins to bind to the phospholipid membrane in the presence of calcium and carry out their functions [90]. Hepatic γ-glutamyl carboxylase (GGCX) and its cofactor, reduced vitamin K (KH2) aids the carboxylation process and in this process vitamin K is converted into vitamin K epoxide [91, 92]. The vitamin K epoxide is recycled to reduced vitamin K by the vitamin K epoxide reductase (VKOR) enzyme complex [91, 92]. GGCX is encoded by the gene located on chromosome 2 and VKORC1 is encoded by the gene present on chromosome 16 [93, 94]. Mutations in these gene cause loss of GGCX or VKOR complex function and lead to vitamin K dependent coagulation factor deficiency [95]. The clinical manifestations of VKCFD include intracranial hemorrhage or umbilical stump bleeding [95]. Viral inactivated frozen fresh plasma is the agent of choice for VKCFD patients, who require surgical procedures or have acute bleeding [95].

6. Thrombosis

Blood clotting occurs at the site of injury to prevent the leakage of the blood However in thrombosis, blood clots are formed in the blood vessel without any damage response and occlude the blood vessel [96]. Thrombosis is classified based on the location of the clot formation, it includes atrial thrombosis, venous thromboembolism (VTE) and pulmonary embolism (PE) [97, 98]. Thrombosis causes high mortality in United States where, annually 900,000 patients develop VTE and 300,000 people die due to PE [99–101]. Atrial emboli is found predominantly in surgical and intensive care patients due to preexisting conditions such as age, hypercoagulability, cardiac abnormalities and atherosclerosis [102]. Most often the clots are found in the veins due to low shear rates in veins (20–200/s) compared to arteries (300–800/s) [103]. Thrombosis found in veins is termed as venous thrombosis. The thrombus formation in the deep veins is termed as deep vein thrombosis. The risk factors for thrombosis are classified by Virchow and they referred as Virchow's Triad [104]. The triad includes endothelial injury, stasis or turbulence of blood flow, and blood hypercoagulability. Endothelial injuries generally happen during surgery, the turbulence of blood flow occurs due to cardiovascular disorders or hypertension [104]. Hypercoagulability is caused by the environment, unhealthy habits and age. The environmental risk factors include exposure to high altitudes and hypoxic environment [103]. The external risk factors for the thrombosis include smoking, chronic alcoholism and consumption of oral contraceptive pills [103]. Similarly, health conditions like cancer, obesity and aging promote the risk of thrombosis [103]. The molecular mechanisms under these risk factors are yet to be understood. Thrombosis is also caused by inherited factors such as mutations in the genes that encode for coagulation factors or anticoagulants.

6.1. Procoagulants - thrombosis

Serine proteases of coagulation cascade play a vital role in the progression of clot formation [3]. Mutations in the proteases convert them into hyper active forms and some of the mutations prevent their degradation and enhance thrombin generation. High levels of FVIII, FIX, FVII and TF are known to cause the thrombosis [105].

6.1.1. FVIII and thrombosis

FVIII is secreted from the hepatocytes, the mature FVIII zymogen circulates in the blood stream at a concentration of 0.1–0.2 μg/ml (<100 IU/dl) [105]. In blood FVIII is bound to vWF produced by the endothelial cells, with a dissociation constant of 0.2–0.4 nM [106]. The complex of vWF-FVIII stabilizes FVIII by preventing the cleavage of inactive FVIII by FXa and APC and it also blocks the procoagulant of FVIII by allowing the selective activation of FVIII by thrombin (**Figure 2**). vWF anchors and multimerizes at the site of tissue damage and helps in the formation of platelet plugs [106]. These vWF multimers are cleaved by ADAMTS13 (ADAMTS13 is a Disintegrin like and Metalloprotease with ThromboSpodin repeats family metalloprotease) [107]. Mutations in vWF or ADAMTS13 increases plasma FVIII levels. Increase in the plasma FVIII above 150 IU/dl increases the risk of thrombosis by 4.8 fold [105, 108]. Further each increase in FVIII level with 10 IU/dl is associated with a 10% increase in the risk of a first event of thrombosis.

6.1.2. FIX and thrombosis

FIX is a key component of intrinsic/contact pathway. Levels of FIX are important to regulate the hemostasis [3]. Lower levels of FIX antigen leads to hemophilia and recently two studies showed that higher levels of FIX lead to thrombosis [109]. Saenko et al. demonstrated that risk of thrombosis increases by 2.3–2.8 fold in the subjects with plasma FIX activity >150 IU/dl and van HylckamaVlieg et al. demonstrated that risk of thrombosis increases by 2.8 fold with plasma FIX levels >129 U/dl [110, 111]. Age, increase in blood lipids and use of oral contraceptive pills are some of the reasons for elevated plasma FIX levels [110, 111]. Some of the mutations in FIX gene lead to increase in FIX activity thereby, increase in the risk of thrombosis. FIX Padua variant is a one among the FIX mutants to show enhanced risk of thrombosis. FIX Padua is a single amino acid substitution variant where arginine 388 is mutated to leucine [112].

6.1.3. Tissue factor and thrombosis

Tissue factor is also known as Factor III (FIII), it is a 47 kDa glycoprotein highly expressed in the pericytes and adventitial fibroblasts, low levels of TF expression are observed in CD14-positive monocytes [113]. TF is expressed in the parenchyma of highly vascularized organs such as placenta, brain, heart, kidneys, and lungs [114]. Circulatory TF is found in macrovesicles produced by apoptotic bodies, smooth muscle cells, monocytes and cancer cells. TF expression is enhanced by pathological conditions such as bacterial infections and cancer [115, 116].

6.1.4. Other procoagulants and thrombosis

FXI levels more than 110 IU/dl increases the chances of thrombosis by 2 fold and inhibition of FXI in thrombosis models rescues the DVT. Prothrombin levels more than 115 IU/dl increases the risk of thrombosis by 2.1 fold. Plasma thrombin levels are reported to increase due to polymorphic variations. FV leiden is one the well-known FV variant that causes high risk of thrombosis. Koster et al. reported increase in fibrinogen levels increases the risk of thrombosis by 2.8 fold [105].

6.2. Anticoagulants - thrombosis

Activated Protein C, Protein S, Protein Z and Tissue factor pathway inhibitor are natural anticoagulants that help in preventing the accidental or pathological thrombi formation. Defects in these clotting factors lead to thrombosis [10].

6.2.1. Protein C (PC)

PC is a vitamin K dependent serine protease majorly synthesized by liver and its expression has also been identified in epididymis, kidney, lung, brain and male reproductive organ. PC is a single polypeptide of 461 amino acids, consist one Gla domain, a helical aromatic segment, two epidermal growth factor (EGF)-like domains, an activation peptide and a trypsin-like serine protease domain [117]. In the presence of Calcium, PC binds to the endothelial membrane through its Gla domain and interacts with its receptor (endothelial PC receptor: EPCR) [117]. The complex of PC-EPCR facilitates the activation of PC by thrombin, thrombomodulin complex where, thrombin cleaves PC at Arg169-Leu170. This cleavage removes activation peptide from PC. Activated Protein C (APC) cleaves FV and FVIII, and inactivates them. Zymogen PC circulates in the blood at a concentration of 63 nM with a half-life of 2–3 hours whereas, plasma APC concentration is 40 pM with a half-life of 20 min. APC function is increased in presence of Protein S (PS) as PS acts as a cofactor for APC. Reduction of plasma APC antigen levels or loss of APC function is one of the causes for thrombosis. Causes for PC deficiency include congenital/ hereditary deficiencies due to mutations in PC gene. Till date 380 mutations are reported in PC gene (http://www.hgmd.cf.ac.uk/ac/gene.php?gene=PROC). Hereditary PC deficiency is treated by a protein C zymogen concentrate derived from human plasma known as Protexel® (Raosevich et al. 2003). Low plasma PC antigen levels (<10 IU/dl) are also caused by acquired PC deficiency. Acquired PC deficiency is caused by consumption of vitamin K antagonist or severe hepatic dysfunction. A recombinant analogue to the physiologic human activated PC (Drotrecogin alpha activated/ Xigris®) is used to treat the acquired PC deficiency. Thrombosis is also observed due to loss of APC function (APC resistance). APC resistance is observed due to mutations in FV (FV leiden) or APC resistance is acquired by smoking, chronic alcoholism and obesity [118].

6.2.2. TFPI

TFPI is a single chain polypeptide with specialized domains called Kuntz domains. It is primarily synthesized in endothelial cells, liver and macrophages [7]. TFPI is mainly bound to the endothelial cell surface through glycosaminoglycans. TFPI circulates in the plasma at a concentration of 1.0–2.5 nM with a half-life of 60–120 min. Major portion of plasma TFPI is bound to LDL and levels of TFPI are regulated by thyroid hormones. TFPI is cleared from the system by liver and kidney. TFPI directly binds to FVIIa, FXa complex and inhibits their function. Inhibitory function of TFPI is enhanced in presence of Protein S [7]. Low levels of TFPI increases the risk of thrombosis by 2 fold [119].

6.2.3. *Protein S*

PS is a vitamin K dependent single chain polypeptide consist of one Gla domain, four EGF like domains and two Laminin G domains. PS is primarily synthesized in liver and it circulates in the plasma at a concentration of 450 nM. 60% of circulatory PS is bound to compliment component binding protein 4b (C4BP) and only 40% of the circulatory PS is free [6, 120]. PS acts as a cofactor for APC and TFPI in inhibiting FVIIIa, FVa, and TF-FVIIa-FXa complex [121, 122]. PS was reported to directly interact with procoagulants such as FV, FIXa and FX and inhibit their function [121, 122]. PS plays a key role in regulating inflammation and clearing the apoptotic bodies from the system. PS deficiency enhances the risk of thrombosis and PS deficiency is classified as hereditary PS deficiency and acquired PS deficiency. Hereditary PS is caused by mutations in the PS gene and till date ~200 mutations are reported in PS gene. Acquired PS deficiency is caused by several factors such as, usage of oral contraceptive pills, pregnancy, consumption of vitamin K antagonists and pathogen infections.

6.2.4. *Protein Z and protein Z dependent protease inhibitor*

Protein Z is a 62 kDa vitamin K dependent plasma protein that acts as a cofactor for 72 kDa serpin family protease inhibitor – Protein Z Dependent Protease Inhibitor (ZPI). ZPI-PZ complex rapidly inhibits FXa and FXIa [8].

6.2.5. *Anticoagulants in the treatment for thrombosis*

Thrombosis is treated by selectively inhibiting the major procoagulant proteins. Major drug targets for the treatment of thrombosis include vitamin K agonists, FXa, FIXa, Thrombin and platelet inhibitors. Current oral anticoagulants approved by FDA are rivaroxaban, Apixaban, dabigatran and endoxaban. Revaroxaban and Apixaban inhibit FXa, whereas dabigatran and endoxaban inhibit thrombin. Several other procoagulant inhibitors such as RNA aptamers are under investigation [123].

7. Acquired coagulation disorders

An individual can acquire coagulation disorders due to several reasons. Infections such as streptococci cause thrombosis by inactivating Protein S [124]. Chronic smoking and chronic alcoholism effect coagulation system by altering the liver functions. Environmental factors like hypoxia, drugs like aspirin, oral contraceptive pills, dietary problems like vitamin K deficiency affect the blood coagulation [12, 56–61].

7.1. Disseminated intravascular coagulation (DIC)

DIC is characterized by activation of clotting system within the vasculature which blocks the micro vessels and can cause further organ dysfunction [125]. In contrast, it can also accelerate fibrinolysis and cause severe bleeding. The international Society of Hematology (ISTH) has defined DIC as *"an acquired syndrome characterized by the intravascular activation of coagulation with loss of localization arising from different causes. It can originate from and cause damage to microvasculature, which if severe, can produce organ dysfunction"* [125–127]. DIC occurs in all ages, races and all genders. DIC is classified as acute DIC, developed due to sudden exposure of procoagulants [125–127]. In acute DIC compensatory hemostatic mechanisms are quickly overwhelmed and leads to hemorrhage development. Chronic DIC is develops due to constant or intermittent exposure of small amounts of tissue factor (TF) [125–127]. DIC is acquired due to several reasons which include external agents such as infections, snake bite, trauma, severe transfusion reactions and environmental changes that cause hemocytopenia [125–127]. Disease conditions leading to DIC include malignancy, organ disfunctions such as hepatic failure and pancreatitis, vascular abnormalities. The phenotypes of DIC include non-symptomatic, bleeding, massive bleeding and organ failure type. If there is no observed phenotype in the patients, whereas the abnormalities were observed in clinical laboratory only, the diagnosis is known as Non-symptomatic DIC [125–127]. In the bleeding type is more predominantly observed phenotype in DIC, the primary symptom is bleeding due to hyperfibrinolysis [125–127]. This phenotype is observed in patients with leukemia, aortic aneurysm and obstetric diseases. Organ failure phenotype is observed in the patients with hypercoagulation, this phenotype is observed in patients with infections. Massive bleeding is observed when the fibrinolysis and hypercoagulation are remarkable. Massive bleeding often leads to death [125–127].

DIC is diagnosed by global tests such as platelet count, prothrombin time (PT), aPTT and the amount of fibrinogen, fibrin and fibrin degradation products. Other diagnostic markers include antithrombin, Protein C, Thrombin-Antithrombin (TAT) complex, VWF propeptide and plasminogen activator inhibitor-1 (PAI-1) (**Table 2**). Treatment of DIC depends on the type of phenotype (**Table 2**) [128]. Heparin treatment is recommended for the treatment of non-symptomatic type whereas, antifibrinolytic treatment is not recommended. The recommended treatment for the organ failure type DIC is natural protease inhibitor whereas, antifibrinolytic treatment is not recommended [128]. Recommended treatments for the bleeding phenotype DIC include blood transfusion, synthetic protease inhibitors and a fibrinolytic treatment, the non-recommended treatments include heparin and anti-Xa [128] (**Figure 3**).

7.2. Vitamin K deficiency and warfarin therapy

Vitamin K is an essential cofactor needed for carboxylation of glutamate residues of Gla domain containing proteins [95]. Dietary deficiency of vitamin K leads to acquired bleeding disorders. Vitamin K oral supplementation is recommended to treat the vitamin K deficiency [95]. Vitamin K deficiency is diagnosed by prolonged prothrombin time, detection of non-carboxylated proteins and measuring the plasma vitamin K by high performance liquid chromatography [129].

Warfarin is a coumarin-based anticoagulant and it is used as an oral anticoagulant. It inhibits vitamin K epoxide reductase (VKOR) thereby prevents vitamin K recycling which in turn limits the availability of vitamin K. Limitation in Vitamin K prevents carboxylation of glutamate residues of Gla domain containing proteins. Preventing Gla domain carboxylation of

Type of DIC	Phenotype	Diagnosis	Causes	Recommended treatments	Non-recommended treatments
Non symptomatic type DIC	No clinical symptoms whereas, abnormalities observed in the dinical examination	Elevation in the fibrin degradation product levels, decreased platelet count, elevation in levels of soluble fibrin and thrombin-anti thrombin complex	Venous thrombosis, operation and bone marrow disorders	Heparin	Afibrinolytic treatment
Organ failure type DIC	Hyper coagulation	Prolonged prothrombin time, elevated fibrinogen and fibrin degradation products, soluble fibrin, thrombin-antithrombin complex, VWF propeptide and plasminogen activator inhibitor-I. reduced platelet count, reduced antithrombin and Protein C levels, ADAMTMS 13	Liver dysfunction, Vitamin K deficiency, venous thromboembolism, operation, bone marrow disorder, capillary leak syndrome, renal disfunction, thrombotic microangiopathy and infection	Natural protease inhibitor	Afibrinolytic treatment
Bleeding type DIC	Hyperfibrinolysis	Prolonged PT, elevated fibrin degradation products, soluble fibrin, thrombin and antithrombin complex and plasmin-plasmin inhibitor complex. Reduced fibrinogen, platelet count.	Liver dysfunction, vitamin K deficiency, venous thromboembolism, operation, liver dysfunction and bone marrow disorder.	Blood transfusion, synthetic protease inhibitor and afibrinolytic treatment	Anti-Xa and heparin
Massive bleeding phenotype	Both hyper coagulation and hyper fibrinolysis	Prolonged PT, reduced fibrinogen and platelet count. Increased soluble fibrin, thrombin-anti thrombin complex and plasmin-plasmin inhibitor complex.	Liver dysfunction, vitamin K deficiency, venous thromboembolism, operation, liver dysfunction and bone marrow disorder.	Blood transfusion, synthetic protease inhibitor and antifibrinolytic treatment	Heparin, Anti-Xa and natural inhibitor

Table 2. DIC phenotypes, diagnosis and treatment.

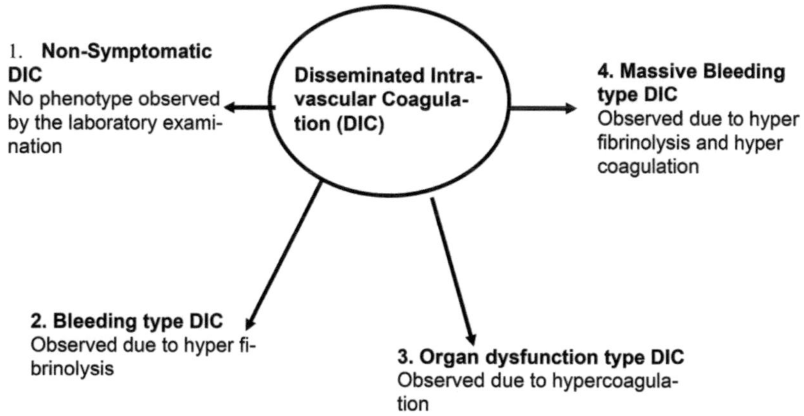

Figure 3. Schematic representation of DIC and its phenotypes.

clotting factors II, VII, IX and X prevents the risk of thrombosis, thereby Warfarin is used as an efficient oral anticoagulant/ blood thinner. Over dosage of Warfarin is lethal as it can cause severe bleeding. 2% of the warfarin consumers are prone to the risk of major hemorrhage [130]. Vitamin K is administered as an antidote for warfarin.

7.3. Acquired disorders of platelet function

Platelet activation and aggregation is essential for clot formation and fibrinolysis [131]. Decrease in platelet number or inhibition of platelet activation impairs blood clotting. Infections such as dengue virus, chickenpox, rubella and bacteria effect the circulating platelet number in the blood [132]. Antiplatelet drugs like aspirin impairs platelet aggregation therefore over dosage of aspirin can cause hemorrhage [133]. Acquired platelet disorders are analyzed by platelet count and their aggregation properties.

7.4. Liver disorders

Liver is the major source of coagulation factors. Chronic alcoholism, smoking and high fat consumption affect the function of liver and there by impact the synthesis of coagulation factors [134]. Blood transfusion is recommended for treating the coagulation defects caused by liver disorders.

8. Diagnosis of coagulation disorders

Coagulation defects are measured by the general assays such as aPTT and PT assays, direct measurement of antigen levels and specific coagulation factor activity assays. Some of the commonly used assays were discussed here.

8.1. Prothrombin time assay (PT assay)

PT assay is used to measure the functional integrity of extrinsic pathway. Clotting is initiated by supplementing tissue factor and calcium chloride to the platelet poor plasma. Elongation of PT indicates the increase in bleeding disorders, similarly shortening of PT indicates the enhanced chances of thrombosis [135].

8.2. Activated prothrombin time assay (aPTT assay)

aPTT assay is used to measure the integrity of intrinsic pathway. In this method the clotting is initiated by supplementing Kontact reagent and calcium chloride to the platelet poor plasma. Similar to PT assay, prolongation of aPTT indicates the risk of bleeding disorders and shortening of the aPTT indicates risk of thrombosis [136].

8.3. Clot waveform analysis (CWA)

CWA is a modified form of aPTT assay, where the light absorbance of the clot measured from the clot initiation to the lysis of the clot and the absorbance is plotted with respect to time using first and second derivates. This assay is more sensitive to measure the changes in FXII, X, IX, VII, V and II levels in the plasma [137, 138].

8.4. Coagulation markers

The coagulation activation and fibrinolysis markers are measured to determine the defects in the coagulation system. One of the diagnostic method to estimate the risk of thrombosis is measuring the D-Dimer antigen levels in the plasma. D-Dimers are the degradation products of cross linked fibrinogen generated during fibrinolysis, increase in the plasma D-Dimer antigen levels directly corresponds to an increase in the risk of thrombosis [139]. Prothrombin fragment 1 + 2 (F1 + 2) are the cleavage products generated from prothrombin and F1 + 2 levels are measured to diagnose the risk of thrombosis, sepsis and DIC [140]. Free thrombin that moves away from the site of clot formation forms a complex with antithrombin III and the complex is known as TAT complex. TAT complex is used to measure the risk of thrombosis in patients with multiple trauma, liver dysfunction and septicemia [141, 142]. Coagulation factors like FXIII, Protein S and Antiphospholipid antibodies are also quantified by immune assays to measure the alterations in coagulation system [141].

9. Conclusions

Coagulation is a complicated biological phenomenon which maintains the hemostasis. Abnormalities in the genes that regulate the coagulation factors cause hereditary coagulation defects such as hemophilia and mutations in genes that encode anticoagulants such as Protein S, Protein Z cause thrombosis. Disruption in the anticoagulant and coagulation factors in the healthy individual causes acquired bleeding disorders. Acquired bleeding disorders include a bleeding disorder or a thrombotic disorder. These disorders can be diagnosed by current methods and can be treated with known methods. There is a high demand for efficient diagnostic and treatment methods for the abnormalities in the coagulation disorders.

Author details

Vijaya S. Pilli

Address all correspondence to: pvssekar@gmail.com

Department of Surgery, University of Wisconsin, Madison, WI, USA

References

[1] Gale AJ. Continuing education course #2: Current understanding of hemostasis. Toxicologic Pathology. 2011;**39**:273-280

[2] Johari V, Loke C. Brief overview of the coagulation cascade. Disease-a-month : DM. 2012;**58**:421-423

[3] Palta S, Saroa R, Palta A. Overview of the coagulation system. Indian Journal of Anaesthesia. 2014;**58**:515-523

[4] Smith SA, Travers RJ, Morrissey JH. How it all starts: Initiation of the clotting cascade. Critical Reviews in Biochemistry and Molecular Biology. 2015;**50**:326-336

[5] Castoldi E, Rosing J. Apc resistance: Biological basis and acquired influences. Journal of thrombosis and haemostasis : JTH. 2010;**8**:445-453

[6] Garcia de Frutos P, Fuentes-Prior P, Hurtado B, Sala N. Molecular basis of protein s deficiency. Thrombosis and Haemostasis. 2007;**98**:543-556

[7] Wood JP, Ellery PE, Maroney SA, Mast AE. Biology of tissue factor pathway inhibitor. Blood. 2014;**123**:2934-2943

[8] Almawi WY, Al-Shaikh FS, Melemedjian OK, Almawi AW. Protein z, an anticoagulant protein with expanding role in reproductive biology. Reproduction. 2013;**146**:R73-R80

[9] Sidelmann JJ, Gram J, Jespersen J, Kluft C. Fibrin clot formation and lysis: Basic mechanisms. Seminars in Thrombosis and Hemostasis. 2000;**26**:605-618

[10] Kesieme E, Kesieme C, Jebbin N, Irekpita E, Dongo A. Deep vein thrombosis: A clinical review. Journal of Blood Medicine. 2011;**2**:59-69

[11] Triplett DA. Coagulation and bleeding disorders: Review and update. Clinical Chemistry. 2000;**46**:1260-1269

[12] Cope G, Kaushik G, O'Sullivan SM, Healy V. Gamma-melanocyte stimulating hormone regulates the expression and cellular localization of epithelial sodium channel in inner medullary collecting duct cells. Peptides. 2013;**47**:54-59

[13] Coppola A, Di Capua M, Di Minno MN, Di Palo M, Marrone E, Ierano P, Arturo C, Tufano A, Cerbone AM. Treatment of hemophilia: A review of current advances and ongoing issues. Journal of Blood Medicine. 2010;**1**:183-195

[14] Konkle BA, Huston H, Nakaya Fletcher S. Hemophilia a. In: Adam MP, Ardinger HH, Pagon RA, Wallace SE, LJH B, Mefford HC, Stephens K, Amemiya A, Ledbetter N, editors. Genereviews(r). Seattle (WA). p. 1993

[15] Konkle BA, Huston H, Nakaya Fletcher S. Hemophilia b. In: Adam MP, Ardinger HH, Pagon RA, Wallace SE, Bean LJH, Mefford HC, Stephens K, Amemiya A, Ledbetter N, eds. Genereviews(r). Seattle (WA); 1993

[16] Shearin-Patterson T, Davidson E. Hemophilia c. JAAPA : official journal of the American Academy of Physician Assistants. 2013;**26**:50

[17] Zimmerman B, Valentino LA. Hemophilia: In review. Pediatrics in Review. 2013;**34**:289-294; quiz 295

[18] Nair PS, Shetty S, Ghosh K. A homozygous female hemophilia a. Indian Journal of Human Genetics. 2012;**18**:134-136

[19] Theophilus BD, Enayat MS, Williams MD, Hill FG. Site and type of mutations in the factor viii gene in patients and carriers of haemophilia a. Haemophilia: The Official Journal of the World Federation of Hemophilia. 2001;**7**:381-391

[20] Albanez S, Ruiz-Saez A, Boadas A, de Bosch N, Porco A. Identification of factor viii gene mutations in patients with severe haemophilia a in Venezuela: Identification of seven novel mutations. Haemophilia: The Official Journal of the World Federation of Hemophilia 2011;**17**:e913-e918

[21] Fomin ME, Zhou Y, Beyer AI, Publicover J, Baron JL, Muench MO. Production of factor viii by human liver sinusoidal endothelial cells transplanted in immunodeficient upa mice. PLoS One. 2013;**8**:e77255

[22] Hollestelle MJ, Geertzen HG, Straatsburg IH, van Gulik TM, van Mourik JA. Factor viii expression in liver disease. Thrombosis and Haemostasis. 2004;**91**:267-275

[23] Fay PJ. Factor viii structure and function. International Journal of Hematology. 2006;**83**: 103-108

[24] Thompson AR. Structure and function of the factor viii gene and protein. Seminars in Thrombosis and Hemostasis. 2003;**29**:11-22

[25] Fay PJ. Activation of factor viii and mechanisms of cofactor action. Blood Reviews. 2004;**18**:1-15

[26] Hill-Eubanks DC, Parker CG, Lollar P. Differential proteolytic activation of factor viii-von willebrand factor complex by thrombin. Proceedings of the National Academy of Sciences of the United States of America. 1989;**86**:6508-6512

[27] Plantier JL, Rolli V, Ducasse C, Dargaud Y, Enjolras N, Boukerche H, Negrier C. Activated factor x cleaves factor viii at arginine 562, limiting its cofactor efficiency. Journal of thrombosis and haemostasis : JTH. 2010;**8**:286-293

[28] Koedam JA, Meijers JC, Sixma JJ, Bouma BN. Inactivation of human factor viii by activated protein c. Cofactor activity of protein s and protective effect of von willebrand factor. The Journal of Clinical Investigation. 1988;**82**:1236-1243

[29] Orfeo T, Elsman R, Gissel M, Mann KG, Butenas S. Activation, activity and inactivation of factor viii in factor viii products. Haemophilia: The Official Journal of the World Federation of Hemophilia. 2016;**22**:462-473

[30] Lieuw K. Many factor viii products available in the treatment of hemophilia a: An embarrassment of riches? Journal of Blood Medicine. 2017;**8**:67-73

[31] Mannucci PM. The choice of plasma-derived clotting factor concentrates. Baillière's Clinical Haematology. 1996;**9**:273-290

[32] Kaufmann JE, Oksche A, Wollheim CB, Gunther G, Rosenthal W, Vischer UM, Vasopressin-induced v. Willebrand factor secretion from endothelial cells involves v2 receptors and camp. The Journal of Clinical Investigation. 2000;**106**:107-116

[33] Vilhardt H, Barth T, Melin P, Aurell CJ. Antidiuretic activity and release of factor viii by vasopressin analogues. European Journal of Pharmacology. 1993;**232**:223-226

[34] Lusher JM, Arkin S, Abildgaard CF, Schwartz RS. Recombinant factor viii for the treatment of previously untreated patients with hemophilia a. Safety, efficacy, and development of inhibitors. Kogenate previously untreated patient study group. The New England Journal of Medicine. 1993;**328**:453-459

[35] Sallah S. Treatment of acquired haemophilia with factor eight inhibitor bypassing activity. Haemophilia: The Official Journal of the World Federation of Hemophilia. 2004;**10**:169-173

[36] Scharrer I. Recombinant factor viia for patients with inhibitors to factor viii or ix or factor vii deficiency. Haemophilia: The Official Journal of the World Federation of Hemophilia. 1999;**5**:253-259

[37] Dooriss KL, Denning G, Gangadharan B, Javazon EH, McCarty DA, Spencer HT, Doering CB. Comparison of factor viii transgenes bioengineered for improved expression in gene therapy of hemophilia a. Human Gene Therapy. 2009;**20**:465-478

[38] High KH, Nathwani A, Spencer T, Lillicrap D. Current status of haemophilia gene therapy. Haemophilia: The Official Journal of the World Federation of Hemophilia. 2014;**20**(Suppl 4):43-49

[39] Buchanan GR, Kevy SV. Use of prothrombin complex concentrates in hemophiliacs with inhibitors: Clinical and laboratory studies. Pediatrics. 1978;**62**:767-774

[40] Wynn TT, Gumuscu B. Potential role of a new pegylated recombinant factor viii for hemophilia a. Journal of Blood Medicine. 2016;**7**:121-128

[41] Peters RT, Toby G, Lu Q, Liu T, Kulman JD, Low SC, Bitonti AJ, Pierce GF. Biochemical and functional characterization of a recombinant monomeric factor viii-fc fusion protein. Journal of thrombosis and haemostasis : JTH. 2013;**11**:132-141

[42] Shetty S, Ghosh K. Why should hemophilia b be milder than hemophilia a? Haematologica. 2016;**101**:e213

[43] Cramer R, Matter M, Loeliger A. Hemophilia b; two familial case of blood disease due to deficiency of a new coagulation factor, christmas factor. Helvetica Paediatrica Acta. 1953;**8**:185-201

[44] Cullen CR, Hubberman P, Kaslow DC, Migeon BR. Comparison of factor ix methylation on human active and inactive x chromosomes: Implications for x inactivation and transcription of tissue-specific genes. The EMBO Journal. 1986;**5**:2223-2229

[45] Gailani D, Geng Y, Verhamme I, Sun MF, Bajaj SP, Messer A, Emsley J. The mechanism underlying activation of factor ix by factor xia. Thrombosis Research. 2014;**133**(Suppl 1): S48-S51

[46] Liu DY, Rosen S. Activation of bovine factor ix by the reaction product of bovine factor vii and human tissue factor. Chinese Medical Journal. 1994;**107**:181-185

[47] Brandstetter H, Bauer M, Huber R, Lollar P, Bode W. X-Ray structure of clotting factor ixa: Active site and module structure related to xase activity and hemophilia b. Proceedings of the National Academy of Sciences of the United States of America. 1995;**92**:9796-9800

[48] Brown PE, Hougie C, Roberts HR. The genetic heterogeneity of hemophilia b. The New England Journal of Medicine. 1970;**283**:61-64

[49] Monahan PE, Sun J, Gui T, Hu G, Hannah WB, Wichlan DG, Wu Z, Grieger JC, Li C, Suwanmanee T, Stafford DW, Booth CJ, Samulski JJ, Kafri T, McPhee SW, Samulski RJ. Employing a gain-of-function factor ix variant r338l to advance the efficacy and safety of hemophilia b human gene therapy: Preclinical evaluation supporting an ongoing adeno-associated virus clinical trial. Human Gene Therapy. 2015;**26**:69-81

[50] Heemskerk JW, Mattheij NJ, Cosemans JM. Platelet-based coagulation: Different populations, different functions. Journal of thrombosis and haemostasis : JTH. 2013;**11**:2-16

[51] Yun SH, Sim EH, Goh RY, Park JI, Han JY. Platelet activation: The mechanisms and potential biomarkers. BioMed Research International. 2016;**2016**:9060143

[52] Song S, Mody M, Freedman J, Ellis J, Lazarus AH. Von willebrand factor (vwf)-dependent human platelet activation: Porcine vwf utilizes different transmembrane signaling pathways than does thrombin to activate platelets, but both require protein phosphatase function. Journal of thrombosis and haemostasis : JTH. 2003;**1**:337-346

[53] Du LM, Nurden P, Nurden AT, Nichols TC, Bellinger DA, Jensen ES, Haberichter SL, Merricks E, Raymer RA, Fang J, Koukouritaki SB, Jacobi PM, Hawkins TB, Cornetta K, Shi Q, Wilcox DA. Platelet-targeted gene therapy with human factor viii establishes haemostasis in dogs with haemophilia a. Nature Communications. 2013;**4**:2773

[54] Montgomery RR, Shi Q. Platelet and endothelial expression of clotting factors for the treatment of hemophilia. Thrombosis Research. 2012;**129**(Suppl 2):S46-S48

[55] Riedl J, Ay C, Pabinger I. Platelets and hemophilia: A review of the literature. Thrombosis Research. 2017;**155**:131-139

[56] Kaushik G, Thomas MA, Aho KA. Psychoactive pharmaceuticals as environmental contaminants may disrupt highly inter-connected nodes in an autism-associated protein-protein interaction network. BMC Bioinformatics. 2015;**16**(Suppl 7):S3

[57] Kaushik G, Zarbalis KS. Prenatal neurogenesis in autism spectrum disorders. Frontiers in Chemistry. 2016;**4**:12

[58] Kaushik G, Huber DP, Aho K, Finney B, Bearden S, Zarbalis KS, Thomas MA. Maternal exposure to carbamazepine at environmental concentrations can cross intestinal and placental barriers. Biochemical and Biophysical Research Communications. 2016;**474**: 291-295

[59] Kaushik G, Xia Y, Yang L, Thomas MA. Psychoactive pharmaceuticals at environmental concentrations induce in vitro gene expression associated with neurological disorders. BMC Genomics. 2016;**17**(Suppl 3):435

[60] Gompers AL, Su-Feher L, Ellegood J, Copping NA, Riyadh MA, Stradleigh TW, Pride MC, Schaffler MD, Wade AA, Catta-Preta R, Zdilar I, Louis S, Kaushik G, Mannion BJ, Plajzer-Frick I, Afzal V, Visel A, Pennacchio LA, Dickel DE, Lerch JP, Crawley JN, Zarbalis KS, Silverman JL, Nord AS. Germline chd8 haploinsufficiency alters brain development in mouse. Nature Neuroscience. 2017;**20**:1062-1073

[61] Kaushik G, Xia Y, Pfau JC, Thomas MA. Dysregulation of autism-associated synaptic proteins by psychoactive pharmaceuticals at environmental concentrations. Neuroscience Letters. 2017;**661**:143-148

[62] Lebreton A, Casini A. Diagnosis of congenital fibrinogen disorders. Annales de Biologie Clinique. 2016;**74**:405-412

[63] Tziomalos K, Vakalopoulou S, Perifanis V, Garipidou V. Treatment of congenital fibrinogen deficiency: Overview and recent findings. Vascular Health and Risk Management. 2009;**5**:843-848

[64] Bell RG. Metabolism of vitamin k and prothrombin synthesis: Anticoagulants and the vitamin k--epoxide cycle. Federation Proceedings. 1978;**37**:2599-2604

[65] Lancellotti S, Basso M, De Cristofaro R. Congenital prothrombin deficiency: An update. Seminars in Thrombosis and Hemostasis. 2013;**39**:596-606

[66] Royle NJ, Irwin DM, Koschinsky ML, MacGillivray RT, Hamerton JL. Human genes encoding prothrombin and ceruloplasmin map to 11p11-q12 and 3q21-24, respectively. Somatic Cell and Molecular Genetics. 1987;**13**:285-292

[67] Stewart JD. Clinical significance of prothrombin deficiency and its treatment. Annals of Surgery. 1941;**114**:907-918

[68] Camire RM. A new look at blood coagulation factor v. Current Opinion in Hematology. 2011;**18**:338-342

[69] Hayward CP, Fuller N, Zheng S, Adam F, Jeimy SB, Horsewood I, Quinn-Allen MA, Kane WH. Human platelets contain forms of factor v in disulfide-linkage with multimerin. Thrombosis and Haemostasis. 2004;**92**:1349-1357

[70] Jenny RJ, Pittman DD, Toole JJ, Kriz RW, Aldape RA, Hewick RM, Kaufman RJ, Mann KG. Complete cdna and derived amino acid sequence of human factor v. Proceedings of the National Academy of Sciences of the United States of America. 1987;**84**:4846-4850

[71] Duga S, Asselta R, Tenchini ML. Coagulation factor v. The International Journal of Biochemistry & Cell Biology. 2004;**36**:1393-1399

[72] Huang JN, Koerper MA. Factor v deficiency: A concise review. Haemophilia: The Official Journal of the World Federation of Hemophilia. 2008;**14**:1164-1169

[73] Millar DS, Kemball-Cook G, McVey JH, Tuddenham EG, Mumford AD, Attock GB, Reverter JC, Lanir N, Parapia LA, Reynaud J, Meili E, von Felton A, Martinowitz U, Prangnell DR, Krawczak M, Cooper DN. Molecular analysis of the genotype-phenotype relationship in factor vii deficiency. Human Genetics. 2000;**107**:327-342

[74] Mulliez SM, Devreese KM. Isolated acquired factor vii deficiency: Review of the literature. Acta Clinica Belgica. 2016;**71**:63-70

[75] Mariani G, Bernardi F. Factor vii deficiency. Seminars in Thrombosis and Hemostasis. 2009;**35**:400-406

[76] Napolitano M, Siragusa S, Mariani G. Factor vii deficiency: Clinical phenotype, genotype and therapy. Journal of Clinical Medicine. 2017;**6**

[77] Hertzberg M. Biochemistry of factor x. Blood Reviews. 1994;**8**:56-62

[78] Rocchi M, Roncuzzi L, Santamaria R, Archidiacono N, Dente L, Romeo G. Mapping through somatic cell hybrids and cdna probes of protein c to chromosome 2, factor x to chromosome 13, and alpha 1-acid glycoprotein to chromosome 9. Human Genetics. 1986;**74**:30-33

[79] Brown DL, Kouides PA. Diagnosis and treatment of inherited factor x deficiency. Haemophilia: The Official Journal of the World Federation of Hemophilia. 2008;**14**: 1176-1182

[80] Uprichard J, Perry DJ. Factor x deficiency. Blood Reviews. 2002;**16**:97-110

[81] Emsley J, McEwan PA, Gailani D. Structure and function of factor xi. Blood. 2010;**115**:2569-2577

[82] Kato A, Asakai R, Davie EW, Aoki N. Factor xi gene (f11) is located on the distal end of the long arm of human chromosome 4. Cytogenetics and Cell Genetics. 1989;**52**:77-78

[83] Kitchens CS. Factor xi: A review of its biochemistry and deficiency. Seminars in Thrombosis and Hemostasis. 1991;**17**:55-72

[84] Wheeler AP, Gailani D. Why factor xi deficiency is a clinical concern. Expert Review of Hematology. 2016;**9**:629-637

[85] Schroeder V, Kohler HP. Factor xiii: Structure and function. Seminars in Thrombosis and Hemostasis. 2016;**42**:422-428

[86] Wolberg AS. Plasma factor xiii: Understanding the 99%. Blood. 2014;**123**:1623-1624

[87] Odame JE, Chan AK, Wu JK, Breakey VR. Factor xiii deficiency management: A review of the literature. Blood Coagulation & Fibrinolysis: An International Journal in Haemostasis and Thrombosis. 2014;**25**:199-205

[88] Josic D, Hoffer L, Buchacher A. Preparation of vitamin k-dependent proteins, such as clotting factors ii, vii, ix and x and clotting inhibitor protein c. Journal of Chromatography. B, Analytical Technologies in the Biomedical and Life Sciences. 2003;**790**:183-197

[89] Nelsestuen GL, Shah AM, Harvey SB. Vitamin k-dependent proteins. Vitamins and Hormones. 2000;**58**:355-389

[90] Huang M, Rigby AC, Morelli X, Grant MA, Huang G, Furie B, Seaton B, Furie BC. Structural basis of membrane binding by gla domains of vitamin k-dependent proteins. Nature Structural Biology. 2003;**10**:751-756

[91] Berkner KL. Vitamin k-dependent carboxylation. Vitamins and Hormones. 2008;**78**: 131-156

[92] Tie JK, Stafford DW. Structure and function of vitamin k epoxide reductase. Vitamins and Hormones. 2008;**78**:103-130

[93] De Vilder EY, Debacker J, Vanakker OM. Ggcx-associated phenotypes: An overview in search of genotype-phenotype correlations. International Journal of Molecular Sciences. 2017;**18**

[94] Garcia AA, Reitsma PH. Vkorc1 and the vitamin k cycle. Vitamins and Hormones. 2008;**78**:23-33

[95] Brenner B, Kuperman AA, Watzka M, Oldenburg J. Vitamin k-dependent coagulation factors deficiency. Seminars in Thrombosis and Hemostasis. 2009;**35**:439-446

[96] Poole JC. Structural aspects of thrombosis. The Scientific basis of Medicine Annual Reviews. 1964:55-66

[97] Previtali E, Bucciarelli P, Passamonti SM, Martinelli I. Risk factors for venous and arterial thrombosis. Blood transfusion = Trasfusione del sangue. 2011;**9**:120-138

[98] Tarbox AK, Swaroop M. Pulmonary embolism. International Journal of Critical Illness and Injury Science. 2013;**3**:69-72

[99] Anderson FA Jr, Wheeler HB, Goldberg RJ, Hosmer DW, Patwardhan NA, Jovanovic B, Forcier A, Dalen JE. A population-based perspective of the hospital incidence and case-fatality rates of deep vein thrombosis and pulmonary embolism. The Worcester dvt study. Archives of Internal Medicine 1991;**151**:933-938

[100] Kopcke D, Harryman O, Benbow EW, Hay C, Chalmers N. Mortality from pulmonary embolism is decreasing in hospital patients. Journal of the Royal Society of Medicine. 2011;**104**:327-331

[101] Silverstein MD, Heit JA, Mohr DN, Petterson TM, O'Fallon WM, Melton LJ, 3rd. Trends in the incidence of deep vein thrombosis and pulmonary embolism: A 25-year population-based study. Archives of Internal Medicine 1998;**158**:585-593

[102] Lyaker MR, Tulman DB, Dimitrova GT, Pin RH, Papadimos TJ. Arterial embolism. International Journal of Critical Illness and Injury Science. 2013;**3**:77-87

[103] Machlus KR, Aleman MM, Wolberg AS. Update on venous thromboembolism: Risk factors, mechanisms, and treatments. Arteriosclerosis, Thrombosis, and Vascular Biology. 2011;**31**:476-478

[104] Kumar DR, Hanlin E, Glurich I, Mazza JJ, Yale SH. Virchow's contribution to the understanding of thrombosis and cellular biology. Clinical Medicine & Research. 2010;**8**:168-172

[105] Bertina RM. Elevated clotting factor levels and venous thrombosis. Pathophysiology of Haemostasis and Thrombosis. 2003;**33**:395-400

[106] Peyvandi F, Garagiola I, Baronciani L. Role of von willebrand factor in the haemostasis. Blood transfusion = Trasfusione del sangue. 2011;**9**(Suppl 2):s3-s8

[107] Zander CB, Cao W, Zheng XL. Adamts13 and von willebrand factor interactions. Current Opinion in Hematology. 2015;**22**:452-459

[108] Kraaijenhagen RA, in't Anker PS, Koopman MM, Reitsma PH, Prins MH, van den Ende A, Buller HR. High plasma concentration of factor viiic is a major risk factor for venous thromboembolism. Thrombosis and Haemostasis 2000;**83**:5-9

[109] Lowe G. Factor ix and deep vein thrombosis. Haematologica. 2009;**94**:615-617

[110] Sweeney JD, Hoernig LA. Age-dependent effect on the level of factor ix. American Journal of Clinical Pathology. 1993;**99**:687-688

[111] van Hylckama Vlieg A, van der Linden IK, Bertina RM, Rosendaal FR. High levels of factor ix increase the risk of venous thrombosis. Blood. 2000;**95**:3678-3682

[112] Simioni P, Tormene D, Tognin G, Gavasso S, Bulato C, Iacobelli NP, Finn JD, Spiezia L, Radu C, Arruda VR. X-Linked thrombophilia with a mutant factor ix (factor ix Padua). The New England Journal of Medicine. 2009;**361**:1671-1675

[113] DelGiudice LA, White GA. The role of tissue factor and tissue factor pathway inhibitor in health and disease states. Journal of Veterinary Emergency and Critical Care. 2009;**19**:23-29

[114] Versteeg HH, Ruf W. Emerging insights in tissue factor-dependent signaling events. Seminars in Thrombosis and Hemostasis. 2006;**32**:24-32

[115] Falanga A, Russo L, Milesi V, Vignoli A. Mechanisms and risk factors of thrombosis in cancer. Critical Reviews in Oncology/Hematology. 2017;**118**:79-83

[116] Kothari H, Rao LV, Vankayalapati R, Pendurthi UR. Mycobacterium tuberculosis infection and tissue factor expression in macrophages. PLoS One. 2012;**7**:e45700

[117] Esmon CT. The protein c pathway. Chest. 2003;**124**:26S-32S

[118] Agrawal N, Kumar S, Puneet, Khanna R, Shukla J, Khanna AK. Activated protein c resistance in deep venous thrombosis. Annals of Vascular Surgery. 2009;**23**:364-366

[119] Dahm A, Van Hylckama Vlieg A, Bendz B, Rosendaal F, Bertina RM, Sandset PM. Low levels of tissue factor pathway inhibitor (tfpi) increase the risk of venous thrombosis. Blood. 2003;**101**:4387-4392

[120] Heeb MJ. Role of the pros1 gene in thrombosis: Lessons and controversies. Expert Review of Hematology. 2008;**1**:9-12

[121] Castoldi E, Hackeng TM. Regulation of coagulation by protein s. Current Opinion in Hematology. 2008;**15**:529-536

[122] Chattopadhyay R, Sengupta T, Majumder R. Inhibition of intrinsic xase by protein s: A novel regulatory role of protein s independent of activated protein c. Arteriosclerosis, Thrombosis, and Vascular Biology. 2012;**32**:2387-2393

[123] Harter K, Levine M, Henderson SO. Anticoagulation drug therapy: A review. The Western Journal of Emergency Medicine. 2015;**16**:11-17

[124] Chen CL, Wu YY, Lin CF, Kuo CF, Han CL, Wang S, Chuang WJ, Chen CY, Wu JJ, Tsai PJ, Liu CC, Lin YS. Streptococcal pyrogenic exotoxin b inhibits apoptotic cell clearance by macrophages through protein s cleavage. Scientific Reports. 2016;**6**:26026

[125] Venugopal A. Disseminated intravascular coagulation. Indian Journal of Anaesthesia. 2014;**58**:603-608

[126] Levi M. Disseminated intravascular coagulation. Critical Care Medicine. 2007;**35**: 2191-2195

[127] Levi M, van der Poll T. Disseminated intravascular coagulation: A review for the internist. Internal and Emergency Medicine. 2013;**8**:23-32

[128] Wada H, Matsumoto T, Yamashita Y. Diagnosis and treatment of disseminated intravascular coagulation (dic) according to four dic guidelines. Journal of Intensive Care. 2014;**2**:15

[129] Isarangkura P, Mahasandana C, Chuansumrit A, Angchaisuksiri P. Acquired bleeding disorders: The impact of health problems in the developing world. Haemophilia: The Official Journal of the World Federation of Hemophilia. 2004;**10**(Suppl 4):188-195

[130] Keeling D, Baglin T, Tait C, Watson H, Perry D, Baglin C, Kitchen S, Makris M. British Committee for Standards in H. Guidelines on oral anticoagulation with warfarin - fourth edition. British Journal of Haematology. 2011;**154**:311-324

[131] Travers RJ, Smith SA, Morrissey JH. Polyphosphate, platelets, and coagulation. International Journal of Laboratory Hematology. 2015;**37**(Suppl 1):31-35

[132] Hassan AA, Kroll MH. Acquired disorders of platelet function. Hematology. American Society of Hematology. Education. Program. 2005:403-408

[133] Zucker ML, Trowbridge C, Woodroof J, Chernoff SB, Reynoso L, Dujovne CA. Low-vs high-dose aspirin. Effects on platelet function in hyperlipoproteinemic and normal subjects. Archives of Internal Medicine. 1986;**146**:921-925

[134] Ng VL. Liver disease, coagulation testing, and hemostasis. Clinics in Laboratory Medicine. 2009;**29**:265-282

[135] Reddy DVS, Venkataramiah C. Prothrombin time in health and disease. (according to quick's method). The. Indian Medical Gazette. 1941;**76**:341-344

[136] Korsan-Bengtsen K. Routine tests as measures of the total intrinsic blood clotting potential. A comparison of whole blood clotting time (wbct), recalcification time of citrated plasma (rtst), partial thromboplastin time (ptt), and activated partial thromboplastin time (aptt). Scandinavian Journal of Haematology. 1971;**8**:359-368

[137] Lance MD. A general review of major global coagulation assays: Thrombelastography, thrombin generation test and clot waveform analysis. Thrombosis Journal. 2015;**13**:1

[138] Shima M, Thachil J, Nair SC, Srivastava A, Scientific, Standardization C. Towards standardization of clot waveform analysis and recommendations for its clinical applications. Journal of thrombosis and haemostasis : JTH. 2013;**11**:1417-1420

[139] Dempfle CE. Use of d-dimer assays in the diagnosis of venous thrombosis. Seminars in Thrombosis and Hemostasis. 2000;**26**:631-641

[140] Bruhn HD, Conard J, Mannucci M, Monteagudo J, Pelzer H, Reverter JC, Samama M, Tripodi A, Wagner C. Multicentric evaluation of a new assay for prothrombin fragment f1+2 determination. Thrombosis and Haemostasis. 1992;**68**:413-417

[141] Kappel A, Ehm M. Immunoassays for diagnosis of coagulation disorders. Hämostaseologie. 2010;**30**:194-201

[142] Seitz R, Wolf M, Egbring R, Havemann K. The disturbance of hemostasis in septic shock: Role of neutrophil elastase and thrombin, effects of antithrombin iii and plasma substitution. European Journal of Haematology. 1989;**43**:22-28

Chapter 8

Sickle Cell Nephropathy: Current Understanding of the Presentation, Diagnostic and Therapeutic Challenges

Baba P.D. Inusa, Lodi Mariachiara,
Palazzi Giovanni and Kenneth I. Ataga

Additional information is available at the end of the chapter

http://dx.doi.org/10.5772/intechopen.76588

Abstract

Sickle cell nephopathy (SCN) begins early in childhood from failure of urinary concentration (hyposthenuria), albuminuria to hyperfiltration, hematuria and progression to falling glomerular filtration to end-stage renal disease and increased mortality. Renal involvement is more severe in homozygous individuals (HbSS) than in compound heterozygous patients (HbSC). The pathogenesis of SCN is multifactorial from hypoxia, acidosis, hemolysis, ischemia-reperfusion injury and albuminuria. The clinical manifestations depend on whether the main pathology is tubular, glomerular or a mixture of both abnormalities. This chapter offers a critical review of the recent literature and will highlight the pathophysiology, epidemiology, clinical manifestations and management of sickle cell nephropathy with particular focus on the major advance in the early diagnosis. *Learning points*: For SCN, the onset of hyperfiltration and albuminuria in infants and childhood is an opportunity to intervene early. There is no diagnostic markertest capable of detecting the onset of these changes. Moreover there is no reliable therapeutic agent to prevent or halt early changes due to SCN. The development of a marker of renal impairment in SCD such as such as Cystatin C assay if validated may be appropriate for wider clinical application.

Keywords: sickle cell disease, sickle cell nephropathy, acute kidney injury, biomarkers

1. Introduction

Sickle cell disease (SCD) is one of the most frequent genetic disorders in the world. It predominantly affects people of African descent as well as individuals from the Middle East, India and

Mediterranean regions. Recent estimates report about 305,800 babies with SCD are born every year in the word and over two-thirds are in sub-Saharan Africa rising to over 404,200 by 2050 [1, 2]. The disease is associated with a high lifetime morbidity and premature mortality [3], as described in the 2013 Global Burden of Disease Study [4]. The age-standardized death rate in sickle cell anemia increased from 1990 to 2013 (median change 28) [5]. The World Health Organization (WHO) has addressed the significant public health implication of sickle cell anemia, urging implementation of equitable and effective programs for the prevention and management of SCD [6]. Furthermore, encouragement was provided for the promotion, support and coordination of much needed research in SCD [6].

The term'sickle cell disease' refers to all genotypes that cause the clinical syndrome. It occurs due to the inheritance of abnormal beta globin S (βS) alleles with the substitution of valine for glutamic acid in position 6 of the beta globin; the most common phenotype is homozygous β^S/β^S which is referred to as sickle cell anemia (SCA). The second most common phenotype, hemoglobin SC disease (HbSC), occurs due to co-inheritance of the β^S and β^C alleles, and presents a more moderate phenotype. HbS/β-thalassemia is the co-inheritance of β^S with a β-thalassemia allele [7], those with a thalassemia null mutation (HbSβ^0) presenting with a phenotype that is clinically indistinguishable from SCA, whereas individuals with HbSβ^+ thalassemia have a milder disorder [8]. The resulting sickle hemoglobin (HbS) polymerizes when the concentration of its deoxygenated form (deoxyHbS) exceeds a critical threshold. Low oxygen levels, increased acidity and cellular dehydration facilitate the polymerization of HbS and the distortion of the red blood cells leading to sickle-shaped erythrocytes [9]. The co-inheritance of genetic factors such as α-thalassemia or hereditary persistence of fetal hemoglobin are known to reduce the rate of HbS polymerization [10]. Sickling of red blood cells results in both obstruction of blood flow leading to organ and tissue ischemia, and hemolytic anemia [2, 11]. Reduced blood flow is mediated via a dynamic interaction between sticky HbS-containing red blood cells, white blood cells and the vessel wall [2]. Chronic intravascular hemolysis leads to the release of free hemoglobin that sequesters nitric oxide, a potent vasodilator and anti-inflammatory molecule, leading to vasoconstriction in different organs. Stroke and pulmonary hypertension are thought to be consequences of the diminished vascular relaxation caused by nitric oxide deficiency [12]. In addition, intravascular hemolysis in SCD leads to high plasma levels of cell-free heme and hemoglobin (Hb), sources of redox active iron. Iron-derived reactive oxygen species are implicated in the pathogenesis of numerous vascular disorders including atherosclerosis, microangiopathic hemolytic anemia, vasculitis and reperfusion injury [13]. Exposure of endothelium to heme greatly potentiates cell death. Recurrent cycles of ischemia-reperfusion injury in the microvasculature might amplify endothelial dysfunction and further organ injury including the stroke, pulmonary hypertension and kidney injury.

2. Sickle cell nephropathy

Renal involvement in SCD is a complex phenomenon resulting from an increased tendency of sickling in the renal medulla due to hypoxia, acidosis and hyperosmolar conditions [13]. Abnormally, high hemodynamic renal blood flow leads to early onset hypertrophic and impaired urinary concentrating ability, distal nephron dysfunction and progressive glomerulopathy. The combination of cortical hyperperfusion, medullary hypoperfusion and vasoconstriction leads to further vasculopathy in the kidney. Sickle cell nephropathy (SCN) is a spectrum of changes resulting from a cascade of events occurring in the kidney. This is triggered by RBC vascular occlusion, infarction and reperfusion injury occurring within the renal medullar, cortex and collecting system. These may present as hyperfiltration, microalbuminuria, impaired urinary concentrating ability complicated by episodes of acute kidney disease (AKD) features early in childhood. In young adults, there is progressive increase in albuminuria and regression of the glomerular filtration rate (GFR). Further deterioration of renal function with the development of chronic kidney disease (CKD) (defined as estimated GFR of less than 90 ml/min/1.73 m^2) eventually leads to end-stage renal disease (ESRD) in adulthood (**Figure 1**).

2.1. Pathobiology/histology

Early stages of SCN are characterized by glomerular hypertrophy, hemosiderin deposits with focal areas of hemorrhage or necrosis. This is followed by interstitial inflammation, edema, fibrosis, tubular atrophy and papillary infarcts [14–16]. Some of these features were reported in a multi-center, retrospective analysis of renal biopsies of 18 SCD patients (16-HbSS, 1-HbSC, 1 HbSβ thalassemia) who presented with proteinuria, acute or progressive impairment of renal function [17]. The study reported focal segmental glomerulosclerosis (FSGS) in seven cases, membranoproliferative glomerulonephritis (MPGN) in five and thrombotic microangiopathic glomerulopathy in three; while glomerular hypertrophy with or without mesangial hypercellularity was reported in three cases. Furthermore immunofluorescence microscopy

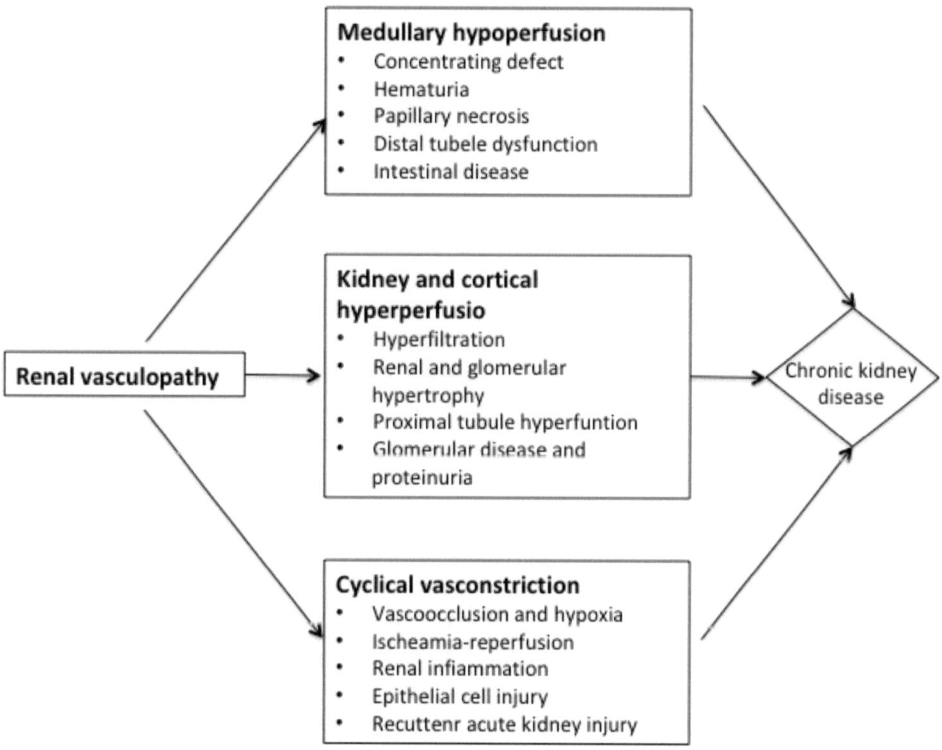

Figure 1. The pathogenetic processes in the development of sickle cell nephropathy [13].

in the patients with FSGS-type lesions showed irregular staining for IgM and C3 in areas of sclerosis [15, 16, 18]. Complement deposition occur in the glomeruli coinciding with various degrees of proteinuria including nephrotic syndrome [19].

2.2. Risk factors for renal impairment in sickle cell disease

2.2.1. *Hemolysis and vasculopathy*

Hemolysis in SCD leads to release of arginase 1, asymmetric dimethylarginine and adenine nucleotides, these promote vasomotor dysfunction and proliferative vasculopathy. Circulating hemoglobin and heme both referred to as erythrocytic danger-associated molecular pattern (eDAMP) molecules activate endothelial inflammatory and angiogenesis. Hemolysis in SCD therefore leads to anemia, increased superoxide anion and reactive oxygen species (ROS) production and low ROS scavenging enzymes activity promote oxidative stress-induced vascular complications. Itokua et al. reported in their study [20] that albuminuria was associated with increased white blood cell (WBC) count and LDH enzyme levels. Oxidative damage may alter both the structure and the function of the glomerulus due to its effects on mesangial and endothelial cells. Activated circulating white blood cells and platelets express adhesion glycoproteins leading to endothelial cell adhesion molecules and endothelial dysfunction.

2.2.2. *Endothelin-A receptor antagonismo retards the progression of sickle cell nephopathy*

Endothelin-1 (ET-1) is a signaling peptide produced by diverse cell types that exerts its physiologic and pathophysiologic actions by binding to two receptor subtypes, ETA and ETB. ETA receptor activation induces vasoconstriction, inflammation and nociception which is abolished by ETB activation in some tissues. ETA receptor signaling produces oxidant stress and the release of cytokines such as NF-kB activate and promote the production of ET-1, the agonist for the ETA receptor. A number of studies have reported increased production of ET-1 in SCD thus promoting sickling and tissue injury. Kasztan et al. reported that by blocking ETA receptor, the progression of SCN in a murine model of SCD was abolished [21]. The introduction of sickle RBCs into murine endothelial cells induces ET-1, leading to ETA-dependent vasoconstriction [22, 23]. It has also been shown that plasma ET-1 levels are elevated in patients with SCD during steady state periods as well as during acute vaso-occlusive crisis. Conversely, plasma ET-1 levels are decreased in SCD patients treated with hydroxyurea [24]. Elevated ET-1 level in SCD is associated with endothelial dysfunction and albuminuria in patients with SCD [25]. Bosentan, a dual ETA/ETB receptor antagonist used in murine models, decreases hypoxia-related injury to renal vessels and lung inflammation [26]. As it has been shown by Kasztan' s studies, administration of ambrisentan (an ETA receptor antagonist), at the time of weaning and continued for 10 weeks, prevented glomerular dysfunction, tubulointerstitial inflammation and fibrosis [24]. The observations of Kasztan et al. support this speculation as the markedly elevated plasma ET-1 levels that occur in this model are normalized by chronic administration of ambrisentan [21]. Long-term administration of ambrisentan significantly reduced the degree of iron deposit in renal tubules. The reduction in tubular iron deposits suggests that ambrisentan reduces hemolysis in murine models. Free heme is a well-known promoter of oxidative stress and the generation of proinflammatory species, for example, ROS. Free heme also stimulates the production of placenta growth factor (PlGF), an angiogenic growth factor that is implicated in the pathogenesis of tissue injury in SCD as well as the production of ET-1 [27–29]. NO is a suppressor of ET-1 synthesis and vascular ET-1 production may also increase when the vascular system is depleted due to NO binding to HbS plasma. ET-1 causes RBC dehydration by activating the Gardos channel present in the plasma membrane of RBCs [30, 31].

2.2.3. Mouse models

Mouse models provide opportunities to explore the mechanisms of globin gene regulation and the feasibility of gene therapy for this condition and the molecular basis of end-organ damage, including SCN [32]. The use of established mouse models is of invaluable help to investigate the pathogenesis of SCD-associated multiple organ complications and to identify targets for prevention and therapy.

Several murine models have been developed to mimic human SCD. Of these, the Berkeley model (BERK mice) has targeted deletions of murine α and β globins ($\alpha^{-/-}$, $\beta^{-/-}$) with a transgene containing human α, β^{s}, $^{A}\gamma$, $^{G}\gamma$ and β globins (Hba0/0 Hbb0/0 TG (Hu-miniLCRα1GγA$\gamma\delta\beta$S) ($\alpha^{-/-}$, $\beta^{-/-}$, transgene +); thus, these mice almost exclusively express human sickle hemoglobin [33]. The BERK mouse model exhibits a wide spectrum of hematologic and histopathologic findings that are similar to those found in humans with SCD. Erythrocyte sickling is significant in BERK mice, and erythrocyte survival is very short resulting in massive amounts of heme being released into the plasma. As seen in humans with SCD, BERK mice showed a wide spectrum of kidney pathologies such as increased cortical hypertrophy, gross and microscopic infarcts, iron deposition, enlarged glomeruli associated with mesangial cell and mononuclear cell hypercellularity are observed in kidneys from BERK mice [34].

Another mouse model of SCD, the transgenic SAD mouse bears the human α-globin gene and the HbS mutation, β^{S}, as well as $\beta^{Antilles}$ and $\beta^{D\text{-}Punjab}$ which greatly enhance the tendency of its hemoglobin to polymerize [35]. The SAD mice display renal hemosiderosis, microvascular occlusions, vascular thrombosis, cortical infarcts and papillary necrosis. Most mice show glomerular hypertrophy and mesangial sclerosis. The glomerular damage is associated with abnormal function, characterized by increased blood urea nitrogen levels and proteinuria [35]. The glomerular lesions of SAD mice faithfully mimic sickle cell glomerulosclerosis, the most severe renal complication observed in individuals with SCD. Therefore, the SAD mouse constitutes a valuable model to investigate the pathophysiology of the thrombotic and glomerulosclerotic complications of human SCD. Ischemic injury contributes to end-organ damage and other complications of SCD. Increased sensitivity of tissues in SCD to ischemic insults has been demonstrated in SCD mice. As it has been showed by Nath et al., after induction of bilateral renal ischemia, transgenic SCD mice exhibited massive vascular congestion, sickling of red blood cells and more prominent capillary congestion in the lungs and heart compared to control mice [36]. These results demonstrated increased susceptibility to vascular congestion and to ischemia in tissues from SCD mice, suggesting that ischemic episodes may contribute to the renal complications observed in SCD. Abnormal leukocyte-endothelium attachment associated with endothelial activation was observed in SCD mice, showing interesting parallels between the vascular injury after reperfusion and kidney damage. In addition, this study suggested that allopurinol, that prevents ischemia-reperfusion generation of reactive oxygen species, might be a potential therapy for SCD [37]. The anti-sickling property of fetal hemoglobin was also demonstrated in SCD mice [38]. Patients with SCD suffer from painful crises associated with vaso-occlusion. Increased circulating erythrocyte membrane microparticles (MPs) have been associated with occlusion of capillaries. Interestingly, MPs triggered immediate renal vaso-occlusion in mice. In vitro studies showed that MPs stimulate the production of reactive oxygen species by endothelial cells, stimulate RBC adhesion and induce endothelial apoptosis. This work introduced a novel concept that associates the shedding of MPs from sickled RBC with vascular disease [39]. An interaction of free heme with TLR4 receptor was shown to mediate the nephrotoxicity of heme, in particular, the effects of heme on renal blood flow and inflammatory responses [40].

2.2.4. Development of sickle cell nephropathy from infancy to adulthood

Glomerular changes in SCD occur early in the first decade of life even though SCD patients remain asymptomatic. These are characterized by high renal blood flow, hyperfiltration and hypertrophy. Current data suggest that infants with SCD develop a hyperfiltration phase, which plateaus during early childhood. As early as the first year, renal enlargement is observed in correlation to hyperfiltration. Hyperfiltration is a well-known phenomenon in SCD even though the pathogenesis and pathophysiology is less well understood. As a result of hyperperfusion, increased amount of fluids is presented to the proximal tubule triggering more tubular reabsorption of sodium and water in order to restore glomerulotubular balance. Increased proximal tubular sodium reabsorption is associated with high metabolism and adaptive cellular response leading to overall renal enlargement. This complex phenomenon might be relevant to the glomerular hypertrophy that occurs in SCD [13]. Some studies show that for children with HbSS, there is an age-related increase in the estimated creatinine clearance in the first decade of life, with a decline toward normal values in the second decade [41–43]. In the study by Etteldorf and colleagues, children with SCD aged 4–11 years had a significantly higher mean measured glomerular filtration rate (mGFR) (169 mL/min/1.73 m^2) than normal controls (128 mL/min/1.73 m^2) [44]. In the BABY HUG trial, 176 children aged 9–19 months had a measured GFR at baseline of 125 mL/min/1.73 m^2 [45], which was significantly higher than published normal values for the same age group [46].

In a cross-sectional study of 410 patients with SCD aged 2–21 (mean age 11) years, 23% of HbSS patients showed elevated urinary albumin excretion (≥30 mg/g), while other investigators have reported a HbSS prevalence of 16–27% in the childhood SCD population [47–49].

Further progressive kidney injury and CKD is reflected in a declining and abnormally low GFR. During adolescence, estimated glomerular filtration rate (eGFR) begins to decline in some patients, and aroud 10% of adolescent patients with SCD develop a GFR of <90 mL/min/1.73 m^2 [50]. Similarly, Bodas et al. recently reported a CKD prevalence of 8% in a cohort of patients with SCD aged 3–17 years [51].

The prevalence of end-stage renal disease (ESRD) in the pediatric SCD population is also not well described; however, childhood SCD accounts for only 0.3% of incident pediatric ESRD [52].

Eventually, renal failure develops in early adulthood (median age 23–37 years) in SCA and in mid-life (median age 50 years) in HbSC disease.

2.2.5. *Proteinuria and chronic kidney disease*

The prevalence of albuminuria in SCD is age dependent. It may be classified as moderately increased albuminuria (previous called microalbuminuria)—urine albumin concentration of 30–300 mg/g creatinine and severely increased albuminuria (macroalbuminuria)—urine albumin concentration of 300 mg/g creatinine. The prevalence of albuminuria in the first three decades of life is up to 27% increasing to 68% in older SCD patients [13]. The understanding of the evolution of CKD in SCD is evolving the extent to which moderate albuminuria progresses to severely increased albuminuria and the relationship with SCN. The development of SCN is likely due to complex interactions between SCD-related risk factors and non-SCD phenotype characteristics. Albuminuria is more likely to occur in patients who express specific single-nucleotide polymorphisms in the MYH9 and APOL1 genes, which are associated with an increased risk of CKD in African Americans [53]. On the other hand, microdeletions in the gene that encodes α-globin (reflecting a form of α-thalassemia trait) leads to a lower prevalence albuminuria [54]. Genetic polymorphisms of bone morphogenetic protein receptor 1B also influence GFR in SCD [55, 56]. SCD patients with albuminuria have increased levels of urinary excretion of markers of tubular injury (KIM-1 and NAG) [57]. The individual contribution of these phenomena to SCN is not clear.

2.2.6. *Chronic kidney disease and end-stage renal disease*

The reported prevalence of ESRD in SCD varies from 5 to 18% depending on the age of the cohort but reamins a significant cause of mortality [58, 59]. Similarly, CKD (defined based on eGFR) which is usually diagnosed between 30 and 40 years is also a risk factor death [47, 60]. In a recent study in Rio de Janeiro, Brazil, 4.3% of patients admitted with SCD had CKD [61]. A lower incidence was observed in a study from Senegal, where CKD was identified in 2.6% of 229 adults with SCD [62]. The manifestations of CKD in SCD include hypertension, proteinuria and anemia. Vaso-occlusive history, legs ulcers, osteonecrosis, retinopathy, proteinuria, hematuria, hypertension and severe anemia were all identified as predictive factors for CKD in SCD [58, 61, 63]. In a recent study from Nigeria, 50% of SCD patients with proteinuria had CKD [64]. Risk factors associated with progression of CKD to ESRD (**Table 1**) include increased blood pressure, low hemoglobin levels, haemolysis, leukocytosis, hematuria, prior vaso-occlusive crisis, the βS Central African Republic (CAR) haplotype, pulmonary hypertension, stroke, acute chest syndrome and infection with parvovirus B19 [65–78]. The mean survival of patients with ESRD and SCD is estimated to be 4 years, even with dialytic treatment [79].

2.2.7. *Urinary concentration abnormalities*

The onset of urinary concentration defects begins in early infancy (6–12 months) and may account for nocturia, polyuria and enuresis in later childhood. The defect in urinary concentration does not respond to vasopressin but it is reported to improve with chronic blood transfusions in young children [47, 63, 64, 80–83]. Further deterioration of the defect in urinary concentration is observed from the second decade of life due to the onset of medullary fibrosis and the loss of the collecting ducts system. High HBF levels are associated with better urinary concentration [84–86]. There may be a role for drugs therapy that enhance the production of HbF such as hydroxyurea and decitabine.

Risk factors associated with progression of CKD to ESRD	Protective factors for the progression of CKD to ESRD
▪ Hypertension ▪ Nephrotic range proteinuria ▪ Severe anemia ▪ Vaso-occlusive crisis ▪ Acute chest syndrome ▪ Stroke ▪ βS CAR haplotype ▪ Genetic variants of MYH9 and APLO1 ▪ Pulmonary hypertension ▪ Parvovirus B19 infection	▪ Co-inheritance with α-thalassemia ▪ Higher fetal hemoglobin level

Table 1. Risk and protective factors associated with progression of CKD to ESRD.

2.2.8. Urinary acidification deficit

The defect in urinary acidification may be a combination of ischemic changes in the medulla and reduced capacity of the collecting duct to maintain hydrogen gradient. It is not clear what is responsioble for this defect but it has been suggested a resistance of the distal nephron to aldosterone may exist [81, 87].

2.2.9. Hematuria

One of the most frequent featurs of SCN is hematuria which is also found in individuals with sickle trait [88], it may be micro or macroscopic and it is usually painless [63, 81]. The mecahanism is not well defined but capillary congestion due to vaso-oclusive and ischemic injury may account for it. It is reported that the left kidney is more likely to be involved due to the fact that the left renal vein is compressed between the aorta and the superior mesenteric artery; also referred to as a "nutcracker-like" phenomenon [37]. Hematuria might also be due to renal papillary necrosis from vaso-occlusion of vasa recta but rarely from renal medullary carcinoma [63]. Nevertheless it is important to exclude other causes such as urinary tract infections, neoplasms, vascular malformations, vasculitis, glomerulonephritis and coagulation disturbances [61, 88].

2.2.10. Sickle cell nephropathy and acute kidney injury

The prevalence of acute kidney injury (AKI) in children with SCD presenting to the hospital emergency room may be as high as 17% [89], AKI is underreported in pediatric SCD patients. In adults, AKI is reported in 4–10% of patients, and in up to 14% of adults with acute chest syndrome. AKI in SCD may also reflect the frequent use of non-steroidal anti-inflammatory drugs (NSAIDs) to treat painful crises in this patient population [52]. A recent retrospective analysis reported 8% of AKI in 149 pediatric patients admitted for acute chest syndrome using the Kidney Disease Improving Global Outcomes (KDIGO) and higher with increased hospital length of stay [90]. The true incidence of AKI in pediatric SCD patients may be underestimated in retrospective studies [89, 90]. In addition, serum creatinine may be an inaccurate marker of renal function in SCD due to the relatively high proximal tubular secretion of creatinine found in this population [91]. Interestingly, a recent adult study showed that even in patients with a normal creatinine level during a pain crisis, acute tubular injury likely occurs, as evidenced by a more than twofold rise in urinary neutrophil gelatinase-associated lipoprotein excretion [92]. NSAID use is common in children with SCD [93], without evidence to support its benefit compared to other less nephrotoxic options. Similarly, the use of non-steroid anti-inflammatory agents (NSAIDS) in children with SCD hospitalized for various indications, including dehydration due to gastroenteritis, was associated with a significant increase in the incidence of AKI [94, 95]. Therefore hemodynamic changes may increase the risk of AKI secondary to NSAIDs, Another contributing factor includes potential toxic tubular effects of free hemoglobin during a sickle crisis. Some SCD patients with CYP2C9 allele variants that alter NSAID metabolism may be at increased risk of toxicity. During vaso-occlusive pain crises and acute chest syndrome, the risk of AKI is increased by the drop in hemoglobin leading to hypoxic-ischemic events, hemolysis or inflammation. In murine SCD models, brief episodes of hypoxic-ischemic events produce profound acute renal injury [36, 96]. The murine model of SCD has shown that an increase in hemolysis or exposure to excess cell-free hemoglobin can also lead to renal injury [97].

3. Assessment of kidney function

The gold standard for assessing how well the kidneys are working is direct measurement of the GFR. CKD is classified based on the eGFR and the level of proteinuria and helps to risk stratify patients (**Table 2A** and **B**). In individuals with SCD, a GFR greater than 120 mL/min/1.73 m^2 is an additional indicator of abnormal kidney function. However, direct measurement of GFR is invasive and time consuming and so estimations of GFR based on the serum creatinine are more commonly used. A number of equations exist, including the `Modification of Diet in Renal Disease' (MDRD), CKD-EPI and Cockcroft-Gault equations [98–100]. Different estimated GFR calculations have been compared to the measured GFR in people with HbSS from the Caribbean and sub-Saharan Africa, the CKD-EPI equation was found to provide the most accurate estimate in two small studies [101, 102]. In individuals with SCD, increased proximal tubule secretion of creatinine results in the serum creatinine level being a poor estimate of GFR [103]. The diagnostic performance of cystatin C in comparison to serum creatinine was analyzed in a meta-analysis of 46 studies, including children and adults. The data compared correlation coefficients between GFR and the reciprocals of serum creatinine and cystatin C in 3703 participants and showed significantly better correlations for cystatin C, suggesting that cystatin is superior to serum creatinine for the detection of impaired GFR in cross-sectional studies [104].

Proteinuria, albumin-to-creatinine ratio (ACR) is greater than 2.5 mg/mmol in men or 3.5 mg/mmol in women, or a protein-to-creatinine ratio (PCR) is greater than 15 mg/mmol is sufficient for a diagnosis of CKD. Proteinuria may be classified as moderately increased albuminuria (3–30 mg/mmol creatinine) or severely increased albuminuria (greater than 30 mg/mmol creatinine) [105].

Table. 2A

GFR categories (mL/min/1.73 m ^{2})	
Stage 1:	Kidney damage with normal or increased GFR (>90 mL/min/1.73 m ^{2})
Stage 2:	Mild reduction in GFR (60-89 mL/min/1.73 m ^{2})
Stage 3a:	Moderate reduction in GFR (45-59 mL/min/1.73 m ^{2})
Stage 3b:	Moderate reduction in GFR (30-44 mL/min/1.73 m ^{2})
Stage 4:	Severe reduction in GFR (15-29 mL/min/1.73 m ^{2})
Stage 5:	Kidney failure (GFR <15 mL/min/ 1.73 m ^{2} or dialysis)

Table. 2B

ACR categories (mg/mmol)	
A1	ACR of less than 3mg/mmol
A2	ACR of 3-30mg/mmol
A3	ACR of more than 30mg/mmo

Table 2. (A) GFR categories in CKD; (B) ACR categories (KDIGO 2012) [105].

4. Novel diagnostic and predictive biomarkers of AKI in children

4.1. Biomarkers used in sickle cell disease

New biomarkers are promising for the early detection of renal function loss in patients with SCD (**Table 3**), including cystatin C, plasma neutrophil gelatinase-associated lipocalin (NGAL), serum liver fatty acid-binding protein (L-FABP), serum kidney injury marker 1 (KIM-1), serum interleukin 18 (IL-18), soluble FMS-like tyrosine kinase-1 (sFLT-1) and N-acetyl-b-D glucosaminidase (NAG) [106].

4.1.1. Serum cystatin C

Cystatin C (CysC) or cystatin 3, a protein encoded by the CST3 gene, is mainly used as a biomarker of kidney function. Recently, it has been studied for its role in predicting new-onset or deteriorating cardiovascular disease (CVD). CysC is a nonglycosylated low molecular weight (13 kDa) basic protein that inhibits cysteine proteases and it has been demonstrated its closely correlation to glomerular filtration rate (GFR) in children [107]. CysC crosses the glomerular membrane, and it is reabsorbed and metabolized in the renal tubules and not returned to the bloodstream. It is not secreted by the tubules, even in cases of reduced GFR, and is not affected by muscle mass, protein intake, metabolic factors, drugs and inflammatory stimuli. It has also been reported that serum CysC correlates with the level of albuminuria [108, 109] and its levels well perform as marker of renal function to detect cardiovascular outcome both in

Biomarker	Source
Cystatin C	All nucleated cells
NGAL	Distal tubule and collecting duct
KIM-I	Proximal tuble
L-FABP	Proximal tuble
IL - 18	Proximal tuble
sFLT-1	Proximal tubular cells
NAG	Proximal tubular

Table 3. Novel urinary biomarkers.

population-based studies and in patients with non-ST-elevation acute coronary syndrome [110]. Therefore CysC is an ideal biomarker for study the renal function in SCD patients which is ongoing hemolysis and inflammation secondary to the sickling phenomenon and in which creatinine clearance is generally increased and serum creatinine is low. Tantawy et al. [111] have found significantly higher serum CysC in patients with SCD compared to healthy controls. In particular, patients of their court of study with nephropathy had higher cystatin levels than those without, and a significant positive correlation was found with ACR. The authors have demonstrated also that patients with SCD treated with hydroxyurea had lower CysC levels than untreated patients, possibly due to the role of hydroxyurea in decreasing inflammation [111]. In agreement with Tantawy's results, Alvarez et al. [108] examined the value of serum CysC as a marker for GFR in small cohort of 20 children with SCD with and without albuminuria, compared to serum creatinine and creatinine clearance. The mean GFR derived from serum cystatin was significantly different among these subgroups, becoming abnormal in the proteinuric cohort (63 mL/min per 1.73 m^2), compared to 94 mL/min per 1.73 m^2 for the microalbuminuric and 103 mL/min per 1.73 m^2 for the normal subgroups. Serum creatinine or creatinine clearance did not change significantly with the level of albuminuria. The authors concluded that serum CysC was higher than serum creatinine in SCD, and this probably relates to the fact that serum CysC is not secreted by the kidney, as creatinine. Moreover other studies have demonstrated the utility of CysC in patients with SCD. Asnani and Reid [109] have proved in 98 adults with SCD that CysC levels were significantly correlated with measured GFR, hemoglobin, serum creatinine, urinary albumin-creatinine ratio (UACR) and systolic blood pressure. In addition to urine, screening for albuminuria may help in the diagnosis of early renal impairment in the patients with SCD before a significant rise in serum creatinine is observed. Receiver-operating characteristic curve (ROC) analysis has revealed that the cut-off value of CysC at 580 ng/mL could differentiate patients having SCD with and without nephropathy with 87.8% sensitivity and 84.6% specificity. Further prospective studies are needed to validate this threshold. On the other hand, Cho et al. [112] have evaluated the significance of serum cystatin C levels in pediatric patients with chronic kidney disease diagnosed by renal biopsy and showed normal serum creatinine levels. The authors have found that 95% of the patients showed only slightly increased cystatin C levels from the upper normal limit of the reference range and suggested that mildly increased cystatin C without increased creatinine might not have clinical significance.

4.1.2. *Urine neutrophil gelatinase-associated lipocalin*

As it has been showed in several preclinical gene expression analyses performed in AKI murine and human models, neutrophil gelatinase-associated lipocalin (NGAL) gene has been revealed the to be one of the most upregulated genes in the kidney soon after an ischemic or a nephrotoxic insult [113, 114]. NGAL is filtered across the glomerulus, is reabsorbed in proximal tubules and its urinary concentration increases early during ischemic insults [115, 116]. The NGAL protein is also highly induced in regenerating and recovering kidney tubule cells. NGAL binds iron; chelation of toxic iron is an important mechanism that protects the kidney tubules from worsening injury. Thus, the biological role of NGAL in AKI is one of enhanced tubule cell proliferation and recovery [117]. Measurement of urinary NGAL (uNGAL) has been demonstrated to be an early, non-invasive marker of AKI due to a variety of etiologies, such as cardiac surgery [118], intravenous contrast administration [119], critical care settings [120] and kidney transplantation [121]. NAGL has an enormous dynamic range, responds in a dose-dependent fashion to injury, responds within 3 h of injury, and responds to a wide range of injuries, easy to measure due to the recent availability of clinical platforms including a new NGAL dipstick. Thus, uNGAL values may then be used to initiate AKI patient care algorithms earlier than serum creatinine alone. Although multiple investigations have demonstrated that uNGAL is a promising AKI biomarkers, a study by Sundaram et al. [57] has not showed any relationship with albuminuria in patients with SCD. This study has also showed that uNGAL levels were significantly subnormal (<50 ng/mL) in most patients with SCA and the overall uNGAL in most patients were well below levels usually seen in patients with acute or chronic renal injury. The authors have explained the results obtained based on the fact that proximal tubular function is supra-normal in SCA, and it is likely that any filtered NGAL may be reabsorbed much more efficiently, resulting in subnormal urinary NGAL levels in SN.

4.1.3. *Soluble FMS-like tyrosine kinase-1*

Soluble FMS-like tyrosine kinase-1 (sFLT-1) is a member of the vascular endothelial growth factor receptor family (VEGFR) and has an antiangiogenic effect. Soluble FLT-1 is increased in SCD due to its over-expression by vascular endothelial cells, vascular smooth muscles, activated blood monocytes and proximal tubular cells of the renal epithelia [122]. A recent study by Youssry et al. [123] investigated the relationship between serum levels of sFLT-1 and other conventional biomarkers of renal damage. The serum level of sFLT-1 in SCD patients was significantly higher than controls and its median level showed no significant difference when comparing patients with SS and Sβ genotypes, hydroxyurea therapy and iron chelation. On the other hand, the authors have found significant positive correlations between serum levels of sFLT-1 and microalbuminuria, LDH and indirect bilirubin. Meanwhile, there were no significant correlations between serum levels of sFLT-1 and creatinine, eGFR, serum ferritin and erythrocyte sedimentation rate (ESR). This association between sFLT-1 levels and microalbuminuria combined with the association of sFLT-1 with soluble vascular cell adhesion molecule (VCAM) in prior studies [124], suggests that sFLT-1 may contribute to the pathogenesis of albuminuria in SCD by promoting endothelial dysfunction.

4.1.4. Serum liver-type fatty acid-binding protein

Serum liver-type fatty acid-binding protein (L-FABP) is an anti-oxidant, renoprotective molecule induced in the proximal tubule early after experimental AKI. It has been reported in children undergoing cardiopulmonary bypass (CPB), the increase in urinary L-FABP maybe occur within 4 h of initiating CPB [125]. However, there are conflicting data about L-FABP, such as a prospective multi-center study of 311 children undergoing cardiac surgery did not show similar increase in L-FABP [106]. In SCD patients, Sundaram et al. [57] reported that urine L-FABP level was highest in the youngest group (6–12 years old) even with little evidence of renal injury. In fact urine L-FABP levels are reduced with increasing albuminuria.

4.1.5. Kidney injury molecule-I

Preclinical studies have identified the kidney injury molecule-I (KIM-1) gene to be induced in the proximal tubule cells of ischemic rat kidneys [114]. KIM-1 protein regulates phagocytosis of damaged cells and thereby limits injury. An extracellular domain of KIM-1 can be detected by enzyme-linked immunosorbent assays and is useful as a urinary biomarker in patients with AKI. In fact, in a study conducted by Han WK et al., it was shown that in 40 children undergoing CPB, urinary KIM-1 levels were markedly increased in those who have developed AKI [126]. On the other hand, a prospective multi-center study of 311 children undergoing cardiac surgery confirmed the delay in upregulation of urinary KIM-1 in AKI patients and showed that KIM-1 was not significantly associated with AKI after adjusting for other injury biomarkers [127]. This data is in contrast with the results published by Sundaram et al. [57]. Indeed when KIM-1 levels, detected in all SCA urine samples, were compared within the different albuminuria groups, they were detected at lowest levels in patients with normal albuminuria, significantly increased in patients with moderately increased albuminuria and further increased in the severely increased albuminuria group, suggesting this may be another biomarker of relevance in sickle nephropathy that needs to be confirmed in longitudinal studies.

4.1.6. Interleukin-18

Interleukin-18 (IL-18) represents a proinflammatory cytokine that might worsen the degree of AKI. Animal studies have shown that IL-18 is induced in the proximal tubule and detectable in the urine following ischemic AKI. Numerous pediatric studies have proved that urine IL-18 obtained 6- to 12-h post-CPB moderately predicts AKI [128–131]. Cerqueira et al. [131] performed a cross-sectional study composed of 45 SCA patients. They founded that IL-18 levels were correlated closely with markers of hemolysis, endothelial dysfunction and others cytokines levels. These findings suggest probable influences of IL-18 in the pathophysiology of vascular occlusion in SCA. In a recent article published by Duarte et al. [132], the author demonstrated that IL18 is associated with diastolic function in SCD patients, and may be involved in the pathogenesis of the disease. Genetic polymorphisms within the IL-18 gene regions are also associated with diastolic function in SCD, likely by affecting expression levels of the genes [132].

4.1.7. N-acetyl-b-D glucosaminidase

N-acetyl-b-D glucosaminidase (NAG) is a lysosomal enzyme produced in proximal tubular epithelial cells. The levels increased during kidney injury, a marker of proteinuria both in patients with diabetes and in patients with SCD [115, 133]. Sundaram et al. [57] showed that urine NAG activity was higher than baseline levels (>2 U/l) and worse in the presence of albuminuria. The elevations in NAG may precede moderately increased albuminuria, a likely diagnostic tool for early renal damage.

4.1.8. Transforming growth factor-b1

Transforming growth factor-b1 (TGF-b1) is a potent fibrogenic growth factor that may play a significant role in pathogenesis of SN [134]. It is a peptide of low molecular weight and has pleiotropic action. In the kidneys, it stimulates fibrogenesis through enhanced production of extracellular matrix proteins and nephron loss by various mechanisms, such as apoptosis of endothelial cells and podocytes [135]. Whether the urinary levels of TGF-b1 has a diagnostic significance in the early prediction of SN in children with SCD is still to be determined [136]. However in the article published by Sundaram et al. [57], urinary TGF-β was present at very low to undetectable levels in their patient population and showed no association with the degree of albuminuria. These data are in contrast with those published by Ghobrial et al. [137]. In their study, the authors have found a strong positive correlation between urinary TGF-b1 and urinary proteins and eGFR in all groups of SCD patients studied.

4.1.9. Neutrophil-to-lymphocyte and platelet-to-lymphocyte ratio

Neutrophil-to-lymphocyte (NLR) and platelet-to-lymphocyte (PLR) ratios, as indicators of subclinical inflammation, rarely were been investigated in SCD patients. Emokpae et al. [138] recently reported a positive association between NLR, PLR and the increase of inflammatory markers in SCD patients such as C-reactive protein (CRP) and fibrinogen. The highest values of NLR and PLR were detected in patients with proteinuria and altered renal function. This data suggest that these markers may be predictive of a proinflammatory state with underlying renal damage.

4.2. Biomarkers not been investigated in sickle cell disease

4.2.1. Markers of cell-cycle arrest

Metalloproteinases-2 (TIMP-2) and insulin-like growth factor-binding protein 7 (IGFBP7) have been identified as a markers of cell-cycle arrest and are induced in renal tubules following AKI. It is supposed that the resulting cell-cycle arrest then limits proliferation of damaged tubule cells. The metabolites of TIMP-2 and IGFBP7 can be measured in the urine. In a small study of children undergoing CPB, the urinary TIMP-1/IGFBP7 product was increased 4 h post-CPB in children who developed AKI [139].

4.2.2. *Urinary excretion of uromodulin*

Urinary excretion of uromodulin (UMOD), also known as Tamm-Horsfall Protein (THP), is the most abundant protein excreted in urine. It is a glycoprotein that is expressed in the thick ascending limb (TAL) of the loop of Henle [140–143]. It has also several roles in salt transport in the tubules, in the innate immunity and in the protection against kidney stones [144]. Recently, UMOD has been studied as a marker of acute renal injury both in mouse models of ischemia-reperfusion injury and in studies conducted in adult and pediatric patients prior to CPB [140, 143, 145]. These encouraging results suggest the possibility of studying UMOD also for the early determination of renal damage in SCD patients.

5. Current treatment

The treatment of renal complication in SCD patients should include an adequate fluid intake in order to avoid dehydration due to hyposthenuria. The chronic use of drugs toxic to the kidneys, such as non-steroidal anti-inflammatory drugs (NSAIDs) should be avoided due to the potential for adverse hemodynamic-related renal function deterioration, precipitation of papillary necrosis, and the development of NSAID-associated interstitial nephritis and glomerulonephropathies.

5.1. Treatment of hematuria

Hematuria in SCD is typically self-limited. Patients with hematuria should be advised to maintain a high urine output by oral hydration and remain at rest. However, in cases of massive hematuria, a high urine output should be maintained with combination of isotonic fluids and loop diuretics, and adopt measures to alkalinize urine, with sodium bicarbonate or acetazolamide. These measures modify the acid and hypertonic environment of the medullar region, which favors erythrocyte dehydration, HbS concentration and its polymerization [80]. Patients are advised to maintain a urinary volume of 2–4 L/day. Also blood transfusion may be necessary in order to reduce HbS level and sickling [146].

In cases of refractory hematuria, high doses of oral urea may be required to achieve blood urea nitrogen levels greater than 100 mg/dL, or treatment with vasopressin or epsilon-aminocaproic acid (EACA) to promote clotting [147].

5.2. Treatment of proteinuria

The benefits of angiotensin-converting enzyme (ACE) inhibitors and angiotensin-II receptor blockers (ARB) in slowing kidney disease progression in many situations are well-known. Improving nocturia has been reported to be an additional beneficial effect of ACE, presumably as a result of reduction in GFR [148]. A recent Cochrane database review, in 2015, reported the potential for reduction in albuminuria and proteinuria with the use of captopril in patients with SCD compared with those without the disease [148]. However, the administration of ACE and ARB should be carried out carefully due to the risk of hypotension and hyperkalemia, the latter condition often present in SCD patients.

The use of hydroxyurea (HU) has been suggested to reduce proteinuria and hyperfiltration as suggested in one prospective study consisting of 26 patients with SCD. However, no effect on microalbuminuria was found [77, 149]. A cross-sectional study of 149 adult patients showed that those using hydroxyurea were less likely to exhibit albuminuria (defined as urinary urinary-creatinine ratios ≥30 mg/g) [149]. A multi-center trial in infants (mean age 13.8 months) demonstrated that treatment with hydroxyurea for 24 months did not influence the GFR. However, it was associated with better urine-concentrating ability and less renal enlargement, suggesting a possible renoprotective effect [41]. In a non-randomized study of children with SCD requiring hydroxyurea for standard indications, treatment for 3 years led to a mean (standard deviation (SD)) decrease in GFR from 167 (SD 46) mL/min/1.73 m^2 to 145 (SD 27) mL/min/1.73 m^2, indicating an improvement in the hyperfiltration [150].

Dietary protein restriction is not recommended, because of the underlying growth failure and decreased energy state in most patients with SCD [151].

5.3. Treatment of anemia

The use of multiple blood transfusions demonstrated to restore the urinary concentrating ability in children with SCD [152, 153]. One study of 120 children with sickle hemoglobinopathies found that chronic red blood cell transfusions before the age of 9 years was protective against the onset of microalbuminuria [154]. Blood transfusion receives HbS, prevent direct sickling in the kidney and vaso-occulsion, reducing glomerular and tubular ischemia damage to the kidney. However, the benefits of transfusion therapy must be balanced against risks including infections, iron overload, acute or delayed hemolytic transfusion reactions [48, 155–158].

5.4. Treatment of end-stage renal disease

Hemodialysis is reportedly the leading form of renal replacement therapy for SCD-ESRD patients, as well as peritoneal dialysis and kidney transplantation. Mortality in SCD patients is approximately 26% during the first year of therapy for ESRD, nearly threefold higher than in ESRD patients without SCD. However, SCD patients who received pre-dialysis nephrology care had a lower death rate than those who did not receive such care [159].

Kidney transplantation may offer survival advantage over dialysis in ESRD. As in the general population, allograft survival for patients with ESRD is greater in those with a living donor than in those with a deceased donor. The post-transplantation one-year graft survival exceeds 60–80% [160]. Complications specific to the SCD population include higher infection risk due to autosplenectomy and precipitation of sickle cell crises with anemia correction following a successful transplant. Kidney transplant may be also complicated by allograft venous thrombosis, deep vein thrombosis, and vaso-occlusive crises [63, 161, 162]. Suggested maneuvers to decrease the incidence of post-transplant complications in these patients include [63, 163] preoperative blood transfusions to decrease hemoglobin S levels, preoperative oxygen supplementation with 40% oxygen, pretransplantation warming of the kidney allograft using 37°C saline, intraoperative and postoperative dopamine infusion at 4 μg/kg/min stem cell transplantation remain as the only curative treatment with good result and survival rates around 90% in 4 years [164, 165].

http://dx.doi.org/10.5772/intechopen.76588

6. Conclusions

SCN represents a new challenge in the treatment of acute and chronic complications in SCD. The underlying pathophysiology it is not completely understood, but it is already known that kidney damage occurs since the first months of life. The onset of hyperfiltration and albuminuria is an opportunity to intervene. The lack of diagnostic test capable of detecting the onset of symptoms remains a barrier to institute therapy. Furthermore, the absence of therapeutic strategy compounds the management of SCN. New markers of renal impairment in SCD such as the use of cystatin C assays may become available for community-based screening in order to identify patients at risk, to treat them and to improve their survival and quality of life.

Acknowledgements

The authors thank Professor Lorenzo Iughetti, Donatella Venturelli and Elena Bigi for their help and suggestions.

Competing interests

The authors declare that they have no competing interests.

Authors' contributions

BI designed the draft of the chapter, BI and ML reviewed the literature and wrote the manuscript, BI, KA and GP reviewed and made the substantial changes the manuscript. All authors discussed, read and approved the manuscript.

Author details

Baba P.D. Inusa[1]*, Lodi Mariachiara[2], Palazzi Giovanni[3] and Kenneth I. Ataga[4]

*Address all correspondence to: baba.inusa@gstt.nhs.uk

1 Paediatric Sickle Cell and Thalassaemia, Evelina London Children's Hospital, Guy's and St Thomas NHS Trust, London, UK

2 Post Graduate School of Pediatrics, Department of Medical and Surgical Sciences for Mothers, Children and Adults, University of Modena and Reggio Emilia, Modena, Italy

3 Oncology and Hematology Pediatric Unit, Department of Medical and Surgical Science for Mothers, Children and Adults, University Hospital of Modena, Modena, Italy

4 UNC Comprehensive Sickle Cell Program, Division of Hematology/Oncology, University of North Carolina at Chapel Hill, Chapel Hill, NC, USA

References

[1] Piel FB, Patil AP, Howes RE, Nyangiri OA, Gething PW, Dewi M, et al. Global epidemiology of sickle haemoglobin in neonates: A contemporary geostatistical model-based map and population estimates. Lancet. 2012;**381**(9861):142-151. DOI: 10.1016/S0140-6736(12)61229-X

[2] Rees DC, Williams TN, Gladwin MT. Sickle-cell disease. Lancet. 2010;**376**(9757):2018-2031. DOI: 10.1016/S0140-6736(10)61029-X

[3] Grosse SD, Odame I, Atrash HK, Amendah DD, Piel FB, Williams TN. Sickle cell disease in Africa: A neglected cause of early childhood mortality. American Journal of Preventive Medicine. 2011;**41**(suppl 4):S398-S405. DOI: 10.1016/j.amepre.2011.09.013

[4] IHME, Human Development Network, World Bank. The Global Burden of Disease: Generating Evidence, Guiding Policy. Sub-Saharan Africa Regional Edition. Seattle, WA: Institute for Health Metrics and Evaluation; 2013

[5] GBD 2013 Mortality and Causes of Death Collaborators. Global, regional, and national life expectancy, all-cause mortality, and cause-specific mortality for 249 causes of death, 1980-2015: A systematic analysis for the Global Burden of Disease Study 2015. Lancet. 2016;**388**:1459-1544. DOI: 10.1016/S0140-6736(16)31012-1

[6] World Health Organization Regional Office for Africa. Sickle-Cell Disease: A Strategy for the WHO African Region. Geneva: WHO; 2010. Report Number AFR/FC60/8

[7] Rumaney MB, Ngo Bitoungui VJ, Vorster AA, Ramesar R, Kengne AP, Ngogang J, et al. The co-inheritance of alpha-thalassemia and sickle cell anemia is associated with better hematological indices and lower consultations rate in Cameroonian patients and could improve their survival. PLoS One. 2014;**9**:e100516. DOI: 10.1371/journal.pone.0100516

[8] Akinsheye I, Alsultan A, Solovieff N, Ngo D, Baldwin CT, Sebastiani P, et al. Fetal hemoglobin in sickle cell anemia. Blood. 2011;**118**(1):19-27. DOI: 10.1182/blood-2011-03-325258

[9] Steinberg MH, Sebastiani P. Genetic modifiers of sickle cell disease. American Journal of Hematology. 2012;**87**(8):795-803. DOI: 10.1002/ajh.23232

[10] Sparkenbaugh E, Pawlinski R. Interplay between coagulation and vascular inflammation in sickle cell disease. British Journal of Haematology. 2013;**162**(1):3-14. DOI: 10.1111/bjh.12336

[11] Frenette PS, Atweh GF. Sickle cell disease: Old discoveries, new concepts, and future promise. Journal of Clinical Investigation. 2007;**117**(4):850-858. DOI: 10.1172/JCI30920

[12] Kato GJ, Hsieh M, Machado R, Taylor J, Little J, Butman JA, et al. Cerebrovascular disease associated with sickle cell pulmonary hypertension. American Journal of Hematology (6th). 2006;**81**(7):503-510

[13] Nath KA, Hebbel RP. Sickle cell disease: Renal manifestations and mechanisms. Nature Reviews Nephrology. 2015;**11**:161-171. DOI: 10.1038/nrneph.2015.8

[14] Ataga KI, Derebail VK, Archer DR. The glomerulopathy of sickle cell disease. American Journal of Hematology. 2014;**88**(9):907-914. DOI: 10.1002/ajh.23762

[15] Falk RJ, Scheinman J, Phillips G, et al. Prevalence and pathologic features of sickle cell nephropathy and response to inhibition of angiotensin-converting enzyme. The New England Journal of Medicine. 1992;**326**:910-915. DOI: 10.1056/NEJM199204023261402

[16] Bhathena DB, Sondheimer JH. The glomerulopathy of homozygous sickle hemoglobin (SS) disease: Morphology and pathogenesis. Journal of the American Society of Nephrology. 1991;**1**:1241-1252

[17] Maigne G, Ferlicot S, Galacteros F, et al. Glomerular lesions in patients with sickle cell disease. Medicine (Baltimore). 2010;**89**:18-27. DOI: 10.1097/MD.0b013e3181ca59b6

[18] Nasr SH, Markowitz GS, Sentman RL, D'Agati VD. Sickle cell disease, nephrotic syndrome, and renal failure. Kidney International. 2006;**69**:1276-1280. DOI: 10.1038/sj.ki.5000234

[19] Pardo V, Strauss J, Kramer H, Ozawa T, McIntosh RM. Nephropathy associated with sickle cell anemia: An autologous immune complex nephritis. II. Clinicopathologic study of seven patients. The American Journal of Medicine. 1975;**59**(5):650-659

[20] Itokua KE, Makulo JR, Lepira FB, Aloni MN, Ekulu PM, Sumaili EK, Bukabau JB, Mokoli VM, Longo AL, Kajingulu FM, Zinga CV, Nlandu YM, Engole YM, Akilimali PZ, Ngiyulu RM, Gini JL, Nseka NM. Albuminuria, serum antioxidant enzyme levels and markers of hemolysis and inflammation in steady state children with sickle cell anemia. BMC Nephrology. 2016;**17**(1):178. DOI: 10.1186/s12882-016-0398-0

[21] Kasztan M, Fox BM, Speed JS, De Miguel C, Gohar EY, Townes TM, Kutlar A, Pollock JS, Pollock DM. Long-term endothelin-A receptor antagonism provides robust renal protection in humanized sickle cell disease mice. Journal of the American Society of Nephrology. 2017;**28**(8):2443-2458. DOI: 10.1681/ASN.2016070711

[22] Phelan M, Perrine SP, Brauer M, Faller DV. Sickle erythrocytes, after sickling, regulate the expression of the endothelin-1 gene and protein in human endothelial cells in culture. The Journal of Clinical Investigation. 1995;**96**:1145-1151. DOI: 10.1172/JCI118102

[23] Ergul S, Brunson CY, Hutchinson J, Tawfik A, Kutlar A, Webb RC, Ergul A. Vasoactive factors in sickle cell disease: In vitro evidence for endothelin-1-mediated vasoconstriction. American Journal of Hematology. 2004;**76**:245-251. DOI: 10.1002/ajh.20107

[24] Fox BM, Kasztan M. Endothelin receptor antagonists in sickle cell disease: A promising new therapeutic approach. Life Sciences. 2016;**159**:15-19. DOI: 10.1016/j.lfs.2016.04.001

[25] Ataga KI, Caughey M, Elsherif L, Shen JH, Jones SK, Maitra P, Pollock DM, Cai J, Archer DR, Hinderliter AL. Albuminuria is associated with endothelial dysfunction and elevated plasma endothelin-1 in sickle cell anemia. PLoS One. 2016;**11**:e0162652. DOI: 10.1371/journal.pone.0162652

[26] Sabaa N, de Franceschi L, Bonnin P, Castier Y, Malpeli G, Debbabi H, Galaup A, Maier-Redelsperger M, Vandermeersch S, Scarpa A, Janin A, Levy B, Girot R, Beuzard Y,

Leboeuf C, Henri A, Germain S, Dussaule JC, Tharaux PL. Endothelin receptor antagonism prevents hypoxia-induced mortality and morbidity in a mouse model of sickle-cell disease. The Journal of Clinical Investigation. 2008;**118**:1924-1933. DOI: 10.1172/JCI33308

[27] Patel N, Gonsalves CS, Malik P, Kalra VK. Placenta growth factor augments endothelin-1 and endothelin-B receptor expression via hypoxia-inducible factor-1 alpha. Blood. 2008;**112**:856-865. DOI: 10.1182/blood-2007-12-130567

[28] Sundaram N, Tailor A, Mendelsohn L, Wansapura J, Wang X, Higashimoto T, Pauciulo MW, Gottliebson W, Kalra VK, Nichols WC, Kato GJ, Malik P. High levels of placenta growth factor in sickle cell disease promote pulmonary hypertension. Blood. 2010;**116**:109-112. DOI: 10.1182/blood-2009-09-244830

[29] Brittain JE, Hulkower B, Jones SK, Strayhorn D, De Castro L, Telen MJ, Orringer EP, Hinderliter A, Ataga KI. Placenta growth factor in sickle cell disease: Association with hemolysis and inflammation. Blood. 2010;**115**:2014-2020. DOI: 10.1182/blood-2009-04-217950

[30] Mendelsohn L, Rogers H, Leitman S, Raghavachari N, Yang Y, Yau YY, Tallack M, Perkins A, Taylor JG 6th, Noguchi CT, Kato GJ. Heme-bound iron activates placenta growth factor in erythroid cells via erythroid Krüppel-like factor. Blood. 2014;**124**:946-954. DOI: 10.1182/blood-2013-11-539718

[31] Rivera A. Reduced sickle erythrocyte dehydration in vivo by endothelin-1 receptor antagonists. American Journal of Physiology. Cell Physiology. 2007;**293**:C960-C966. DOI: 10.1152/ajpcell.00530.2006

[32] McColl B, Vadolas J. Animal models of β-hemoglobinopathies: Utility and limitations. Journal of Blood Medicine. 2016;**7**:263-274. DOI: 10.2147/JBM.S87955

[33] Pászty C, Brion CM, Manci E, Witkowska HE, Stevens ME, Mohandas N, Rubin EM. Science. 1997;**278**(5339):876-878

[34] Manci EA, Hillery CA, Bodian CA, Zhang ZG, Lutty GA, Coller BS. Pathology of Berkeley sickle cell mice: Similarities and differences with human sickle cell disease. Blood. 2006;**107**(4):1651-1658. DOI: 10.1182/blood-2005-07-2839

[35] De Paepe ME, Trudel M. The transgenic SAD mouse: A model of human sickle cell glomerulopathy. Kidney International. 1994;**46**:1337-1345

[36] Nath KA, Grande JP, Croatt AJ, Frank E, Caplice NM, Hebbel RP, Katusic ZS. Transgenic sickle mice are markedly sensitive to renal ischemia-reperfusion injury. The American Journal of Pathology. 2005;**166**:963-972. DOI: 10.1016/S0002-9440(10)62318-8

[37] Osarogiagbon UR, Choong S, Belcher JD, Vercellotti GM, Paller MS, Hebbel RP. Reperfusion injury pathophysiology in sickle transgenic mice. Blood. 2000;**96**(1):314-320

[38] Dasgupta T, Fabry ME, Kaul DK. Antisickling property of fetal hemoglobin enhances nitric oxide bioavailability and ameliorates organ oxidative stress in transgenic-knockout sickle mice. American Journal of Physiology. Regulatory, Integrative and Comparative Physiology. 2010 Feb;**298**(2):R394-R402. DOI: 10.1152/ajpregu.00611.2009

[39] Camus SM, Gausserès B, Bonnin P, Loufrani L, Grimaud L, Charue D, De Moraes JA, Renard JM, Tedgui A, Boulanger CM, Tharaux PL, Blanc-Brude OP. Erythrocyte microparticles can induce kidney vaso-occlusions in a murine model of sickle cell disease. Blood. 2012;**120**(25):5050-5058. DOI: 10.1182/blood-2012-02-413138

[40] Nath KA, Belcher JD, Nath MC, Grande JP, Croatt AJ, Ackerman AW, Katusic ZS, Vercellotti GM. The Role of TLR4 Signaling in the Nephrotoxicity of Heme and Heme Proteins. Am J Physiol Renal Physiol. 2017 Oct 4:ajprenal.00432.2017. DOI: 10.1152/ajprenal.00432.2017. [Epub ahead of print]

[41] Alvarez O, Miller ST, Wang WC, Luo Z, McCarville MB, Schwartz GJ, et al. Effect of hydroxyurea treatment on renal function parameters: Results from the multi-center placebo-controlled BABY HUG clinical trial for infants with sickle cell anemia. Pediatric Blood & Cancer. 2012;**59**(4):668-674. DOI: 10.1002/pbc.24100

[42] Aygun B, Mortier NA, Smeltzer MP, Hankins JS, Ware RE. Glomerular hyperfiltration and albuminuria in children with sickle cell anemia. Pediatric Nephrology. 2011;**26**:1285-1290. DOI: 10.1007/s00467-011-1857-2

[43] Lebensburger JD, Miller ST, Howard TH, Casella JF, Brown RC, Lu M, Iyer RV, Sarnaik S, Rogers ZR, Wang WC, BABY HUG Investigators. Influence of severity of anemia on clinical findings in infants with sickle cell anemia: Analyses from the BABY HUG study. Pediatric Blood & Cancer. 2012;**59**:675-678. DOI: 10.1002/pbc.24037

[44] Etteldorf JN, Tuttle AW, Clayton GW. Renal function studies in pediatrics. 1. Renal hemodynamics in children with sickle cell anemia. American Journal of Diseases of Children. 1952;**83**:185-191

[45] Ware RE, Rees RC, Sarnaik SA, Iyer RV, Alvarez OA, Casella JF, Shulkin BL, Shalaby-Rana E, Strife CF, Miller JH, Lane PA, Wang WC, Miller ST, Investigators BABYHUG. Renal function in infants with sickle cell anemia: Baseline data from the BABY HUG trial. The Journal of Pediatrics. 2010;**156**:66-70. DOI: 10.1016/j.jpeds.2009.06.060

[46] Piepsz A, Tondeur M, Ham H. Revisiting normal (51) Cethylenediaminetetraacetic acid clearance values in children. European Journal of Nuclear Medicine and Molecular Imaging. 2006;**33**:1477-1482. DOI: 10.1007/s00259-006-0179-2

[47] Becker AM. Sickle cell nephropathy: Challenging the conventional wisdom. Pediatric Nephrology. 2011 Dec;**26**(12):2099-2109. DOI: 10.1007/s00467-010-1736-2

[48] Alvarez O, Montane B, Lopez G, Wilkinson J, Miller T. Early blood transfusions protect against microalbuminuria in children with sickle cell disease. Pediatric Blood & Cancer. 2006;**47**:71-76. DOI: 10.1002/pbc.20645

[49] Dharnidharka VR, Dabbagh S, Atiyeh B, Simpson P, Sarnaik S. Prevalence of microalbuminuria in children with sickle cell disease. Pediatric Nephrology. 1998;**12**:475-478

[50] Lebensburger JD, Cutter GR, Howard TH, Muntner P, Feig DI. Evaluating risk factors for chronic kidney disease in pediatric patients with sickle cell anemia. Pediatr Nephrol. 2017 Sep;**32**(9):1565-1573. DOI: 10.1007/s00467-017-3658-8

[51] Bodas P, Huang A, O'Riordan MA, Sedor JR, Dell KM. The prevalence of hypertension and abnormal kidney function in children with sickle cell disease—A cross sectional review. BMC Nephrology. 2013;**14**:237. DOI: 10.1186/1471-2369-14-237

[52] Mammen C, Bissonnette ML, Matsell DG. Acute kidney injury in children with sickle cell disease-compounding a chronic problem. Pediatric Nephrology. 2017;**32**(8):1287-1291. DOI: 10.1007/s00467-017-3650-3

[53] Nolan VG, Ma Q, Cohen HT, Adewoye A, Rybicki AC, Baldwin C, Mahabir RN, Homan EP, Wyszynski DF, Fabry ME, Nagel RL, Farrer LA, Steinberg MH. Estimated glomerular filtration rate in sickle cell anemia is associated with polymorphisms of bone morphogenetic protein receptor 1B. American Journal of Hematology. 2007;**82**:179-184. DOI: 10.1002/ajh.20800

[54] Guasch A, Zayas CF, Eckman JR, Muralidharan K, Zhang W, Elsas LJ. Evidence that microdeletions in the alpha globin gene protect against the development of sickle cell glomerulopathy in humans. Journal of the American Society of Nephrology. 1999;**10**:1014-1019

[55] Schmitt F, Martinez F, Brillet G, Giatras I, Choukroun G, Girot R, Bachir D, Galacteros F, Lacour B, Grünfeld JP. Early glomerular dysfunction in patients with sickle cell anemia. American Journal of Kidney Diseases. 1998;**32**:208-214

[56] Guasch A, Cua M, Mitch WE. Early detection and the course of glomerular injury in patients with sickle cell anemia. Kidney International. 1996;**49**:786-791

[57] Sundaram N, Bennett M, Wilhelm J, Kim MO, Atweh G, Devarajan P, Malik P. Biomarkers for early detection of sickle nephropathy. American Journal of Hematology. 2011;**86**:559-566. DOI: 10.1002/ajh.22045

[58] Saborio P, Schneinman JI. Sickle cell nephropathy. Journal of the American Society of Nephrology. 1999;**10**:187-192

[59] Audard V, Homs S, Habibi A, Galacteros F, Bartolucci P, Godeau B, Renaud B, Levy Y, Grimbert P, Lang P, Brun-Buisson C, Brochard L, Schortgen F, Maitre B, Mekontso Dessap A. Acute kidney injury in sickle patients with painful crisis or acute chest syndrome and its relation to pulmonary hypertension. Nephrology, Dialysis, Transplantation. 2010;**25**:2524-2529. DOI: 10.1093/ndt/gfq083

[60] Powars DR, Chan LS, Hiti A, Ramicone E, Johnson C. Outcome of sickle cell anemia: A 4-decade observational study of 1056 patients. Medicine (Baltimore). 2005;**84**:363-376

[61] Loureiro MM, Rozenfeld S, Portugal RD. Acute clinical events in patients with sickle cell disease: Epidemiology and treatment. Revista Brasileira de Hematologia e Hemoterapia. 2008;**30**:95-100. DOI: 10.1590/S1516-84842008000200005

[62] Diop S, Diop D, Seck M, Guèye Y, Faye A, Dièye TN, Touré Fall AO, Sall Diallo A, Thiam D, Diakhaté L. Facteurs prédictifs des complications chroniques de la drépanocytose homozygote chez l'adult à Dakar (Sénégal). Medecine Tropicale. 2010;**70**:471-474

[63] Schneinman JI. Sickle cell disease and the kidney. Nature Clinical Practice. Nephrology. 2009;**5**:78-88. DOI: 10.1038/ncpneph1008

[64] Abdu A, Emokpae MA, Uadia PO, Kuliya-Gwarzo A. Proteinuria among adult sickle cell anemia patients in Nigeria. Annals of African Medicine. 2011;**10**:34-37. DOI: 10.4103/1596-3519.76578

[65] Ataga KI, Brittain JE, Moore D, Jones SK, Hulkower B, Strayhorn D, Adam S, Redding-Lallinger R, Nachman P, Orringer EP. Urinary albumin excretion is associated with pulmonary hypertension in sickle cell disease: Potential role of soluble fms-like tyrosine kinase-1. European Journal of Haematology. 2010;**85**:257-263. DOI: 10.1111/j.1600-0609.2010.01471.x

[66] Becker AM, Goldberg JH, Henson M, Ahn C, Tong L, Baum M, Buchanan GR. Blood pressure abnormalities in children with sickle cell anemia. Pediatric Blood & Cancer. 2014;**61**:518-522. DOI: 10.1002/pbc.24843

[67] Thompson J, Reid M, Hambleton I, Serjeant GR. Albuminuria and renal function in homozygous sickle cell disease: Observations from a cohort study. Archives of Internal Medicine. 2007;**167**:701-708. DOI: 10.1001/archinte.167.7.701

[68] Gordeuk VR, Sachdev V, Taylor JG, Gladwin MT, Kato G, Castro OL. Relative systemic hypertension in patients with sickle cell disease in associated with risk of pulmonary hypertension and renale insufficiency. American Journal of Hematology. 2008;**83**:15-18. DOI: 10.1002/ajh.21016

[69] Aygum B, Mortier NA, Smeltzer MP, Hakis JS, Ware RE. Glomerular hyerfiltration and albuminuria in children with sickle cell anemia. Pediatric Nephrology. 2011;**26**:128. DOI: 10.1007/s00467-011-1857-2

[70] Faulkner M, Turner EA, Deus J, Phillips K, Weaver C, Taiwo O, Omitowoju O. Severe anemia: A risk factor for glomerular injury in sickle cell disease. Journal of the National Medical Association. 1995;**87**:209-213

[71] Lebensburger J, Johnson SM, Askenazi DJ, Rozario NL, Howard TH, Hilliard LM. Protective role of hemoglobin and fetal hemoglobin in early kidney disease for children with sickle cell anemia. American Journal of Hematology. 2011;**86**:430-430. DOI: 10.1002/ajh.21994

[72] Gurkan S, Scarponi KJ, Hotchkiss H, Savage B, Drachtman R. Lactate dehydrogenase as a predictor of kidney involvement in patients with sickle cell anemia. Pediatric Nephrology. 2010;**25**:2123-2127. DOI: 10.1007/s00467-010-1560-8

[73] Day TG, Drasar ER, Fulford T, Sharpe CC, Thein SL. Association between hemolysis and albuminuria in adults with sickle cell anemia. Hema. 2012;**97**:201-205. DOI: 10.3324/haematol.2011.050336

[74] Hamideh D, Raj V, Harrington T, Li H, Margolles E, Amole F, Garcia-Buitrago M, Ruiz P, Zilleruelo G, Alvarez O. Albuminuria correlates with hemolysis and NAG and KIM-1 in patients with sickle cell anemia. Pediatric Nephrology. 2014;**29**:1997-2003. DOI: 10.1007/s00467-014-2821-8

[75] Wigfall DR, Ware RE, Burchinal MR, Kinney TR, Foreman JW. Prevalence and clinical correlates of glomerulopathy in children with sickle cell disease. The Journal of Pediatrics. 2000;**136**:749-753

[76] Powars DR, Elliott-Mills DD, Chan L, Niland J, Hiti AL, Opas LM, Johnson C. Chronic renal failure in sickle cell disease: Risk factors, clinical course, and mortality. Annals of Internal Medicine. 1991;**115**:614-620

[77] Laurin LP, Nachman PH, Desai PC, Ataga KI, Derebail VK. Hydroxyurea is associated with lower prevalence of albuminuria in adults with sickle cell disease. Nephrology, Dialysis, Transplantation. 2014;**29**:1211-1218. DOI: 10.1093/ndt/gft295

[78] Wierenga KJ, Pattison JR, Brink N, Griffiths M, Miller M, Shah DJ, Williams W, Serjeant BE, Serjeant GR. Glomerulonephritis after human parvovirus infection in homozygous sickle-cell disease. Lancet. 1995;**346**:475-476

[79] Kanso AA, Hassan NMA, Badr KF. Microvascular and macrovascular diseases of the kidney. In: Brenner BM, editor. Brenner & Rector's the Kidney. 8th ed. Saunders: Philadelphia; 2007. pp. 1147-1173

[80] Saunthararajah Y, Vichinsky EP. Sickle cell disease—Clinical features and management. In: Hoffman, editor. Hematology: Basic Principles and Practice. 5th ed. Oxford: Churchill Livingstone; 2008. pp. 577-601

[81] Da Silva GB Jr, Libório AB, Daher Ede F. New insights on pathophysiology, clinical manifestations, diagnosis, and treatment of sickle cell nephropathy. Annals of Hematology. 2011;**90**(12):1371-1379. DOI: 10.1007/s00277-011-1327-8

[82] Noguchi CT, Gladwin M, Diwan B, Merciris P, Smith R, Yu X, Buzard G, Fitzhugh A, Keefer LK, Schechter AN, Mohandas N. Pathophysiology of a sickle cell trait mouse model: Human αβS transgenes with one mouse β-globin allele. Blood Cells, Molecules & Diseases. 2001;**27**(6):971-977. DOI: 10.1006/bcmd.2001.0469

[83] Arogundade FA, Sanusi AA, Hassan MO, Salawu L, Durosinmi MA, Akinsola A. An appraisal of kidney dysfunction and its risk factors in patients with sickle cell disease. Nephron. Clinical Practice. 2011;**118**(3):c225-c231. DOI: 10.1159/000321138

[84] Ataga KI, Orringer EP. Renal abnormalities in sickle cell disease. American Journal of Hematology. 2000;**63**:205-211

[85] Burry A, Cross R, Axelsen R. Analgesic nephropathy and the renal concentrating mechanism. Pathology Annual. 1977;**12**:1-31

[86] De Jong PE, Statius Van Eps LW. Sickle cell nephropathy: New insights into its pathophysiology. Kidney International. 1985;**27**:711-717

[87] Maurel S, Stankovic Stojanovic K, Avellino V, Girshovich A, Letavernier E, Grateau G, Baud L, Girot R, Lionnet F, Haymann JP. Prevalence and correlates of metabolic acidosis among patients with homozygous sickle cell disease. Clinical Journal of the American Society of Nephrology. 2014;**9**(4):648-653. DOI: 10.2215/CJN.09790913

[88] Sens YAS, Miorin LA, Silva HGC, Jabur P. Hematúria em portadores de traço falciforme. In: Cruz J, Barros RT, editors. Atualidades em Nefrologia 4. São Paulo: Sarvier; 1996. pp. 138-142

[89] Baddam S, Aban I, Hilliard L, Howard T, Askenazi D, Lebensburger JD. Acute kidney injury during a pediatric sickle cell vaso-occlusive pain crisis. Pediatric Nephrology. 2017;**32**(8):1451-1456. DOI: 10.1007/s00467-017-3623-6

[90] Lebensburger JD, Palabindela P, Howard TH, Feig DI, Aban I, Askenazi DJ. Prevalence of acute kidney injury during pediatric admissions for acute chest syndrome. Pediatric Nephrology. 2016;**31**:1363-1368. DOI: 10.1007/s00467-016-3370-0

[91] De Jong PE, de Jong-Van Den Berg TW, Sewrajsingh GS, Schouten H, Donker AJ, Statius van Eps LW. The influence of indo-methacin on renal haemodynamics in sickle cell anaemia. Clinical Science. 1980;**59**:245-250

[92] Audard V, Moutereau S, Vandemelebrouck G, Habibi A, Khellaf M, Grimbert P, Levy Y, Loric S, Renaud B, Lang P, Godeau B, Galacteros F, Bartolucci P. First evidence of subclinical renal tubular injury during sickle-cell crisis. Orphanet Journal of Rare Diseases. 2014;**9**:67. DOI: 10.1186/1750-1172-9-67

[93] Cacciotti C, Vaiselbuh S, Romanos-Sirakis E. Pain management for sickle cell disease in the pediatric emergency department: Medications and hospitalization trends. La Clinica Pediatrica. 2017 Oct;**56**(12):1109-1114. DOI: 10.1177/0009922816674521

[94] Hardwick WE Jr, Givens TG, Monroe KW, King WD, Lawley D. Effect of ketorolac in pediatric sickle cell vaso-occlusive pain crisis. Pediatric Emergency Care. 1999;**15**:179-182

[95] Balestracci A, Ezquer M, Elmo ME, Molini A, Thorel C, Torrents M, Toledo I. Ibuprofen-associated acute kidney injury in dehydrated children with acute gastroenteritis. Pediatric Nephrology. 2015;**30**:1873-1878. DOI: 10.1007/s00467-015-3105-7

[96] Juncos JP, Grande JP, Croatt AJ, Hebbel RP, Vercellotti GM, Katusic ZS, Nath KA. Early and prominent alterations in hemodynamics, signaling, and gene expression following renal ischemia in sickle cell disease. American Journal of Physiology. Renal Physiology. 2010;**298**:F892-F899. DOI: 10.1152/ajprenal.00631.2009

[97] Chintagari NR, Nguyen J, Belcher JD, Vercellotti GM, Alayash AI. Haptoglobin attenuates hemoglobin-induced heme oxygenase-1 in renal proximal tubule cells and kidneys of a mouse model of sickle cell disease. Blood Cells, Molecules & Diseases. 2015;**54**:302-306. DOI: 10.1111/bjh.14280

[98] Botev R, Mallie´JP, Couchoud C, Schück O, Fauvel JP, Wetzels JF, Lee N, De Santo NG, Cirillo M. Estimating glomerular filtration rate: Cockcroft-Gault and modification of diet in renal disease formulas compared to renal inulin clearance. Clinical Journal of the American Society of Nephrology. 2009;**4**(5):899-906. DOI: 10.2215/CJN.05371008

[99] Levey AS, Greene T, Beck GJ, Caggiula AW, Kusek JW, Hunsicker LG, et al. Dietary protein restriction and the progression of chronic renal disease: What have all of the results of the MDRD study shown? Modification of diet in renal disease study group. Journal of the American Society of Nephrology. 1999;**10**(11):2426-2439

[100] Levey AS, Stevens LA, Schmid CH, Zhang YL, Castro AF 3rd, Feldman HI, Kusek JW, Eggers P, Van Lente F, Greene T, Coresh J. A new equation to estimate glomerular filtration rate. Annals of Internal Medicine. 2009;**150**(9):604-612

[101] Arlet JB, Ribeil JA, Chatellier G, et al. Determination of the best method to estimate glomerular filtration rate from serum creatinine in adult patients with sickle cell disease: A prospective observational cohort study. BMC Nephrology. 2012;**13**:83. DOI: 10.1186/1471-2369-13-83

[102] Asnani MR, Lynch O, Reid ME. Determining glomerular filtration rate in homozygous sickle cell disease: Utility of serum creatinine based estimating equations. PLoS One. 2013;**8**(7):e69922. DOI: 10.1371/journal.pone.0069922

[103] Asnani MR, Reid ME. Renal function in adult Jamaicans with homozygous sickle cell disease. Hematology. 2015;**20**(7):422-428. DOI: 10.1179/1607845414Y.0000000213

[104] Dharnidharka VR, Kwon C, Stevens G. Serum cystatin C is superior to serum creatinine as a marker of kidney function: A meta-analysis. American Journal of Kidney Diseases. 2002;**40**(2):221-226. DOI: 10.1053/ajkd.2002.34487

[105] National Kidney Foundation. KDIGO 2012 clinical practice guideline for the evaluation and management of chronic kidney disease. Kidney International Supplements. 2013;**3**(1):1-163

[106] Ciccia E, Devarajan P. Pediatric acute kidney injury: Prevalence, impact and management challenges. International Journal of Nephrology and Renovascular Disease. 2017;**10**:77-84. DOI: 10.2147/IJNRD.S103785

[107] Bökenkamp A, Domanetzki M, Zinck R, Schumann G, Byrd D, Brodehl J. Cystatin C—A new marker of glomerular filtration rate in children independent of age and height. Pediatrics. 1998;**101**(5):875-881

[108] Alvarez O, Zilleruelo G, Wright D, Montane B, Lopez-Mitnik G. Serum cystatin C levels in children with sickle cell disease. Pediatric Nephrology. 2006;**21**(4):533-537. DOI: 10.1007/s00467-006-0033-6

[109] Asnani M, Reid M. Cystatin C: A useful marker of glomerulopathy in sickle cell disease? Blood Cells, Molecules & Diseases. 2015;**54**(1):65-70. DOI: 10.1016/j.bcmd.2014.07.018

[110] Mariani M, Mariani G, De Servi S. Clinical significance of cystatin c in acute coronary syndrome: Something more than a marker of renal function? Inflammation and Cell Signaling. 2014;**1**(4):e229. DOI: 10.14800/ics.229

[111] Tantawy AAG, Adly AAM, Ismail EAR, Abdelazeem M. Clinical predictive value of cystatin C in pediatric sickle cell disease: A marker of disease severity and subclinical cardiovascular dysfunction. Clinical and Applied Thrombosis/Hemostasis. 2017;**23**(8):1010-1017. DOI: 10.1177/1076029616665921

[112] Cho SY, Lee HJ, Suh JT, et al. The significance of serum cystatin C accompanied by a normal serum creatinine level in pediatric patients with chronic kidney disease. Science. 2011;**42**(9):549-552. DOI: 10.1309/LM4DVIAKEL35WRGU

[113] Supavekin S, Zhang W, Kucherlapati R, Kaskel FJ, Moore LC, Devarajan P. Differential gene expression following early renal ischemia/reperfusion. Kidney International. 2003;**63**(5):1714-1724. DOI: 10.1046/j.1523-1755.2003.00928.x

[114] Devarajan P. Genomic and proteomic characterization of acute kidney injury. Nephron. 2015;**131**(2):85-91. DOI: 10.1159/000437237

[115] Koyner JL, Vaidya VS, Bennett MR, et al. Urinary biomarkers in the clinical prognosis and early detection of acute kidney injury. Clinical Journal of the American Society of Nephrology. 2010;**5**:2154-2165. DOI: 10.2215/CJN.00740110

[116] Devarajan P. Review: Neutrophil gelatinase-associated lipocalin: A troponin-like biomarker for human acute kidney injury. Nephrology (Carlton). 2010;**15**:419-428, 59. DOI: 10.1111/j.1440-1797.2010.01317.x

[117] Mishra J, Mori K, Ma Q, Kelly C, Yang J, Mitsnefes M, Barasch J, Devarajan P. Amelioration of ischemic acute renal injury by neutrophil gelatinase-associated lipocalin. Journal of the American Society of Nephrology. 2004;**15**(12):3073-3082. DOI: 10.1097/01.ASN.0000145013.44578.45

[118] Wagener G, Gubitosa G, Wang S, Borregaard N, Kim M, Lee HT. Urinary neutrophil gelatinase-associated lipocalin and acute kidney injury after cardiac surgery. American Journal of Kidney Diseases. 2008;**52**(3):425-433. DOI: 10.1053/j.ajkd.2008.05.018

[119] Ling W, Zhaohui N, Ben H, Leyi G, Jianping L, Huili D, et al. Urinary IL-18 and NGAL as early predictive biomarkers in contrast-induced nephropathy after coronary angiography. Nephron. Clinical Practice. 2008;**108**(3):c176-c181. DOI: 10.1159/000117814

[120] Siew ED, Ware LB, Gebretsadik T, Shintani A, Moons KG, Wickersham N, Bossert F, Ikizler TA. Urine neutrophil gelatinase associated lipocalin moderately predicts acute kidney injury in critically ill adults. Journal of the American Society of Nephrology. 2009;**20**(8):1823-1832. DOI: 10.2215/CJN.09061209

[121] Parikh CR, Jani A, Mishra J, Ma Q, Kelly C, Barasch J, et al. Urine NGAL and IL-18 are predictive bio-markers for delayed graft function following kidney transplantation. American Journal of Transplantation. 2006;**6**(7):1639-1645. DOI: 10.1111/j.1600-6143.2006.01352.x

[122] Carmeliet P. Angiogenesis in life, disease and medicine. Nature. 2005;**438**:932-936. DOI: 10.1038/nature04478

[123] Youssry I, Makar S, Fawzy R, Wilson M, AbdAllah G, Fathy E, Sawires H. Novel marker for the detection of sickle cell nephropathy: Soluble FMS-like tyrosine kinase-1 (sFLT-1). Pediatric Nephrology. 2015 Dec;**30**(12):2163-2168. DOI: 10.1007/s00467-015-3172-9

[124] Ataga KI, Brittain JE, Desai P, Delaney J, Jones SK, Strayhorn D, Redding-Lallinger R, Orringer EP. Association of soluble FMS-like tyrosine kinase-1 with pulmonary hypertension and hemolysis in sickle cell disease. British Journal of Haematology. 2011;**152**:485-449. DOI: 10.1111/j.1365-2141.2010.08410.x

[125] Portilla D, Dent C, Sugaya T, Nagothu KK, Kundi I, Moore P, Noiri E, Devarajan P. Liver fatty acid-binding protein as a biomarker of acute kidney injury after cardiac surgery. Kidney International. 2008;73(4):465-472. DOI: 10.1038/sj.ki.5002721

[126] Han WK, Waikar SS, Johnson A, Betensky RA, Dent CL, Devarajan P, Bonventre JV. Urinary biomarkers in the early diagnosis of acute kidney injury. Kidney International. 2008;**73**(7):863-869

[127] Parikh CR, Thiessen-Philbrook H, Garg AX, Kadiyala D, Shlipak MG, Koyner JL, Edelstein CL, Devarajan P, Patel UD, Zappitelli M, Krawczeski CD, Passik CS, Coca SG, TRIBE-AKI Consortium. Performance of kidney injury molecule-1 and liver fatty acid-binding protein and combined biomarkers of AKI after cardiac surgery. Clinical Journal of the American Society of Nephrology. 2013;**8**(7):1079-1088. DOI: 10.2215/CJN.10971012

[128] Parikh CR, Devarajan P, Zappitelli M, Sint K, Thiessen-Philbrook H, Li S, Kim RW, Koyner JL, Coca SG, Edelstein CL, Shlipak MG, Garg AX, Krawczeski CD, TRIBE-AKI Consortium. Postoperative biomarkers predict acute kidney injury and poor outcomes after pediatric cardiac surgery. Journal of the American Society of Nephrology. 2011;**22**(9):1737-1747. DOI: 10.1681/ASN.2010111163

[129] Parikh CR, Coca SG, Thiessen-Philbrook H, Shlipak MG, Koyner JL, Wang Z, Edelstein CL, Devarajan P, Patel UD, Zappitelli M, Krawczeski CD, Passik CS, Swaminathan M, Garg AX, TRIBE-AKI Consortium. Postoperative biomarkers predict acute kidney injury and poor outcomes after adult cardiac surgery. Journal of the American Society of Nephrology. 2011;**22**(9):1748-1757. DOI: 10.1681/ASN.2010121302

[130] Krawczeski CD, Goldstein SL, Woo JG, Wang Y, Piyaphanee N, Ma Q, Bennett M, Devarajan P. Temporal relationship and predictive value of urinary acute kidney injury biomarkers after pediatric cardiopulmonary bypass. Journal of the American College of Cardiology. 2011;**58**(22):2301-2309. DOI: 10.1016/j.jacc.2011.08.017

[131] Cerqueira BA, Boas WV, Zanette AD, Reis MG, Goncalves MS. Increased concentrations of IL-18 and uric acid in sickle cell anemia: Contribution of hemolysis, endothelial activation and the inflammasome. Cytokine. 2011;**56**(2):471-476. DOI: 10.1016/j.cyto.2011.08.013

[132] Duarte JD, Desai AA, Sysol JR, Abbasi T, Patel AR, Lang RM, Gupta A, Garcia JG, Gordeuk VR, Machado RF. Genome-wide analysis identifies IL-18 and FUCA2 as novel genes associated with diastolic function in African Americans with sickle cell disease. PLoS One. 2016;**11**(9):e0163013. DOI: 10.1371/journal.pone.0163013

[133] Voskaridou E, Terpos E, Michail S, et al. Early markers of renal dysfunction in patients with sickle cell/beta-thalassemia. Kidney International. 2006;**69**:2037-2042. DOI: 10.1038/sj.ki.5000248

[134] Wolf G. Renal injury due to renin-angiotensin-aldosterone system activation of the transforming growth factor-beta pathway. Kidney International. 2006;**70**:1914e9. DOI: 10.1681/ASN.2006040356

[135] Blumenberg M, Gao S, Dickman K, Grollman AP, Bottinger EP, Zavadil J. Chromatin structure regulation in transforming growth factor-beta-directed epithelial-mesenchymal transition. Cells, Tissues, Organs. 2007;**185**:162e74. DOI: 10.1159/000101317

[136] Mohtat D, Thomas R, Du Z, Boakye Y, Moulton T, Driscoll C, et al. Urinary transforming growth factor beta-1 as a marker of renal dysfunction in sickle cell disease. Pediatric Nephrology. 2011;**26**:275e80. DOI: 10.1007/s00467-010-1677-9

[137] Ghobrial EE, Abdel-Aziz HA, Kaddah AM, Mubarak NA. Urinary transforming growth factor β-1 as a marker of renal dysfunction in sickle cell disease. Pediatrics and Neonatology. 2016;**57**(3):174-180. DOI: 10.1016/j.pedneo.2015.05.001

[138] Emokpae MA, Abdu A, Gwaram BA. Neutrophil-to-lymphocyte, platelet-to-lymphocyte ratios and their association with atherogenic index of plasma in sickle cell nephropathy. Journal of Applied Hematology. 2016;**7**:24-29. DOI: 10.4103/1658-5127.181109

[139] Negishi K, Noiri E, Maeda R, Portilla D, Sugaya T, Fujita T. Renal L-type fatty acid-binding protein mediates the bezafibrate reduction of cisplatin-induced acute kidney injury. Kidney International. 2008;**73**(12):1374-1384. DOI: 10.1038/ki.2008.106

[140] Garimella PS, Jaber BL, Tighiouart H, Liangos O, Bennett MR, Devarajan P, El-Achkar TM, Sarnak MJ. Association of preoperative urinary uromodulin with AKI after cardiac surgery. Clinical Journal of the American Society of Nephrology. 2017;**12**:10-18. DOI: 10.2215/CJN.02520316

[141] Tamm I, Horsfall FL Jr. A mucoprotein derived from human urine which reacts with influenza, mumps, and Newcastle disease viruses. The Journal of Experimental Medicine. 1952;**95**:71-97

[142] Pruijm M, Ponte B, Ackermann D, Paccaud F, Guessous I, Ehret G, Pechère-Bertschi A, Vogt B, Mohaupt MG, Martin P-Y, Youhanna SC, Nägele N, Vollenweider P, Waeber G, Burnier M, Devuyst O, Bochud M. Associations of urinary uromodulin with clinical characteristics and markers of tubular function in the general population. Clinical Journal of the American Society of Nephrology. 2016;**11**:70-80. DOI: 10.2215/CJN.04230415

[143] El-Achkar TM, Wu XR, Rauchman M, McCracken R, Kiefer S, Dagher PC. Tamm-Horsfall protein protects the kidney from ischemic injury by decreasing inflammation and altering TLR4 expression. American Journal of Physiology. Renal Physiology. 2008;**295**:F534-F544. DOI: 10.1152/ajprenal.00083.2008

[144] Rampoldi L, Scolari F, Amoroso A, Ghiggeri G, Devuyst O. The rediscovery of uromodulin (Tamm-Horsfall protein): From tubulointerstitial nephropathy to chronic kidney disease. Kidney International. 2011;**80**:338-347. DOI: 10.1038/ki.2011

[145] Bennett MR, Pyles O, Ma Q, Devarajan P. Preoperative levels of urinary uromodulin predict acute kidney injury after pediatriccardiopulmonary bypass surgery. Pediatric Nephrology. 2017. DOI: 10.1007/s00467-017-3823-0

[146] Pham PC, Pham PT. Sickle cell nephropathy. In: Lerma E, Sparks M, Topf J, editors. Nephrology Secrets. 4th ed. Mosby Elsevier

[147] Kaye JD, Smith EA, Kirsch AJ, Cerwinka WH, Elmore JM. Preliminary experience with epsilon aminocaproic acid for treatment of intractable upper tract haematuria in children with haematological disorders. The Journal of Urology. 2010;**184**(3):1152-1157. DOI: 10.1016/j.juro.2010.05.020

[148] Sasongko TH, Nagalla S, Ballas SK. Angiotensin-converting enzyme (ACE) inhibitors for proteinuria and microalbuminuria in people with sickle cell disease. Cochrane Database of Systematic Reviews 2015, Issue 6. Art. No.: CD009191. DOI: 10.1002/14651858.CD009191.pub3

[149] Silva Junior GB, Vieira AP, Couto Bem AX, Alves MP, Meneses GC, Martins AM, et al. Proteinuria in adults with sickle-cell disease: The role of hydroxycarbamide (hydroxyurea) as a protective agent. International Journal of Clinical Pharmacy. 2014;**36**(4):766-770. DOI: 10.1007/s11096-014-9955-4

[150] Aygun B, Mortier NA, Smeltzer MP, Shulkin BL, Hankins JS, Ware RE. Hydroxyurea treatment decreases glomerular hyperfiltration in children with sickle cell anemia. American Journal of Hematology. 2013;**88**(2):116-119. DOI: 10.1002/ajh.23365

[151] Singhal A, Davies P, Wierenga KJ, Thomas P, Serjeant G. Is there an energy deficiency in homozygous sickle cell disease? The American Journal of Clinical Nutrition. 1997;**66**(2):386-390

[152] Howard J, Hart N, Roberts-Harewood M, Cummins M, Awogbade M, Davis B. Guideline on the management of acute chest syndrome in sickle cell disease. British Journal of Haematology. 2015;**169**(4):492-505. DOI: 10.1111/bjh.13348

[153] McKie KT, Hanevold CD, Hernandez C, Waller JL, Ortiz L, McKie KM. Prevalence, prevention, and treatment of microalbuminuria and proteinuria in children with sickle cell disease. Journal of Pediatric Hematology/Oncology. 2007;**29**(3):140-144. DOI: 10.1097/MPH.0b013e3180335081

[154] Marsenic O, Couloures KG, Wiley JM. Proteinuria in children with sickle cell disease. Nephrology, Dialysis, Transplantation. 2008;**23**(2):715-720. DOI: 10.1093/ndt/gfm858

[155] Chou ST. Transfusion therapy for sickle cell disease: A balancing act. Hematology. American Society of Hematology. Education Program. 2013;**2013**:439-446. DOI: 10.1182/asheducation-2013.1.439

[156] Chou ST, Jackson T, Vege S, Smith-Whitley K, Friedman DF, Whesthoff CM. High prevalence of red blood cell alloimmunization in sickle cell disease despite transfusion from Rh-matched minority donors. Blood. 2013;**122**(6):1062-1071. DOI: 10.1182/blood-2013-03-490623

[157] Porter J, Garbowski M. Consequences and management of iron overload in sickle cell disease. ASH Education Program Book. 2013;**1**:447-456. DOI: 10.1182/asheducation-2013.1.447

[158] Scheunemann LP, Ataga KI. Delayed hemolytic transfusion reaction in sickle cell disease. American Journal of the Medical Sciences. 2010;**339**(3):266-269

[159] McClellan AC, Luthi JC, Lynch JR, Soucie JM, Kulkarni R, Guasch A, et al. High one year mortality in adults with sickle cell disease and end-stage renal disease. British Journal of Haematology. 2012;**159**(3):360-367. DOI: 10.1111/bjh.12024

[160] Huang E, Parke C, Mehrnia A, Kamgar M, Pham PT, Danovitch G, et al. Improved survival among sickle cell kidney transplant recipients in the recent era. Nephrology, Dialysis, Transplantation. 2013;**28**(4):1039-1046. DOI: 10.1093/ndt/gfs585

[161] Scheinman JI. Sickle cell disease and the kidney. Nature Clinical Practice Nephrology. 2009 Feb;**5**(2):78-88. DOI: 10.1038/ncpneph1008

[162] Okafor UH, Aneke E. Outcome and challenges of kidney transplant in patients with sickle cell disease. Journal of Transplantation. 2013;**2013**:614610. DOI: 10.1155/2013/614610

[163] Miner DJ, Jorkasky DK, Perloff LJ, Grossman RA, Tomaszewski JE. Recurrent sickle cell nephropathy in a transplanted kidney. American Journal of Kidney Diseases. 1987;**10**(4):306-313

[164] Walters MC, De Castro LM, Sullivan KM, et al. Indications and results of HLA-identical sibling hematopoietic cell transplantation for sickle cell disease. Biology of Blood and Marrow Transplantation. 2016;**22**:207-211

[165] Gluckman E, Cappelli B, Bernaudin F, et al. Sickle cell disease: An international survey of results of HLA-identical sibling hematopoietic stem cell transplantation. Blood. 2017 Mar 16;**129**(11):1548-1556. DOI: 10.1182/blood-2016-10-745711

Idiosyncratic Drug-Induced Severe Neutropenia and Agranulocytosis: State of the Art

Emmanuel Andrès and Rachel Mourot-Cottet

Additional information is available at the end of the chapter

http://dx.doi.org/10.5772/intechopen.78769

Abstract

In this chapter, we report and discuss the diagnosis and management of idiosyncratic drug-induced, or drug-associated, severe neutropenia, and agranulocytosis (neutrophil count of $<0.5 \times 10^9/L$). In this setting, neutropenia remains a potentially serious adverse event due to the frequency of severe sepsis, with severe deep tissue infections (e.g., pneumonia), life-threatening infections, septicemia, and septic shock in two-thirds of all hospitalized patients. Recently, several poor prognostic factors, impacting the hematological recovery, the duration of hospitalization, and the outcome have been identified that may be helpful when identifying "frailty" patients. These factors include: old age, poor performance status, septicemia or shock, comorbidities such as renal failure, and a neutrophil count below $0.1 \times 10^9/L$. recovery. In this situation, modern management, with broad-spectrum antibiotics in case of any sepsis sign and hematopoietic growth factors (HGF) (particularly G-CSF), is likely to improve the prognosis, with a current mortality rate around 5%.

Keywords: agranulocytosis, neutropenia, drugs, infections, pneumonia, antibiotics, hematopoietic growth factor

1. Introduction

White blood cells, as granulocytes or leukocytes, are an important component of the host defense system, responsible for protection against bacteria, viruses, fungi, and invading parasites [1]. The white blood cells constitute only 1% of the total blood volume. The term neutropenia describes an absolute decrease in neutrophil numbers [1].

Neutropenia is defined by a neutrophil count <1.5 × 10^9/L (<1.2 × 10^9/L in black people). The degree of neutropenia predicts the risk of serious bacterial infections. Severe neutropenia is characterized by a profound decrease of circulating neutrophils in case of an absolute lack of circulating neutrophils, classically resulting in a neutrophil count of <0.5 × 10^9/L [1, 2].

Schultz first introduced the term "agranulocytosis" in 1922, for cases of acute and severe pharyngeal infections, associated with a lack of granulocytes in the blood in relation to drug intake [2]. Such unpredictable event, named "idiosyncratic," is typically serious, with around 50% of cases exhibiting severe sepsis, and a mortality rate of 10–20% [2, 3].

In this chapter, we report and discuss the diagnosis and management of idiosyncratic drug-induced, or drug-associated, severe neutropenia, and agranulocytosis.

2. Search strategy

A literature search was performed on the *PubMed* database of the *US National Library of Medicine* and *Scholar Google*. We searched for articles published between January 2010 and March 2018, using the following keywords or associations: *"drug-induced neutropenia," "drug-induced agranulocytosis," "idiosyncratic neutropenia"* and *"idiosyncratic agranulocytosis"*; restrictions included: English- or French-language publications; published from January 1, 2010 to February 31, 2018; human subjects; clinical trials, review articles or guidelines. All of the English and French abstracts were reviewed by at least two senior researchers from our work group (*GRoupes d'Etudes des Agranulocytoses médicamenTeuses* (GREAT) des *Hôpitaux Universitaires de Strasbourg* (HUS), Strasbourg, France). After rigorous selection, only 15 papers were selected and analyzed. The latter was used to write this paper in the form of a short narrative review.

American Society of Hematology educational books, textbooks of Hematology and Internal medicine, and information gleaned from international meetings were also used.

3. Etiologies of severe neutropenia

In adults, the diagnosis of acute and severe neutropenia (neutrophil count of <0.5 × 10^9/L includes a limited number of conditions [1]. In fact, the main differential diagnoses outside the context of treatment of cancer with chemotherapy (e.g., alkylating agents, antimetabolites, etc.) or radiotherapy, include myelodysplastic syndromes, especially in elderly patients, and acute leukemia.

All other conditions induced moderate neutropenia, with an absolute neutrophil count between 1.5 and 0.5 × 10^9/L. These conditions mainly include: neutropenia secondary to sepsis, particularly viral infections or bacterial infections (severe Gram-negative infections with Salmonella sp., tuberculosis, Brucella sp.); and neutropenia associated with hypersplenism [2]. Other rarer differential diagnoses include neutropenia secondary to alcoholism, nutritional deficiencies (folic acid, vitamin B12, cooper, etc.), Felty's syndrome, systemic lupus erythematosus or Sjögren's syndrome, and lastly aplastic anemia or paroxysmal nocturnal hemoglobinuria [2].

In the literature, acute and severe neutropenia has been shown to be attributable to drugs in 70–90% of cases [2]. Thus, in practice, idiosyncratic drug-induced neutropenia or agranulocytosis should be discussed routinely (considered in first) even if there is a context moving toward another condition.

4. Definition

To date, drug-induced, or drug associated, severe neutropenia, or agranulocytosis is defined at least by a neutrophil count of $<0.5 \times 10^9/L$, which occurs as a result of exposure to drugs [3]. The presence of fever and sepsis signs is usual, even required, for some authors. In the majority of patients, the neutrophil count is under $0.1 \times 10^9/L$.

All drugs may be the causative agents, particularly: chemotherapy, immune modulator agents or biotherapies. Other daily drugs may also be more rarely incriminated. Such event is called "idiosyncratic" drug-induced neutropenia and agranulocytosis [2, 3]. Either the drug itself or one of its metabolites may be the causative agent.

Currently, the recommended criteria for diagnosing blood cytopenias and for implicating a drug as a causative agent in neutropenia are derived from an international consensus meeting [2, 4]. These criteria are outlined in **Table 1**. As idiosyncratic severe neutropenia and agranulocytosis are life-threatening conditions, no patient was re-challenged with the incriminated drug ("theoretical method of reference").

Definition of agranulocytosis	Criteria of drug imputability
Neutrophil count $<0.5 \times 10^9/L$ ± existence of a fever and/or any signs of infection	Onset of agranulocytosis during treatment or within 7 days of exposure to the drug, with a complete recovery in neutrophil count of more than $1.5 \times 10^9/L$ within one month of discontinuing the drug
	Recurrence of agranulocytosis upon re-exposure to the drug (this is rarely observed, as the high risk of mortality contra-indicates new administration of the drug)
	Exclusion criteria: history of congenital neutropenia or immune mediated neutropenia, recent infectious disease (particularly recent viral infection), recent chemotherapy and/or radiotherapy and/or immunotherapy* and existence of an underlying hematological disease

*Immunoglobulins, interferon, anti-TNF antibodies, anti-CD20 (rituximab).

Table 1. Criteria for idiosyncratic drug-induced agranulocytosis.

5. Epidemiology and causative drugs

Idiosyncratic agranulocytosis is a rare disorder. In Europe, the annual incidence of such events is between 1.6 and 9.2 cases per million populations [2, 4]. In the USA, reported ranges from 2.4 to 15.4 per million per year. In our experience, the incidence remains unchanged, despite the withdrawn of incriminated drugs (which carry a high-risk), and increased levels of medical awareness and pharmacovigilance [5]. Older patients are thought to be at greater risk for to drug-induced neutropenia, probably because of increased medication use.

Almost all classes of drugs have been implicated as "causative," but for the majority, the risk appears to be very small (**Table 2**) [2, 5]. However, for drugs such as antithyroid drugs, ticlopidine, clozapine, phenothiazines, sulfasalazine, trimethoprim-sulfametoxazole (cotrimoxazole), and dipyrone or sulfasalazine, the risk may be higher. For antithyroid drugs (propyl-thiouracil and méthimazole), a risk of 3 per 10,000 users has been reported. For

Family drug	Drugs
Analgesics and nonsteroidal anti-inflammatory drugs:	Acetaminophen, acid acetylsalicylic (aspirin), aminopyrine, benoxaprofen, diclofenac, diflunisal, dipyrone, fenoprofen, indomethacin, ibuprofen, naproxen, phenylbutazone, piroxicam, sulindac, tenoxicam, tolmetin
Antipsychotics, hypnosedatives and antidepressants:	Amoxapine, chlomipramine, chlorpromazine, chlordiazepoxide, clozapine, diazepam, fluoxetine, haloperidol, levopromazine, imipramine, indalpin, meprobamate, mianserin, olanzapine, phenothiazines, risperidone, tiapride, ziprasidone
Antiepileptic drugs:	Carbamazepine, ethosuximide, phenytoin, trimethadione, valproic acid (sodium valproate)
Antithyroid drugs:	Carbimazole, methimazole, potassium perchlorate, potassium thiocyanate, propylthiouracil
Cardiovascular drugs:	Acid acetylsalicylic, amiodarone, aprindine, bepridil, captopril, coumarins, dipyridamole, digoxin, flurbiprofen, furosemide, hydralazine, lisinopril, methyldopa, nifedipine, phenindione, procainamide, propafenone, propanolol, quinidine, ramipril, spironolactone, thiazide diuretics, ticlopidine, vesnarinone
Anti-infective agents:	Abacavir, acyclovir, amodiaquine, atovaquone, cephalosporins, chloramphenicol, chloroguanine, chloroquine, ciprofloxacin, clindamycin, dapsone, ethambutol, flucytosine, fusidic acid, gentamicin, hydroxychloroquine, isoniazid, levamizole, lincomycin, linezolid, macrolids, mebendazole, mepacrine, metronidazole, minocycline, nitrofurantoin, norfloxacin, novobiocin, penicillins, pyrimethamine, quinine, rifampicin, streptomycin, terbinafine, tetracycline, thioacetazone, tinidazole, trimethoprim-sulfametoxazole (cotrimoxazole), vancomycin, zidovudine
Miscellaneous drugs:	Acetazolamide, acetylcysteine, allopurinol, aminoglutethimide, arsenic compounds, benzafibrate, brompheniramine, calcium dobesilate, chloropheniramine, cimetidine, colchicine, dapsone, deferiprone, famotidine, flutamide, gold, glucocorticoids, hydroxychloroquine, mesalazine, metapyrilène, methazolamide, metoclopramide, levodopa, olanzapine, omeprazole, oral hypoglycemic agents (glibenclamide), mercurial diuretics, penicillamine, ranitidine, riluzole, sulfasalazine, most sulfonamides, tamoxifen, thenalidine, tretinoid, tripelennamine

Table 2. Drugs implicated in the occurrence of idiosyncratic agranulocytosis.

ticlopidine, the risk is more than 100-fold higher. Clozapine induces agranulocytosis in almost 1% of patients, particularly in the first three months of treatment, with older patients and females being at a higher risk [2, 5].

In our single-center cohort from the GREAT team (n = 203), the most frequent causative drugs are: antibiotics (49.3%), especially ß-lactams and cotrimoxazole; antithyroid drugs (16.7%); neuroleptic and anti-epileptic agents (11.8%); antiviral agents (7.9%); and platelet aggregation inhibitors (6.9%), especially ticlopidine [5]. Since 1990–2000, no case of noramidopyrine- and ticlopidine-induced agranulocytosis is reported in the literature. Recently, several new drugs have been listed as causative agents for severe neutropenia and agranulocytosis, for example, acyclovir, ganciclovir, lamotrigine, terbinafine or deferiprone [2, 5].

6. Mechanisms of idiosyncratic drug-induced neutropenia

The pathogenesis of drug-induced neutropenia is a heterogeneous process, which is not yet fully understood [2, 3]. Clinical observations, studies in volunteers and laboratory experiments have suggested that this disorder is mediated by immune allergic and toxic mechanisms. In many cases, neutropenia occurs after prolonged drug exposure, resulting in decreased granulocyte production by hypoplastic bone marrow. In other cases repeated, intermittent exposure is implicated. This suggests an immune mediated mechanism, although this hypothesis is not entirely confirmed.

Direct damage, either to the microenvironment of the bone marrow or myeloid precursors, plays a significant role in most other cases [3]. Complex metabolic pathways that metabolize drugs and other chemicals are regulated by genetic factors. Genetic polymorphism results in heterogeneity of expression of the various enzymes, which generate or destroy intermediate toxic compounds [3].

Other mechanisms, involving cytotoxic T cells, haptens, auto-immunity, and oxidative modification of the drug have also been considered [3]. The impact of myeloperoxidase and NADPH-oxidase polymorphism in drug-induced neutropenia and agranulocytosis have also been studied. Clozapine appears to accelerate the process of apoptosis, thought to be due to depletion of ATP and reduced glutathione, which renders the neutrophils highly susceptible to oxidant-induced apoptosis [3].

7. Clinical manifestations

Initially, symptomatic patients with idiosyncratic drug-induced severe neutropenia or agranulocytosis usually present with fever, which often is the earliest and sometimes the only sign during evolution. This later is often associated with general malaise, often including chills [2, 3]. In this setting, symptoms may appear either immediately or insidiously, depending on the time course of neutropenia development. Symptomatic patients are commonly present at discovery a non-specific sore throat, acute tonsillitis or sinusitis. More rarely, patients have first, as a not expected and brutal event, a severe deep and potentially life-threatening infection [2].

It is important to note that without medical intervention, particularly immediate antibiotics administration, natural history of agranulocytosis include severe and potentially life-threatening infections with often signs of general sepsis and septicemia (fever, chills, hypotension, etc.). During the evolution, documented pneumonia as well as anorectal, skin or oropharyngeal infections and septic shock were the most reported infections [2, 3]. To date, classical manifestations as necrotic tonsillitis and perinea gangrene or are exceptional.

In our experience (203 patients), the clinical manifestations include: isolated fever (unknown origin) (26.3%); septicemia (13.9%); documented pneumonia (13.4%); sore throat and acute tonsillitis (9.3%); and septic shock (6.7%) [5]. While in hospital 19.2% of the patients worsened clinically and exhibited features of severe sepsis, septic shock, or systemic inflammatory response syndrome (SIRS).

However, besides these "loud" clinical manifestations, clinicians must keep in mind that the signs of these infections may be sometimes crude and atypical because of the neutropenia (**Figure 1**). For practitioners, it is to note that pneumonia is often asymptomatic because of the lack of neutrophil cells. In this situation, thoracic CT-scan may be proposed with much better results than X-ray (**Figure 2**). Similarly, when antibiotics are administered prophylactically, or at the beginning of this adverse event, both the patient's complaints and the physical findings may be "masked," and fever is often the only clinical sign detected [2].

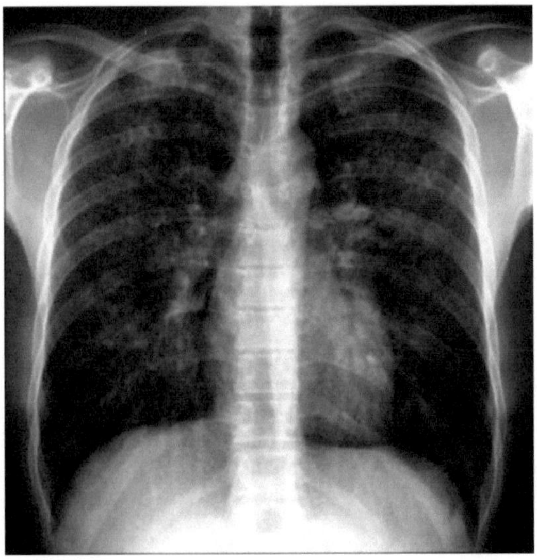

Figure 1. Chest radiography in a patient with absolute neutrophil count $<0.1 \times 10^9$/L: "Masked" pneumonia.

http://dx.doi.org/10.5772/intechopen.78769

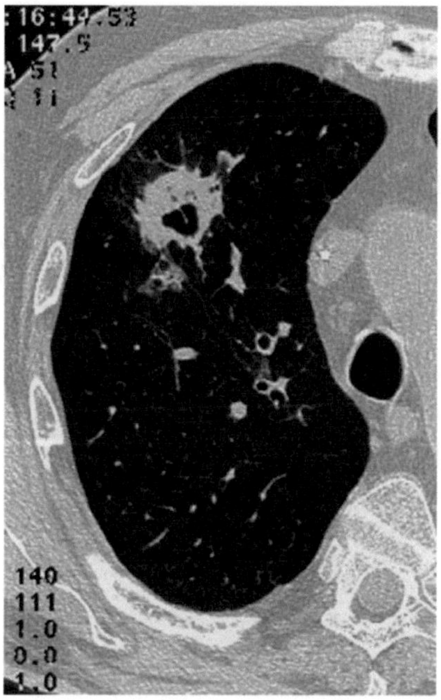

Figure 2. CT-scan in a patient with absolute neutrophil count $<0.1 \times 10^9/L$: Lung aspergillosis.

8. Biological data

Theoretically, acute neutropenia is classically diagnosed in a blood sample, resulting in a neutrophil count of $<0.5 \times 10^9/L$ [3, 5]. In this setting, monocyte and basophile counts may be increased. In the majority of patients, the neutrophil count is under $0.1–0.2 \times 10^9/L$.

In this setting, bone marrow examination may not be required in for all patients but is pivotal to exclude an underlying pathology, particularly in the elderly to rule out myelodysplastic disorders and malignant hematological diseases [1, 2]. Bone marrow examination may be particularly required in case of associated anemia, thrombocytopenia or abnormal blood cells. In such patients with idiosyncratic drug-induced agranulocytosis, the bone marrow typically shows a lack of mature myeloid cells, whereas in other cases, immature cells from the myelocyte stage are preserved. This latter appearance is described as "myeloid maturation arrest" [2, 3].

In severe neutropenia, multiple microbiological specimens should be taken, as in the case of post-chemotherapy neutropenia. With such multiple microbial samples, a causative pathogen, typically Gram-negative bacilli or Gram-positive cocci (mainly Staphylococcus spp.), was isolated in 30% of cases [3]. Fungi are also involved as secondary infective agents (>10%), however, in a few percent of cases regarding neutropenia related to chemotherapy. To date, modern molecular techniques have further facilitated identification of microbial pathogens, allowing for aggressive interventions that appear to improve patient outcomes as documented later in the paper.

9. Prognosis and mortality rate

Idiosyncratic drug-induced severe neutropenia usually resolves over time, with supportive care and management of infection [2, 3]. The time to neutrophil recovery has typically been reported to range from 4 to 24 days.

In our aforementioned cohort study (n = 203), the mean duration of hematological recovery (neutrophil count ≥1.5 × 10^9/L) is 7.8 days (range: 2–20) [5]. The median duration for neutrophil count ≥0.5 × 10^9/L is 6.8 days (range: 1–24).

In this context, the mortality rate for idiosyncratic agranulocytosis has recently fallen from 10 to 16 to 5% (range 2.5–10%) [2, 3]. This is likely due to improved recognition, management, and treatment of the condition. The highest mortality rate is observed in "frailty" patients: older patients (>65 years), with poor performance status, as well as those with several comorbidities as renal failure (defined as serum creatinine level > 120 μmol/L), chronic heart failure; bacteremia septicemia at diagnosis; or shock at diagnosis (**Table 3**); or low neutrophil count levels [2, 6].

Previously, we have found demonstrated that several variables were significantly associated with a longer neutrophil recovery time (>1.5 × 10^9/L), as: that an absolute neutrophil count of <0.1 × 10^9/L at diagnosis, as well as septicemia and/or shock [7], were variables that were significantly associated with a longer neutrophil recovery time. In our cohort, bone marrow showing a lack of myeloid cells was not found to be associated with a delayed recovery (using uni- and multivariate analysis) [5].

It is worth noting, that in elderly patients, clinical manifestations were generally more severe, with septicemia or septic shock in at least two-thirds of patients, as we have previously published [8]. It is also the case in patients with associated morbidities as chronic cardiac failure, chronic obstructive pulmonary disease, renal failure and immune disorders. In our experience, the depth of the neutropenia impacts the severity of the clinical, manifestations [7].

Age > 65 years	Negative impact on duration of hematological recovery**, duration of hospitalization and antibiotherapy
Neutrophil count at diagnosis: ≤0.1 × 10^9/L	Negative impact on duration of hematological recovery, duration of hospitalization and antibiotherapy
Clinical status: Deep severe infections or bacteremia or septic shock (versus isolated fever)	Negative impact on duration of hospitalization and antibiotherapy and of mortality
Severe underlying disease or severe co-morbidity: Renal failure, cardiac or respiratory failure, systemic auto-inflammatory diseases	Negative impact on duration of hematological recovery and hospitalization
Management with pre-established procedures and hematopoietic growth factor for use in severe conditions	Positive impact on duration of hematological recovery, duration of hospitalization and of mortality

*Prognosis: hematological recovery, duration of hospitalization and antibiotherapy, mortality).

**Hematological recovery: absolute neutrophil count >1.5 × 10^9/L.

Table 3. Impact factors for the prognosis* of idiosyncratic drug-induced agranulocytosis.

At the opposite side, some patients (<20%) (not-well identified characteristics or profile) remained asymptomatic [3]. This supports the case for routine monitoring of blood counts in individuals receiving high-risk medications such as, for example, antithyroid drugs [2, 3]. This also supports not consensual home management of such an event in certain patients (young, without medical history, and with fever as the sole sign) [3].

10. General management

The management of idiosyncratic drug-induced severe neutropenia and agranulocytosis begins with the immediate withdrawal of any medications, which may potentially be responsible [2, 3]. Thus, the patient's medication history must be carefully obtained in chronological order so that the suspected agent(s) may be identified.

For experts, routine monitoring for agranulocytosis is required in some high-risk drugs, such as clozapine, ticlopidine, and antithyroid drugs [2, 3]. All cases of drug-induced neutropenia must be notified to the pharmacovigilance center. All febrile patients should be admitted to hospital, without any delay [2, 3].

Concomitant measures include realization of multiple microbial samples (blood, urine, stool, and sputum cultures) and aggressive treatment of confirmed or potential sepsis, as well as the prevention of secondary infections. It should be noted that as a result of neutrophil deficiency, both the patient's symptoms and the physical findings may be altered, and fever may be the only clinical sign [3]. Preventive measures include good hygiene and infection control, paying particular attention to high-risk areas such as the mouth, skin, and perineum [2, 3].

Patients with a low-risk of infection, and good performance status may be managed in home with intensive supervision and monitoring! The occurrence of sepsis requires prompt management, without any delay, including the administration of broad-spectrum intravenous antibiotic therapy [2, 3].

In case of fever or for "frailty" patients, prompt hospitalization without delay may be required [2, 3]. In this setting, patient isolation and the use of prophylactic antibiotics (e.g., for the gastrointestinal tract) have been proposed, but their usefulness in limiting the risk of infection has not been documented or at least, has not been clinically proven [3].

11. Antimicrobial therapy

In case of sepsis, we commonly combine in first-line therapy, new cephalosporins and quinolones or aminoglycosides. It is important to note that a great part of these recommendations is adapted from the evidence-based medicine recommendations for the management of chemotherapy-induced neutropenia (field of oncology) [3]. Of course ureidopenicillins beta-lactam/beta-lactamase inhibitor combinations, as carbapenems, or imipenem can be safely used in these antibiotic combinations. The addition of intravenous vancomycin or teicoplanin is considered in patients at high-risk of serious Gram-positive infections or after 48 hours of continued fever despite first-line of antibiotics with at least cephalosporins [2, 3].

In patients with persistent fever despite broad-spectrum antibiotics against Gram-negative bacilli or Gram-positive cocci or systematically after 1 week of persistent fever, the addition of empirical antifungal agents should be considered, as amphotericin B or related derivates (e.g., liposomal preparation of amphotericin), and voriconazol or caspofungin [2, 3].

12. Hematopoietic growth factors (HGF)

Since 1985, two-thirds of reported cases of idiosyncratic agranulocytosis have been treated with HGF, especially *granulocyte-colony stimulating factor* (G-CSF) [9]. The most recent, major studies on hematopoietic growth factors (HGF) use in drug-induced agranulocytosis are described in **Table 4** [2, 5, 10–15]. In our aforementioned cohort, a faster hematological non-significantly recovery (neutrophil count >1.5 × 10^9/L) was observed in the HGF group: 2.1 days

Type of study and target population	Main results
Systematic review of all published cases (n = 492); all patients with idiosyncratic drug-induced agranulocytosis [2]	Treatment with hematopoietic growth factors was associated with a statistically significantly lower rate of infectious and fatal complications, in cases with a neutrophil count <0.1 × 10^9/L
Meta-analysis (n = 118); all patients with idiosyncratic drug-induced agranulocytosis [10]	*G-CSF* or *GM-CSF* (100 to 600 μg/day) reduced the mean time to neutrophil recovery (neutrophil count >0.5 × 10^9/L) from 10 to 7.7 days, in cases with a neutrophil count <0.1 × 10^9/L, and reduced the mortality rate from 16 to 4.2%
Case control study, retrospective analysis (n = 70); all patients with idiosyncratic drug-induced agranulocytosis [11]	*G-CSF* and *GM-CSF* (100 to 600 μg/day) reduced the recovery of neutrophil count from 7 to 4 days, particularly in patients with a neutrophil count <0.1 × 10^9/L
Cohort study, retrospective analysis (n = 54); patients with idiosyncratic drug-induced agranulocytosis >65 years of age, with poor prognostic factors [12]	*G-CSF* (300 μg/day) significantly reduced the mean duration for hematological recovery from 8.8 to 6.6 days ($p < 0.04$). *G-CSF* reduced the global cost
Cohort study, retrospective analysis (n = 20); patients with antithyroid drug-induced agranulocytosis and poor prognostic factors [13]	*G-CSF* (300 μg/day) significantly reduced the mean durations of hematological recovery, antibiotic therapy and hospitalization from: 11.6 to 6.8 days, 12 to 7.5 days and 13 to 7.3 days, respectively ($p < 0.05$ in all cases). *G-CSF* reduced the global cost
Cohort study, retrospective analysis (n = 145); all patients with idiosyncratic drug-induced agranulocytosis [14]	*G-CSF* shortens time to recovery in patients with agranulocytosis
Cohort study, retrospective analysis (n = 201); all patients with idiosyncratic drug-induced agranulocytosis [5]	*G-CSF* (300 μg/day) reduced the mean durations of hematological recovery for 2.1 days ($p = 0.057$).
Prospective randomized study (n = 24); all patients with antithyroid drug-induced agranulocytosis [15]	*G-CSF* (100 to 200 μg/day) did not significantly reduce the mean duration for hematological recovery

G-CSF: Granulocyte-Colony Stimulating factor; GM-CSF: Granulocyte-Macrophage-Colony Stimulating factor

Table 4. Recent studies on the use of hematopoietic growth factors in idiosyncratic drug-induced agranulocytosis.

http://dx.doi.org/10.5772/intechopen.78769

(p = 0.057) [5]. Thus, for certain hematologist, the usefulness of HGF remains controversy in such patients. To support this view, the only available prospective randomized study (based on 24 patients with antithyroid-related agranulocytosis) did not confirm the benefit of G-CSF [10]. Nevertheless, this negative result may be related to inappropriate G-CSF doses (100–200 μg/day).

To date, no data is available on the use of pegfilgrastim (a long-acting recombinant G-CSF) in idiosyncratic drug-induced neutropenia [2, 3].

In this setting, it is important to keep in mind that transfusion of granulocyte concentrates should only be used in exceptional circumstances, and only then for the control of life-threatening infections with antibiotic resistance such as perineal gangrene [2].

13. Conclusions

In conclusion, it is important to keep in mind that idiosyncratic drug-induced or drug-associated, severe neutropenia and agranulocytosis remains a potentially serious adverse event due to the frequency of severe sepsis, with severe deep tissue infections (e.g., pneumonia), life-threatening infections, septicemia, and septic shock in two-thirds of all hospitalized patients. In this setting, several poor prognostic factors, impacting the hematological recovery, the duration of hospitalization, and the outcome have been documented: old age, poor performance status, septicemia or shock, comorbidities such as renal failure, and a neutrophil count below 0.1×10^9/L. In this situation, modern management, with broad-spectrum antibiotics in case of any sepsis sign and HGF is likely to improve the prognosis, with a currently mortality rate around 5%.

Acknowledgements

The authors have no conflicts of interest that are directly relevant to the content of this manuscript. E. Andrès is recipient of a grant from CHUGAI, AMGEN, ROCHE, GSK, and NOVARTIS but these sponsors had no part in the research or writing of the present manuscript.

Funding

No sources of funding were used to assist the preparation of this manuscript.

Author details

Emmanuel Andrès* and Rachel Mourot-Cottet

*Address all correspondence to: emmanuel.andres@chru-strasbourg.fr

Departments of Internal Medicine, University Hospital of Strasbourg, Strasbourg, France

References

[1] Stock W, Hoffman R. White blood cells 1: Non-malignant disorders. Lancet. 2000; **355**:1351-1357

[2] Andersohn F, Konzen C, Garbe E. Non-chemotherapy drug-induced agranulocytosis: A systematic review of case reports. Annals of Internal Medicine. 2007;**146**:657-665

[3] Andrès E, Zimmer J, Mecili M, Weitten T, Alt M. Clinical presentation and management of drug-induced agranulocytosis. Expert Review of Hematology. 2011;**4**:143-151

[4] Bénichou C, Solal-Celigny P. Standardization of definitions and criteria for causality assessment of adverse drug reactions. Drug-induced blood cytopenias: Report of an international consensus meeting. Nouvelle Revue Française d'Hématologie. 1993;**33**:257-262

[5] Andrès E, Mourot-Cottet R, Maloisel F, Séverac F, Keller O, Vogel T, et al. Idiosyncratic drug-induced neutropenia & agranulocytosis. The Quarterly Journal of Medicine. 2017; **110**:299-305

[6] Julia A, Olona M, Bueno J, Revilla E, Rosselo J, Petit J, et al. Drug-induced agranulocytosis: Prognostic factors in a series of 168 episodes. British Journal of Haematology. 1991;**79**:366-372

[7] Maloisel F, Andrès E, Kaltenbach G, Noel E. Prognostic factors of hematological recovery in nonchemotherapy drug-induced agranulocytosis. Haematologica. 2003;**88**:470-471

[8] Andrès E, Mourot-Cottet R, Maloisel F, Keller O, Séverac F, Vogel T, et al. Idiosyncratic drug-induced severe neutropenia and agranulocytosis in elderly patients (≥75 years): A monocentric cohort study of 61 cases. Drugs - Real World Outcomes. 2016;**3**:393-399

[9] Andrès E, Maloisel F, Zimmer J. The role of haematopoietic growth factors G-CSF and GM-CSF in the management of drug-induced agranulocytosis. British Journal of Haematology. 2010;**150**:3-8

[10] Beauchesne MF, Shalansky SJ. Nonchemotherapy drug-induced agranulocytosis: A review of 118 patients treated with colony-stimulating factors. Pharmacotherapy. 1999; **19**:299-305

[11] Sprikkelman A, de Wolf JTM, Vellenga E. Application of haematopoietic growth factors in drug-induced agranulocytosis: A review of 70 cases. Leukemia. 1994;**8**:2031-2036

[12] Andrès E, Kurtz JE, Martin-Hunyadi C, Kaltenbach G, Alt M, Weber JC, et al. Nonchemotherapy drug-induced agranulocytosis in elderly patients: The effects of granulocyte colony-stimulating factor. The American Journal of Medicine. 2002;**112**:460-464

[13] Andrès E, Kurtz JE, Perrin AE, Dufour P, Schlienger JL, Maloisel F. The use of haematopoietic growth factors in antithyroid-related drug-induced agranulocytosis: A report of 20 patients. The Quarterly Journal of Medicine. 2001;**94**:423-428

[14] Ibáñez L, Sabaté M, Ballarín E, Puig R, Vidal X, Laporte JR, et al. Use of granulocyte colony-stimulating factor (G-CSF) and outcome in patients with non-chemotherapy agranulocytosis. Pharmacoepidemiology and Drug Safety. 2008;**8**:48-57

[15] Fukata S, Kuma K, Sugawara M. Granulocyte colony-stimulating factor (G-CSF) does not improve recovery from antithyroid drug-induced agranulocytosis: A prospective study. Thyroid. 1999;**9**:29-31